MW00679626

SPECIALTY BOARD REVIEW

General Surgery

Fourth Edition

Charles G. Rob, MD, MChir
Professor of Surgery
Uniformed Services
University of the Health Sciences
F. Edward Hebert School of Medicine
Bethesda, Maryland

Gary G. Wind, MD
Professor of Surgery
Uniformed Services
University of the Health Sciences
F. Edward Hebert School of Medicine
Bethesda, Maryland

APPLETON & LANGE
Norwalk, Connecticut/San Mateo, California

0-8385-8638-4

The opinions or assertions contained herein are the private views of the authors and are not to be construed as official or as reflecting the views of the Uniformed Services University or the Department of Defense.

Notice: Our knowledge in clinical sciences is constantly changing. As new information becomes available, changes in treatment and in the use of drugs become necessary. The author(s) and the publisher of this volume have taken care to make certain that the doses of drugs and schedules of treatment are correct and compatible with the standards generally accepted at the time of publication. The reader is advised to consult carefully the instruction and information material included in the package insert of each drug or therapeutic agent before administration. This advice is especially important when using new or infrequently used drugs.

Copyright © 1991 by Appleton & Lange, a Publishing Division of Prentice Hall; © 1986 by Appleton-Century-Crofts; © 1981 by Arco Publishing

All rights reserved. This book, or any parts thereof, may not be used or reproduced in any manner without written permission. For information, address Appleton & Lange, 25 Van Zant Street, East Norwalk, Connecticut 06855.

91 92 93 94 / 10 9 8 7 6 5 4 3 2 1

Prentice Hall International (UK) Limited, *London*
Prentice Hall of Australia Pty. Limited, *Sydney*
Prentice Hall Canada, Inc., *Toronto*
Prentice Hall Hispanoamericana, S.A., *Mexico*
Prentice Hall of India Private Limited, *New Delhi*
Prentice Hall of Japan, Inc., *Tokyo*
Simon & Schuster Asia Pte. Ltd., *Singapore*
Editora Prentice Hall do Brasil Ltda., *Rio de Janeiro*
Prentice Hall, *Englewood Cliffs, New Jersey*

Library of Congress Cataloging-in-Publication Data

Rob, Charles.
  Specialty board review, general surgery / Charles G. Rob, Gary G.
Wind.—4th ed.
     p.   cm.
  Bibliography: p.
  ISBN 0-8385-8638-4
  1. Surgery—Examinations, questions, etc. I. Wind, Gary, G.
II. Title.
  [DNLM: 1. Surgery—examination questions. WO 18 R628s]
RD37.2.R63 1990
617′.0076—dc20
DNLM/DLC
                                                        89-17493
  for Library of Congress   CIP

Editor: R. Craig Percy
Production Editor: Charles F. Evans

PRINTED IN THE UNITED STATES OF AMERICA

Contents

Introduction

The American Board of Surgery was organized and chartered in 1937. It was the eleventh Board to be chartered, the first being the American Board of Ophthalmology in 1916. The American Board of Surgery is composed of about forty members elected from nominees provided by the following organizations:

The American Surgical Association
The American College of Surgeons
The American Medical Association
The Society of University Surgeons
The Southern Surgical Association
The Western Surgical Association
The Pacific Coast Surgical Association
The New England Surgical Society
The Central Surgical Association
The American Pediatric Surgical Association
The Society for Surgery of the Alimentary Tract
The American Board of Colon and Rectal Surgery
The American Board of Pediatrics
The American Board of Plastic Surgery
The American Board of Thoracic Surgery

Certification by the Board indicates that you have completed an approved United States or Canadian Chief Residency in General Surgery and have satisfied members of the Board that your skills, knowledge, judgment and other attributes qualify you to be a Diplomate of the American Board of Surgery. At the present this certification is limited to ten years. You can be recertified by passing a written examination if the Board is satisfied with your credentials.

APPLICATION FOR EXAMINATION FOR GENERAL CERTIFICATION IN SURGERY

If you are within six months of completing one full year as chief resident in an approved United States or Canadian General Surgery Residency Program you should request an *Evaluation Form* from:

American Board of Surgery, Inc.
Suite 1561
1617 John F. Kennedy Boulevard
Philadelphia, PA 19103-1847

To ensure assignment for the *Qualifying Examination* at the earliest possible date you should request this form no later than March 1, or four months before you will have completed your educational requirements. Candidates who complete the educational requirements after September 30th will not be considered for admission to the Qualifying Examination that year.

After you return the *Evaluation Form* you will be advised whether or not it appears you have met or will meet the requirements. If you have not, you will be informed of any additional requirements. Do not submit documents, testimonials, letters of recommendation, or other information unless requested by the Board.

If you are eligible for examination you will receive the formal *Application for Examination*. To be eligible for examination in that year submit the application and the required registration fee by August 1.

Acceptability for examination is determined by information available to the Board regarding the applicant's professional maturity, surgical judgment, technical capabilities, and ethical standing.

The In-Training Examination

The American Board of Surgery offers its In-Training Examination each year to Program Directors of approved residencies. The Program Directors of 309 of the 311 accredited residency programs made this examination available to residents in 1985, and it was administered to just under 8000 residents. This examination is composed of multiple choice questions similar to the types of question on the Qualifying Examination. The results inform the resident of his areas of strength and weakness and of how well he has performed in comparison with other residents. The best preparation for both the In-Training Examination and the Qualifying Examination is the study of a good, current textbook of surgery.

The Qualifying Examination

The Qualifying Examination is a written examination offered once a year, usually in November. Shortly before the date of the examination you will receive an *Admission Card* which indicates the reporting times and location for your examination. You will also receive a pamphlet describing the examination and the types of multiple choice questions to be expected. The examination is administered in two parts, morning and afternoon, but is graded as a single examination. The questions test your fund of cognitive information relevant to the specialty of Surgery.

You must pass the Qualifying Examination to be designated an "Active Candidate for Certification" before you are admitted to the Certifying Examinations.

Rules governing opportunities for taking the Qualifying Examination after having once failed it differ for candidates who have been approved prior to 1985 and those approved in 1985 or who will be approved in subsequent years. The latter candidates may take the Qualifying Examination three times within the five-year period following approval of the formal application. Failure to complete the Qualifying Examination within five years of approval results in additional requirements before one can become a "New Applicant."

The Certifying Examination

The Certifying Examinations are oral. You will be examined by a team of two examiners during each of three sessions. The Certifying Examinations are offered to those who have passed the Qualifying Examination and have thus become "Candidates for Certification."

Each year the Certifying Examinations are given in six or seven major cities within the continental United States. Candidates receive an announcement of the examination to which they may be assigned approximately two months prior to the examination date. *IMPORTANT:* You must return the reply card immediately to be included in that examination. If you

fail to return the card or if you return it late you will have forfeited one of the three opportunities you have to be offered the examination. When your assignment for examination is firm you will receive an Admission Card stating the specific time and place for you to report.

You have only three opportunities to appear for examination following completion of the Qualifying Examination. The expiration date for admission to a Certifying Examination is June 30th of the fifth calendar year after the Qualifying Examination.

If you fail the Certifying Examination three times or if you fail to accept or appear at the three opportunities offered to you, you will lose your status as a "Candidate for Certification." When you lose this status additional requirements must be fulfilled before you are offered a fourth opportunity for examination. If you fail at the fourth opportunity there are still more requirements before you can again be considered for admission to the examination. Candidates for Certification who have failed the Certifying Examination four times and those who have not become Certified within five academic years after becoming a "Candidate for Certification" shall be considered to be "New Applicants."

THE QUALIFYING EXAMINATION

Contents of the Qualifying Examination

The Board's interpretation of the term "general surgery" indicates the breadth of the examinations.

1. A central core of knowledge common to all surgical specialties: for example, anatomy, physiology, metabolism, pathology, wound healing, shock and resuscitation, neoplasia and nutrition.
2. Comprehensive knowledge of the diagnosis and care of patients with disorders of:
   A. The alimentary tract
   B. The abdomen and its contents
   C. The breast
   D. The head and neck
   E. The vascular system (including *diagnosis* of anomalies and diseases of the heart and great vessels)
   F. The endocrine system
   G. The total management of trauma

Preparation for the Qualifying Examination

Read one good, current textbook of surgery. Give extra attention to areas to which you have been least exposed. Each year the In-Training Examination helps identify your weaker areas. The examinations in this book also help you identify gaps in your knowledge and the answers and the explanations of the answers will help you with both the Qualifying and the Certifying Examinations.

Most of the questions in the Qualifying Examination are designed to find out how much you know—not how good you are at using your knowledge—and will require you to recall a great deal of information. Some questions will test your knowledge of recent advances.

The majority of questions will deal with adult and pediatric surgical problems of the alimentary tract, diseases of the breast and endocrine system, peripheral vascular disease, shock, trauma, neoplasia, general thoracic surgery, and diseases of the head and neck. The examination will also test your knowledge of surgical anatomy and physiology, congenital anomalies, nutrition, and fluid and electrolyte balance.

Questions in orthopedics, cardiac surgery, urology, neurosurgery, plastic surgery, gynecology and anesthesiology are often based on what a general surgeon should know about the diagnosis and management of injuries, anomalies, or neoplasms.

In answering the questions try to pace yourself so that you complete the examination in the alloted time. If you want to reconsider some of your answers you can mark the questions and, if time permits, return to them later.

THE CERTIFYING EXAMINATION

The Certifying Examination is oral. Each candidate is examined during three separate sessions during the course of one day. Two examiners, at least one of whom is a member of the American Board of Surgery, conduct each session. Most of the examiners try to put the candidate at ease. They try to find out as much about his understanding of clinical problems, surgical judgment and problem-solving ability as can be done in the time available. The manner in which a candidate conducts himself can affect an examiner's behavior. Don't bluff and don't stall.

Each examiner conducts the questions for about half the time, but at any time the other may interrupt to pursue a point. Most examiners will take notes because they want to remind themselves what questions they have asked and what answers you have given. This note-taking does not indicate to you whether your answer is correct or not. Many times you will have little indication from the examiners whether you are doing well or poorly. They may at times persist in questioning you on some point to see if you are certain of your answer and will stick to your response or may try to get you to come up with a better answer.

Toward the end of each session the questioning may be turned back to the first examiner. He may then either bring up an entirely new area of inquiry or use this time to decide what you really know about an area already covered.

After you leave the room, each examiner will give you a grade. This grade indicates one of three things. In the opinion of the examiner: (1) you have passed (with marginal, medium or high score), (2) you have failed, or (3) it is not entirely clear whether or not you should pass. The examiner notes the last alternative by a "flag."

How to and How Not to Answer

Most candidates who pass the examination should pass and most candidates who fail should fail, but there are exceptions to the latter half of this statement and there are reasons for the exceptions. Why might a worthy candidate fail? A few surgeons (probably very few) are so discomfited by the oral examinations that they cannot express themselves intelligently. If you are this rare sort of person, ask your friends or teachers to give you practice oral examinations which may help you summon sufficient composure. Some knowledgeable candidates fail because they are not properly responsive, and here is a typical example. The examiner gives a brief description of a clinical situation and asks you what you would *do*. At that moment, all he is interested in is what you would do. If you try to give him a long-winded discourse on the differential diagnosis, he is justified in not thinking well of your answer.

Here are some useful suggestions:

1. Answer the question which is asked. Don't ramble on about side-related issues.

2. Be as concise as possible but as thorough as necessary. Examiners are well acquainted with the tactic of trying to prolong an answer to decrease the number of questions asked.

3. Don't say you would call in a consultant. If you don't know the answer, "I don't know" is the correct and acceptable response. This answer will get you into trouble only if you have to use it too often. Sometimes the examiner will indicate he wants to know what *you* would do by telling you all of your colleagues are out of town and the telephones aren't functioning.

4. Give what you think is the correct answer. Don't try to guess what answer might please the examiner.

5. At the end of the day each candidate is discussed after his grades are announced.

If a candidate has received any marginal or failing grades his performance is discussed thoroughly. The discussion includes the questions asked and the answers given.

The Content of the Certifying Examination

The oral examination may cover the full range of subjects in the General Surgery domain. There do seem to be some areas that examiners favor more heavily than others and a knowledge of these patterns may help guide you in the amount of time you devote to each area in your studies. Some broad patterns are obvious and logical. The largest major category, of course, is gastrointestinal. In a sampling of 700 oral board questions asked over the past 17 years, over half the questions dealt with the subjects of colon, stomach and duodenum, liver/biliary, vascular, head and neck, trauma, cardiothoracic, and esophagus. The distribution of all subject areas covered in these 700 questions is listed by percent below with the gastrointestinal subcategories listed individually:

Head and Neck	7.6%	Hernia	2.7%
Colon	7.3%	Pancreas	2.4%
Vascular	7.0%	Pediatrics	2.1%
Trauma	6.6%	Endocrine	1.9%
Stomach/duodenum	6.6%	Shock	1.9%
Liver/biliary	6.1%	Organ failure	1.6%
Cardiothoracic	5.6%	Fluid/electrolytes	1.4%
Esophagus	5.6%	Appendix	1.3%
Breast	4.3%	Coagulation	1.1%
Spleen	3.9%	Nutrition	.9%
Infection	3.7%	Burns	.7%
Small bowel	3.6%	Anesthesia	.7%
Genitourinary	3.3%	Rectum	.4%
Soft tissue	3.1%	Neurosurgery	.4%
Orthopedics	3.1%	Plastic surgery	.3%
GYN	3.0%		

The Focus of the Questions

Most of the questions in the certifying/oral examination fall into one of the following four categories:

1. **Identifying a surgical problem.** These questions take the form of "What is the presentation of . . .", "How would you evaluate . . .", "How would you work up . . .", "What is the differential diagnosis of . . .".
2. **How does a surgical problem behave?** These often begin "What is the natural history of . . .", "What is the physiology of . . .".
3. **Treatment.** You will be asked "What are your treatment options . . .", "How would you manage . . .", "What are the indications for . . .". In this category you will also be asked technical questions, "How do you do . . .".
4. **Results.** These questions are a follow up to your choice of treatment: "What is the prognosis of . . .", "What are the complications of . . .", "How would you follow up on . . .", "How would you treat a recurrence . . .".

These categories are obviously sequential and you may be quizzed on a topic in logical order to test your organization and thought process or you may be asked questions out of context to test spot knowledge. The latter usually occurs toward the end of a session as a time filler.

Listen carefully to the question. It usually takes the form "How would *you* . . .". Do not describe a spectrum of approaches unless asked to do so. If you have no experience with the entity, SAY SO, but whatever you do, do not try to fake it. You may lose half a point for your ignorance, but you won't be flunked for your stupidity. Dishonesty is not a trait an examiner would like to see in a candidate he or she certifies.

After you describe what you would do, you may at times want to ask the results of your actions if this information is not volunteered, for example: "I would perform a Pringle maneuver. . . . does the bleeding slow down?"

Answer the question thoroughly and concisely, but do not volunteer extraneous information. Number one, you may get nailed on it, and number two, when you *do not* volunteer additional information on the next question the examiner will *know* you are not as well informed on that subject and pursue it to your discomfort.

Preparation for the Certifying Examination

A good residency program with a wide clinical experience is the best preparation for the Certifying Examination. The following are useful adjuncts to improve your performance.

The American College of Surgeons periodically makes available a Surgical Education and Self-Assessment Program (SESAP). The current program and the past ones provide a convenient and reliable way to expand your knowledge, test your clinical judgment, and learn your deficiencies. The clinical photographs and reproductions of x-ray films and electrocardiograms are excellent. The correct answers to the questions are explained clearly and the references are useful and current.

The review sections of Selected Readings provide a convenient summary of consensus and controversy about a wide range of surgical problems. If you are particularly weak in some area read most of the sections on the subject.

Postgraduate courses are conducted at the October Annual Clinical Congress of the American College of Surgeons and at the College's Spring Meeting. The symposia and the scientific exhibits provide current, useful information.

Tapes of conferences, symposia and panel discussions presented at the Annual Clinical Congress of the American College of Surgeons provide current information and point out areas of controversy.

EXAMPLES OF CERTIFYING EXAMINATIONS

The following questions and sequences will give you a reasonable idea of what to expect during the Certifying Examination. The Roman numerals indicate one complete session of the three that comprise the examination.

I.

1. A middle-aged woman has a 3-cm tumor above the angle of the mandible.

   (A) What kind of work-up would you do? (A few, brief, pertinent questions from the examinee established that this was not a skin lesion but rather, most likely, a tumor in the parotid gland.)
   (B) Would you biopsy a parotid tumor?
   (C) What operation would you do?
   (D) What technique would you use to perform a superficial parotidectomy?
   (E) It is adherent to the nerve. Would you take the nerve?
   (F) Would you do a radical neck?
   (G) If the diagnosis comes back mucoepidermoid carcinoma rather than mixed tumor, would you do anything different?
   (H) What if it is an adenocarcinoma?

2. (A) What is the safest way to do a cholecystectomy?
   (B) What would you do if the patient is jaundiced?
   (C) You can't get a stone out of the distal common duct; what would you do?
   (D) After duodenotomy and sphincterotomy, you still can't remove the stone; what would you do?
   (E) What if the gallbladder is markedly inflamed and it is very difficult to remove?
   (F) How would you initially treat a patient with acute cholecystitis?
   (G) Hydrops of the gallbladder was described. What would the fluid in the gallbladder look like? Why is it clear?

3. During the course of a colectomy, you discover you have transected the ureter.

   (A) What would you do?
   (B) What size T-tube could you use?
   (C) Would you use a ureteric catheter as a splint?
   (D) Where would you put it in the ureter?
   (E) Where would you bring it out?
   (F) How long would you leave it in?
   (G) What if you had removed a whole section of ureter?
   (H) How does the ureter get its blood supply?

4. A 46-year-old woman has symptoms of gastroesophageal reflux.

   (A) How would you work up the patient?
   (B) How would you treat?
   (C) The patient's symptoms persist despite your medical regimen. How would you proceed?
   (D) What operation would you do?
   (E) How do you do that?
   (F) How would you follow up the patient?

5. An elderly alcoholic is seen in the ER with severe chest and abdominal pain after an episode of drinking and vomiting.

   (A) What are you concerned about?
   (B) How would you diagnose Boerhaave's syndome?
   (C) Where is the esophagus most likely to rupture?
   (D) How would you treat this?
   (E) How would you approach it surgically?
   (F) What interspace would you use to open the chest?

II.

1. A patient has an upper, outer quadrant carcinoma of the breast.

   (A) What operation would you advise?
   (B) Why would you do that instead of an alternative procedure?
   (C) Would you consider just doing a wide local excision (lumpectomy)?
   (D) What if the patient insisted on only having a lumpectomy?

2. A young girl has a fibroadenoma removed. Later, when you examine her, she has five breast nodules. What would you do?

3. What are your indications for partially interrupting or ligating the vena cava?

   (A) Where would you place the filter or clip?
   (B) Would you consider ligating any other veins at the same time?

4. At laparotomy you discover a 7-cm cyst of the ovary.

   (A) What types might it be?
   (B) What would you do?

5. There is a rectal lesion just above the internal sphincter. It is 2 inches in diameter but is very superficial. How would you remove this?

6. A 72-year-old patient is admitted in shock with signs and symptoms that lead to the diagnosis of a ruptured abdominal aneurysm.

   (A) How would you treat?
   (B) What kind of incision?
   (C) How do you obtain proximal control of the aorta?

7. A 70-year-old man with well-controlled congestive heart failure. He has a 6-cm asymptomatic infrarenal abdominal aortic aneurysm.

   (A) What would you advise?
   (B) What is the likely mortality rate of operating?
   (C) What is the chance it will rupture?

8. An elderly man with venous thrombosis of the calves has a pulmonary embolus. What would you do?

9. What do you do with someone who develops a pulmonary embolus on heparin therapy?

   (A) Would you clip the iliac vein?
   (B) Why not?

10. Would you heparinize before operating for saddle embolus of the aorta?

11. The patient had a myocardial infarction 3 weeks ago and now has impending gangrene of one leg What would you do?

12. An elderly man with atrial fibrillation develops a cold, pulseless right leg. What would you do?

III.

1. A child grabs a live electric wire and suffers an electrical burn of the thenar web space.

   (A) How would you treat this?
   (B) Would the tendon be involved?

2. A patient suffers burns from a gasoline fire of 30% of his body. The burns are on the legs and abdomen.

   (A) Describe your treatment.

3. (A) How do you treat an intertrochanteric fracture of the femur in an elderly woman?
   (B) What is the blood supply to the neck of the femur?

4. How do you set a Colles' fracture?

5. What is a Bennett's fracture?

6. A lesion on the foot of a woman is described. The candidate concludes the examiner is describing a melanoma.

   (A) How would you treat?
   (B) Inguinal nodes are not palpable.
   (C) Five years later there is recurrence at the site of the graft on the foot. What would you do?

7. What would you do for a little girl with pectus excavatum?

8. What are the indications for hyperalimentation?

   (A) Discuss the complications of hyperalimentation.

IV.

1. A patient with a lesser curvature gastric ulcer is referred to you. The ulcer has been demonstrated by an upper GI series.

   (A) What work-up would you do?
   (B) What technique of gastroscopy would you recommend?
   (C) Biopsies show no tumor. How would you manage the patient?

(D) One month later this ulcer appears on x-ray examination to be healed but the patient still has abdominal pain and is losing weight. What would you do?

(E) What incision would you use to explore this patient?

(F) You feel a mass in the lesser curvature of the stomach. What would you do?

(G) If you biopsy the ulcer and it shows tumor what is the extent of the resection you would perform?

(H) What tissue in addition to the stomach would you remove?

2. A middle-aged woman has a history strongly suggestive of chronic cholecystitis. The gallbladder is not seen on oral cholecystogram.

(A) What would you do to work this patient up?

(B) An IV cholangiogram is performed. The common duct appears to be normal? At operation, how would you evaluate the common duct?

(C) Do you leave a drain in following cholecystectomy?

(D) What are the indications for common duct exploration?

(E) Six weeks later she still has abdominal pain and indigestion after eating fatty foods. A brief discussion of per-oral cannulation of the common bile duct followed.

3. A 25-year-old male is brought into the ER after a severe motor vehicle accident, complaining of abdominal pain.

(A) What are the first steps you would take?

(B) On abdominal exam there are signs of peritonitis. What would you do next?

(C) Peritoneal lavage is grossly bloody.

(D) On opening the abdomen there is a large supcapsular hematoma of the right lobe of the liver.

(E) On exploration there are no other sources of bleeding.

(F) No, the hematoma is not expanding. Would you open the hematoma?

(G) What are the potential complications of not opening it?

(H) Are there any things you can do to prevent those complications?

(I) At 8 hours after surgery, profuse bleeding occurs through your drains. You re-explore and find the hematoma has ruptured. What would you do?

(J) On evacuating the clot you find a deep stellate laceration of the dome of the right lobe.

(K) Your local measures are inadequate.

(L) Your Pringle maneuver fails to control the bleeding.

(M) How do you do a right hepatic lobectomy?

4. The man in the car wreck just discussed is found to have a large retroperitoneal hematoma. Would you open the hematoma?

5. A known cirrhotic, middle-aged man has massive upper GI bleeding.

(A) How would you manage this patient?

(B) The role of endoscopy, arteriography, and vasopressin infusion into the superior mesenteric artery were discussed.

(C) Emergency portacaval decompression, indications and mortality rate, were discussed. What type of portacaval decompression would you do?

V.

1. You are exploring a young man for an acute abdomen and you find Crohn's disease of the distal ilium only.

(A) What would you do?

(B) Under what circumstances would you do an appendectomy?

(C) Would you ever consider doing a right colectomy in such a patient?

2. A man has a known carcinoma of the large bowel 12 cm from the anal verge. There is no obstruction.

(A) What operative procedure would you choose?

(B) Describe the steps of your operation.

(C) What portion of the colon receives its blood supply from the inferior mesenteric artery?

(D) After resection, the distal segment of rectum is 2 inches in diameter. The proximal colon is 3 inches away from the distal end. What would you do?

(E) How would you handle a size discrepancy of the two segments of large intestine?

3. You perform an incidental appendectomy following a cholecystectomy. The appendix contains a carcinoid.

(A) What would you do?
(B) How would you follow this patient?
(C) What if there were multiple nodules in the liver which could not be resected?
(D) Suppose there were nodules in the distal ileum?

4. A 48-year-old male has signs of claudication after three blocks and can no longer play tennis.

(A) How would you evaluate him?
(B) How would you obtain an ankle pressure index? What does it mean?
(C) He follows your advice, stops smoking nd loses weight without relief. What then?
(D) What are the risks of arteriogram?
(E) What are the risks of surgery in your hands?
(F) What are the chances of a patient like this ending up with an amputation if you bypass him?
(G) What would you use to bypass him?
(H) What is the minimum vein size you would consider adequate?
(I) What if the saphenous is unsuitable?
(J) What other options might you consider beside bypass (balloon angioplasty)?

5. A 12-year-old boy has multiple episodes of abdominal pain. He has circumoral pigmentation.

(A) What do you think of?
(B) At exploration, it seems that there are multiple intestinal polyps. There is a local intussusception.
(C) In Peutz-Jegher's syndrome, what are the intestinal lesions?
(D) How would you treat this patient?

6. A 16-year-old girl has a nodule in the breast. On clinical examination it seems to be a fibroadenoma.

(A) What would you do?
(B) Would you do a mammogram?

7. A 55-year-old woman presents to your clinic with a solitary nodule in the right breast.

(A) What points in the history would raise your suspicion for malignancy?
(B) What physical findings would make you suspect malignancy?
(C) How would you manage the lump?
(D) Aspiration yields no fluid. What would you do next?
(E) Describe your outpatient biopsy procedure (include sending tissue for estrogen receptors).
(F) Describe how you do a modified radical mastectomy.
(G) What is the prognosis if no nodes are positive? If 15 nodes are positive?
(H) If estrogen receptors are positive how would you treat the patient? If ER negative?
(I) The patient returns in three years with a local chest wall recurrence. How would you proceed?
(J) The patient then develops a pulmonary nodule. How would you work it up? It proves to be consistent with breast carcinoma. What would you do now?

8. An 82-year-old woman has an epidermoid carcinoma of the vulva. The groin nodes are not palpable.

(A) What would you do?
(B) What would you do if the nodes in the groin were suspicious for tumor?
(C) What is a serious complication of groin dissection?

9. A young man has a small stab wound just under the sternum. He is markedly hypotensive.

(A) What would you do?
(B) With IV therapy, the blood pressure continues to drop. What would you do?
(C) What technique would you use to withdraw blood from the pericardial sac?
(D) What size syringe would you use?
(E) After removing 30 cc of blood, the blood pressure improves. What is going on?
(F) If a stab wound of the heart requires operative repair, how would you approach it?

10. Three days after anterior colon resection for carcinoma of the sigmoid colon the patient develops fever and more abdominal tenderness.

(A) What would you do?

11. A patient who is being treated with anticoagulants (subcutaneous heparin) has had the clotting time poorly controlled. He develops symptoms and signs of a pulmonary embolus.

    (A) What would you do?
    (B) What technique of heparinization would you advise?
    (C) How do you determine if heparinization is adequate?
    (D) He has more hemoptysis. What would you do?
    (E) A lung scan shows multiple defects. What would you do?
    (F) Suppose the scan did not show clear evidence of further embolization.

12. A patient has a high output small intestinal fistula.

    (A) How would you treat?
    (B) Describe exactly the method you would use for intravenous parenteral hyperalimentation.
    (C) After 1 week of therapy the patient begins to get a little hazy, is intermittently confused and appears dehydrated. What is going on?
    (D) What blood chemistries would you investigate?

VI.

1. A patient is found to have a serum calcium of 13.5 mg%.

    (A) How would you work this patient up?
    (B) If a parathormone level is normal, does this rule out parathyroid adenoma?

2. A patient has hypertension and hypercalcemia.

    (A) How do you work this patient up?
    (B) She is found to have a pheochromocytoma and a parathyroid adenoma. Discuss this.

3. What would you look for in your examination of a 30-year-old male who sustained blunt chest trauma in a motor vehicle accident?

    (A) Several ribs on the left are broken in more than one place and the patient does not appear to be in severe respiratory distress. What would you do?
    (B) One hour later the P_{CO_2} has gone up to 50 and the P_{O_2} has dropped to 60. What now?
    (C) Describe the respirator and the settings you would use.

    (D) What is the pathophysiology of flail chest?
    (E) Once on the respirator, ventilatory resistance increases and gases deteriorate. You hear no breath sounds on the left.
    (F) Describe how you place a chest tube.
    (G) Your x-ray after tube placement shows a widened mediastinum. How do you proceed?
    (H) Angiogram shows a disruption of the aorta distal to the arch, how would you proceed?
    (I) At 1 day post trauma the chest x-ray shows increased lung density near the flail segment. How would you manage pulmonary contusion?

VII.

1. A 42-year-old man presents with a pigmented lesion of the left anterior chest. What would you do?

    (A) It is a Clark's level II melanoma. What do you do next? What is Clark's level II?
    (B) There is no axillary adenopathy. Would you do a prophylactic node dissection?
    (C) What is the prognosis for this patient?

2. A 28-year-old man presents with a perforated duodenal ulcer. He has no ulcer history.

    (A) What would you do?
    (B) How would you close the ulcer?
    (C) If he had a long ulcer history and his perforation was 3 hours old what would you do? If 10 hours old?
    (D) Describe types of pyloroplasty.
    (E) What is the mortality for antrectomy versus pyloroplasty?
    (F) You do an antrectomy and find you cannot easily close the duodenum. What would you do?

3. How would you work an elderly man with painless obstructive jaundice?

    (A) At surgery you find what appears to be a carcinoma of the head of the pancreas. How do you determine resectability?
    (B) Would you biopsy the mass? How?

4. A 75-year-old man has an ulcerating lesion on his lower lip.

    (A) How would you treat it?
    (B) After you wedge it out, what layers need to be approximated?
    (C) What is the blood supply of the lower lip?

5. How would you work up hypercalcemia in a young man?

    (A) You find one enlarged gland and three normal-sized glands on exploration. What would you do?
    (B) The enlarged gland and a biopsy of a normal-sized gland are indistinguishable. What do you do?
    (C) Three weeks later the patient returns with persistent hyperparathyroidism. What do you do?
    (D) How would you re-explore the neck?
    (E) How would you deal with the remaining glands?

6. 15 years after cholecystectomy, a 45-year-old woman presents with fever, chills, jaundice, and abdominal pain.

    (A) How would you work her up?
    (B) Ultrasound shows dilated bile ducts.
    (C) What incision would you use to explore?
    (D) How would you locate and identify the common duct?
    (E) How would you explore the common duct?
    (F) You find some sludge and two stones. What would you do next?
    (G) How do you perform choledochoscopy?
    (H) You see a stone in a hepatic radical. What would you do?
    (I) Describe your options for biliary bypass.

EXAMPLES OF QUESTIONS ASKED DURING RECENT PART II EXAMINATIONS

1. The management of pulmonary contusion.

2. Intra-operative bleeding after a 7-unit transfusion.

3. A child has an inguinal hernia. Do you explore the other side?

4. How do you manage a strawberry hemangioma in an infant?

5. How do you manage infarcted bowel in a strangulated inguinal hernia?

6. During IV hyperalimentation, the patient has *Candida* sepsis. How do you manage it?

7. How much blood loss does it take to produce shock?

8. The fluid therapy for a severe burn.

9. The work-up of a GI bleeder.

10. Techniques for dealing with retained common duct stones.

11. The use of chenodeoxycholic acid to dissolve cholesterol stones.

12. Large bowel trauma.

13. Splenic artery aneurysms.

14. Penetrating wounds of the abdomen.

15. Staging for Hodgkin's disease.

16. Medical or operative treatment for bleeding peptic ulcer. In what percentage of operated patients does bleeding recur? How do you handle recurrent bleeding?

17. How do you manage trauma to the head of the pancreas with retroperitoneal hematoma?

18. How do you manage disruption of the common duct near the pancreas?

19. Indications for surgery for hiatus hernia. Technique of the operative repair.

20. The workup for a mass in the liver of a 23-year-old girl. Technique for resecting a hemangioma of the right lobe of the liver.

21. The workup for destructive jaundice in a 64-year-man. At operation a pancreatic mass is palpated. What would you do?

22. A 14-year-old boy has hematuria following a football game. IVP shows extravasation of urine from the left kidney. At operation, there is a small laceration in the upper pole. What would you do?

23. A patient has an attack of acute pancreatitis. After the attack subsides, how do you work this patient up? An oral cholecystogram shows gallstones. What would you do? What abnormalities on cholangiogram might cause you to do more than a simple cholecystectomy?

24. How would you assess whether a jejunal diverticulum was the cause of gastrointestinal bleeding?

25. During an operation, the patient develops a bleeding disorder. How would you investigate this?

26. A 65-year-old man has fever, left lower quadrant pain, and blood in his stool. How would you manage this patient initially? At operation he has an abscess, apparently from diverticulitis. What would you do?

27. The treatment for cholecystitis which develops in the postoperative period.

28. An elderly man has a fungating carcinoma of the anus. Would you advise radiation or abdominoperineal resection?

29. A similar patient has an adenocarcinoma 10 cm above the anal verge. What is your recommendation? How do you decide when to do a low anterior resection rather than an abdominoperineal resection?

30. Would you do an incidental appendectomy in conjunction with

    (A) hysterectomy?
    (B) cholecystectomy?
    (C) hernia repair?

31. The management of a patient in shock following a stab wound of the left chest.

32. The best anesthesia for pheochromocytoma.

33. The advantages and disadvantages of different types of anesthesia.

34. A 1-year-old male has intermittent groin swelling. What would you do?

35. Differential diagnosis of hypercalcemia.

36. How do you explore the neck for parathyroid adenoma or hyperplasia? Normal and abnormal location of the parathyroids.

37. List the surgically correctable causes of hypertension.

38. What would you advise for an enlarging, crusting lesion on the malar area of a 55-year-old man? It is a senile keratosis. Any further treatment recommended?

39. The treatment for a 1-cm melanoma on the cheek.

40. How would you treat a basal cell carcinoma of the cheek? Several cervical nodes are palpable. What do you think about that?

41. Six days after a puncture wound of the little finger the patient has a swollen tender, red hand. What would you do?

42. How would you prepare a thyrotoxic patient for thyroid surgery?

43. A 50-year-old man has a 1-2 cm nodule in the mid-portion of the anterior neck. How would you treat if it needs treatment? Why examine the axillae and groins?

44. A 43-year-old man who is a heavy drinker is admitted to Emergency because of nausea and vomiting. He is dehydrated.

    (A) Your work-up?
    (B) Your treatment?

    You find acute pyloric stenosis. What is your treatment? Management of peptic ulcer disease.

45. Diagnosis and management of a 19-year-old male with sudden onset of right chest pain. How do *you* insert a chest tube?

46. Work-up for retained common duct stone in a cholecystectomy patient. Treatment if a retained stone is present.

47. 69-year-old woman with hypotension, tachycardia, fever and rigid abdomen.

    (A) Initial treatment?
    (B) Swan-Ganz catheter?
    (C) Dopamine? Other pressors?
    (D) Work-up?
    (E) Treatment and management of perforated sigmoid diverticulitis

48. Twenty-three-old woman who was in a motor vehicle accident has chest pain.

    (A) Management
    (B) Chest films show a hemopneumothorax. What would you do?
    (C) The chest film shows a widened mediastinum. What is your work-up?
    (D) What would lead you to suspect aorta rupture?
    (E) There is rupture of the thoracic aorta. What is your management?

49. Work-up and management of a 6-month-old infant with

    (A) Inguinal hernia
    (B) Umbilical hernia

50. An adult patient has a incarcerated femoral hernia.

    (A) Work-up and management
    (B) Strangulated bowel is present. What operation would you do to repair the hernia?
    (C) Antibiotics indicated?
    (D) Drains indicated?
    (E) If you can't readily reduce the incarcerated hernia what do you do to permit reduction?

51. A 26-year-old nurse becomes dizzy when fasting. She is hypoglycemic. Symptoms are relieved after glucose ingestion.

    (A) Work-up
    (B) Insulinoma is suspected. List other possibilities of the cause of hypoglycemia/hyperinsulinism
    (C) Management of this patient
    (D) Do all lesions of the head of the pancreas require a Whipple's procedure?
    (E) What is Whipple's triad?
    (F) At operation how do you expose the pancreas?
    (G) How will you locate the tumor or tumors?

52. Eight days following cholecystectomy the patient has chest pain and dyspnea.

    (A) How would you work this patient up?
    (B) A diagnosis of pulmonary embolus is made. What is your treatment?
    (C) Would your treatment be the same if the patient had undergone an abdominoperineal resection 8 days earlier?
    (D) What are the indications for the placement of an inferior vena cava umbrella?
    (E) Indications for ligation or clipping the inferior vena cava.
    (F) How do you reverse heparin?
    (G) After cessation of heparin treatment what is the risk of a clot, what is the rate of propagation of a clot?

53. A patient has a perforated diverticulum of the sigmoid colon which has caused peritonitis.

    (A) List the bacteria likely to be present.
    (B) What antibiotic treatment would you prescribe?
    (C) Which antibiotic are you prescribing for which bacteria?
    (D) What operation would you perform?

54. What types of operation would you consider for repair of a recurrent inguinal hernia?

55. Six hours following resection of an abdominal aortic aneurysm in a high risk patient the right leg is cold.

    (A) What would you do?
    (B) What type of anesthesia?
    (C) What size Fogarty catheter?
    (D) Probable cause of patient's cold leg.

56. The management of a patient, not in shock, who has sustained a stab wound of the base of the neck on the left side.

57. Diagnosis and management of a melanoma of the face.

58. What is your management of a perforated peptic ulcer?

59. Indications for operation on Crohn's disease.

    (A) What operation would you perform for Crohn's disease of the colon?
    (B) For Crohn's disease of the ileum and jejunum?

60. Carcinoma of the head of the pancreas.

    (A) Diagnostic studies prior to operation
    (B) At operation how do you decide whether or not to resect the carcinoma?

61. A patient has receive prednisone for 10 months.

    (A) Describe how you would prescribe steroids preoperatively?
    (B) How would you prescribe steroids in the postoperative period?

62. Coin lesion of the lung.

    (A) Work-up
    (B) Likely diagnosis
    (C) At operation how do you determine the type of operation to perform?

References

Below is a numbered list of reference books pertaining to the material in the book.

On the last line of each test item at the right-hand side, there appears a number combination that identifies the reference source and the page or pages where the information relating to the question and the correct answer may be found. The first number refers to the textbook or journal in the list and the second number refers to the page of that textbook or journal.

For example: (2:345) is a reference to the second book in the list, page 345 of Schwartz's *Principles of Surgery*.

1. Way LW. *Current Surgical Diagnosis and Treatment*. 8th ed. Norwalk, Conn: Appleton and Lange, 1988

2. Schwartz SI (ed). *Principles of Surgery*. 4th ed. New York: McGraw-Hill, 1984

3. Sabiston DC Jr (ed). *Textbook of Surgery*. 13th ed. Philadelphia: WB Saunders Co, 1986

4. Rutherford RB. *Vascular Surgery*. 2nd ed. Philadelphia: WB Saunders Co, 1984

5. Moore WS. *Vascular Surgery: A Comprehensive Review*. New York: Greene and Stratton, 1983

6. Hardy JD. *Textbook of Surgery*. 2nd ed. Philadelphia: JB Lippincott, 1988

7. Rob CG. The extraperitoneal approach to the abdominal aorta. *Surgery*. 53:87, 1963

8. Sanford JP. *Guide to Antimicrobial Therapy*. 1986, p 41–46

9. *Advanced Trauma Life Support Course Instructor's Manual*. Chicago: American College of Surgeons, 1984

10. Wilson SE, Veith FJ, Hobson RW, Williams RA. *Vascular Surgery*. New York: McGraw-Hill, 1987

11. *Encyclopedia Britannica*. Chicago: University of Chicago Press, 1987

12. Resnick RH, Chalmers JG, Ishihara AM, et al. Controlled study of the prophylactic porta-caval shunt. *Ann Int Med*. 70:675, 1969

13. Fogarty TJ, Cranley JJ, Krause RJ, et al. A method for extraction of arterial emboli and thrombi. *Surg Gynecol Obstet*. 116:241, 1963

14. May AG, DeWeese JA, Rob CG. Changes in sexual function following operation on the abdominal aorta. *Surgery*. 65:41, 1969

15. Gray H. *Anatomy of the Human Body*. 30th ed. Philadelphia: Lea and Febiger, 1985

16. Lucas A, Max MH. Emergency laparotomy immediately after coronary bypass. *JAMA*. 244:1829, 1980

17. McDonald AP, Howard RJ. Pyogenic liver abscesses. *World J Surg*. 4:369, 1980

18. Symposium on Antimicrobial Agents. *Mayo Clin Proc*. 62:916, 1987

19. Mallory A, Schaefer JW, Cohen JR, Holt SA. Selective intra-arterial vasopressin infusion for upper gastrointestinal tract hemorrhage. *Arch Surg* 115:30, 1980

20. Mulholland MW, Debas HT. Physiology and pathophysiology of gastrin. *Surgery*. 103:135, 1988

21. Ellis FG, Olsen AM. *Achalasia of the Esophagus* Philadelphia: WB Saunders Co, 1969

22. Cameron JL, Brawley RK, Bender HW, Zuidema GD. The treatment of pancreatic ascites. *Ann Surg*. 170:668, 1969

23. Sabiston DC Jr. *Essentials of Surgery*. Philadelphia: WB Saunders Co, 1987

24. Bunnell S. Surgery of the nerves of the hand. *Surg Gynecol Obstet*. 44:145, 1927

First Examination
Questions

DIRECTIONS (Questions 1 through 91): Each of the numbered items or incomplete statements in this section is followed by answers or by completions of the statement. Select the ONE lettered answer or completion that is BEST in each case.

1. One of the following statements concerning an infant's abdominal wall is NOT correct.

   (A) gastroschisis is herniation of abdominal contents through a small defect to the right of the umbilical cord
   (B) omphalocele is a huge hernia into the umbilical cord
   (C) 90% of umbilical hernias in infants close spontaneously by the age of 5 years
   (D) an inguinal hernia in a newborn should be repaired after the age of 6 months
   (E) persistence of the vitelline duct may result in a fistula between the distal ilium and the umbilicus   (3:1279, 1293)

2 Traumatic rupture of the thoracic aorta is associated with all of the following EXCEPT

   (A) history of an accident with severe deceleration
   (B) fractures of the first and second ribs
   (C) cardiac tamponade
   (D) severe pain in the upper chest
   (E) widening of the mediastinum on a chest x-ray   (3:1813)

3. In lymphogranuloma venereum, which of the following statements is UNTRUE?

   (A) rectal strictures occur
   (B) inguinal lymph nodes enlarge
   (C) adenocarcinoma of the rectum often occurs
   (D) treatment with tetracyclines often is effective

   (E) Frei skin test and complement-fixation tests both assist the diagnosis   (2:1235)

4. At operation, a carcinoma of the head of the pancreas is found. It is adherent in the portal and superior mesenteric veins, and the duodenum is partially obstructed. The best operative procedure is

   (A) pancreaticoduodenectomy
   (B) cholecystojejunostomy and gastroenterostomy
   (C) cholecystojejunostomy
   (D) gastroenterostomy
   (E) splanchnic neurectomy   (1:535)

5. The treatment of frostbite should begin as soon as possible and should include all of the following EXCEPT

   (A) rapid rewarming in water at 42°C that is circulated if possible
   (B) slow rewarming in water at 36°F that is circulated if possible
   (C) removing all wet and constricting clothing
   (D) relief of pain with narcotics
   (E) wrapping the patient in warm blankets and giving hot fluids by mouth if possible   (3:238)

6. An adult male aged 55 has a blood serum calcium of 11.5 mg/100 ml. Causes of this abnormality include all of the following EXCEPT

   (A) hypothyroidism
   (B) hyperparathyroidism
   (C) sarcoidosis
   (D) multiple myeloma
   (E) thiazide diuretics   (3:630)

7. Allen's test may assist in the diagnosis of

   (A) occlusion of the radial or ulnar arteries distal to the wrist
   (B) thoracic outlet compression syndrome
   (C) aortic arch syndrome
   (D) carpal tunnel syndrome
   (E) Volkmann's ischemic contracture   *(4:693)*

8. The treatment of acute toxic cholangitis should include all of the following EXCEPT

   (A) medical treatment with antibiotics and full support in an intensive care unit
   (B) operative relief of the underlying common bile duct obstruction
   (C) vigorous use of the appropriate antibiotics
   (D) adequate fluid replacement based on urine output and central venous pressure measurements
   (E) monitoring in an intensive care unit
   (3:1158)

9. All of the following statements about tracheo-esophageal fistula (TEF) are correct EXCEPT

   (A) in the most common form, the esophagus ends as a dilated blind pouch and the distal esophagus originates from a small fistulous communication with the trachea
   (B) other congenital abnormalities are infrequent
   (C) the diagnosis is suggested by excessive secretions from the mouth because the infant cannot swallow saliva
   (D) bronchoscopy at the time of repair removes the need for barium x-ray studies and aids anesthetic tube placement and localization of the TEF
   (E) initial treatment is directed toward minimizing complications from aspiration of saliva.   *(3:1264)*

10. Intussusception is the telescoping of one portion of the bowel into the segment just distal to it. Which of the following statements is correct?

    (A) the typical patient is a healthy infant who suddenly develops intermittent severe abdominal pain
    (B) a lead point, such as a polyp, is usually present in children
    (C) bloody (red currant jelly) stools are rarely seen
    (D) a sausage-shaped mass is palpable in less than half of these patients
    (E) barium enema reduction is unsafe   *(3:1282)*

11. Acute appendicitis occurs approximately once in every 2000 pregnancies. Which of the following statements concerning this problem is INCORRECT?

    (A) the enlarging uterus carries the appendix away from McBurney's point
    (B) the inflammatory reaction often initiates premature labor, with loss of the fetus
    (C) treatment should be conservative without operation when possible
    (D) flaccidity of the abdominal wall in the last trimester means that there will be little rigidity
    (E) regional anesthesia if used for an appendectomy must be placed higher than usual   *(1:57)*

12. A patient is diagnosed as suffering from shock, but his cardiac index, when measured, is found to be increased, and his extremities are warm and dry. Which type of shock is he experiencing?

    (A) hypovolemic shock
    (B) septic shock
    (C) burn shock
    (D) cardiogenic shock
    (E) spinal shock—peripheral pooling of blood
    (3:48)

13. A patient with an extensive burn will require adequate exogenous calories and nitrogen to prevent prolonged catabolism. This is best monitored by accurate daily measurement of the body weight. Such nutrition is best provided by

    (A) enteral nutrition
    (B) intravenous hyperalimentation
    (C) intravenous nutrition by a Broviac or Hickman catheter
    (D) central total parenteral nutrition
    (E) peripheral total parenteral nutrition   *(2:280)*

14. A ruptured lumbar intervertebral disc is associated with all of the following EXCEPT

    (A) herniation of the L4-5 disc compresses the L5 nerve root
    (B) the aim of surgical treatment is to provide relief of nerve compression
    (C) the disc herniates in an anterior and lateral direction
    (D) nearly 95% of disc herniations occur at the L5-S1 of L4-5 levels
    (E) the initial treatment of acute symptoms should be conservative   *(3:1395-1396)*

15. Vomiting is an important symptom that is associated frequently with acute abdominal problems. In all of the following conditions, vomiting is usually not a feature EXCEPT for one in which it is frequent.

(A) perforated duodenal ulcer
(B) many patients with acute appendicitis
(C) ruptured spleen
(D) proximal small bowel obstruction
(E) recent large intestinal obstruction   *(3:907)*

16. A middle-aged woman is diagnosed as suffering from Hashimoto's disease, or lymphadenoid goiter. One of the following statements concerning this patient's problem is INCORRECT.

(A) in the well-established case, hyperthyroidism is present
(B) the thyroid gland is nodular, firm, and rubbery
(C) subtotal thyroidectomy should not be performed
(D) open biopsy is an accepted way by which the diagnosis can be established
(E) there is a strong possibility that this is an autoimmune disease   *(3:593)*

Questions 17 through 19

A 57-year-old white male executive entered the hospital because of hematemesis for 24 hours. Two days before admission, he had a very rich evening meal of wild duck and a considerable amount of whiskey. Some hours later, he noted epigastric distress. Later, he felt faint, became sweaty, and vomited coffeeground material. He repeated the vomiting and passed a dark, tarry stool. He later vomited red blood and came to the hospital by ambulance. Soon after admission, he vomited again. This was accompanied by severe retching, during which he complained of severe epigastric pain radiating to the flanks and back. The abdomen at this time was rigid throughout but remained nontender, and no rebound was present. Peristalsis was present. The temperature was 100°F, pulse 108, respiration 20, and blood pressure 130/84. His pain became unbearable at times and was accompanied by swallowing of air and a complaint of fullness. The abdomen became distended, but gastric aspiration revealed only small quantities of blood-stained fluid and air. Although not constant, the lack of abdominal tenderness in the face of boardlike rigidity was quite striking. The white blood count was 14,000; hematocrit 33.

17. What is the most likely diagnosis?

(A) perforated peptic ulcer
(B) esophageal varices
(C) spontaneous perforation of the esophagus
(D) coronary thrombosis
(E) strangulated diaphragmatic hernia
     (3:750–752)

18. The single best diagnostic procedure for the patient described in the preceding question is

(A) water soluble x-ray contrast examination of the upper gastrointestinal tract
(B) esophagoscopy
(C) chest x-ray films
(D) abdominal x-ray films
(E) electrocardiogram   *(3:750–752)*

19. The treatment of the patient described in the preceding two questions should be

(A) laparotomy
(B) left thoracotomy
(C) gastric aspiration, antibiotics, and supportive care
(D) right thoracotomy
(E) transfer to coronary care unit   *(3:750–752)*

Questions 20 through 22

A 54-year-old woman had an abdominal hysterectomy for uterine fibroids 10 years before. She has suffered from several episodes of crampy central and lower abdominal pain. The recent episode is more severe than previous attacks, and she is admitted to the hospital. She has slight abdominal distention, and she vomits a little. After a night's rest, she is relieved of her symptoms, and the abdomen is not tender.

20. The most likely diagnosis is

(A) stricture of the ureter secondary to the hysterectomy
(B) cholecystitis
(C) partial intestinal obstruction from adhesions
(D) mesenteric angina
(E) pancreatitis   *(1:569–571)*

21. The best method of establishing the diagnosis in the preceding question would be

    (A) intravenous pyelogram
    (B) abdominal films (supine and upright abdominal)
    (C) barium enema
    (D) cholecystogram
    (E) aortogram including lateral views

    (1:569–571)

22. The best method of treatment of the patient discussed in the preceding two questions is

    (A) cholecystectomy
    (B) laparotomy and division of adhesions
    (C) aortomesenteric bypass graft
    (D) sphincterotomy
    (E) continued observations   *(1:569–571)*

23. Which of the following systemic collagen diseases most frequently involves the esophagus?

    (A) periarteritis nodosa
    (B) rheumatoid arthritis
    (C) lupus erythematosus
    (D) scleroderma
    (E) erythema multiforme   *(2:1074)*

24. The symptoms and signs produced by congenital hypertrophic pyloric stenosis include all of the following EXCEPT

    (A) bile is present in the vomitus
    (B) vomiting usually starts at 1 to 2 weeks of age
    (C) the baby is hungry
    (D) the hypertrophied pylorus is palpable as an olive-shaped tumor
    (E) gastric peristaltic waves can be seen in the upper abdomen   *(3:1269)*

25. A patient is diagnosed as suffering from an acute occlusion of the popliteal artery due to fracture-dislocation of the knee. The care while waiting for operation should include all of the following EXCEPT

    (A) placing the involved limb in a dependent position
    (B) warming the ischemic foot
    (C) maintaining satisfactory blood pressure
    (D) relief of pain
    (E) splinting the fracture-dislocation   *(4:446)*

26. In paraesophageal hiatal hernia, which of the following does NOT apply?

    (A) is associated with reflux esophagitis
    (B) may cause gastric obstruction and bleeding
    (C) surgical repair often is indicated
    (D) surgical repair gives satisfactory results
    (E) may cause necrosis of the stomach

    (1:385–386)

27. Of the following statements concerning carcinoembryonic antigen (CEA), which one is correct?

    (A) the level of CEA in the bloodstream is important as a diagnostic test for colon cancer before clinical evidence of the disease appears
    (B) the level of CEA in the bloodstream accurately predicts cancer of the alimentary tract or pancreas
    (C) the level of CEA is not raised in patients with nonmalignant conditions, such as alcoholic cirrhosis and pancreatitis
    (D) study of the CEA level is of value in following the clinical course of patients with known carcinoma of the colon
    (E) the CEA level is not raised in patients with liver metastasis from colon carcinoma   *(2:326)*

28. It has been stated that morbid obesity that is refractory to medical treatment should be treated surgically. Which of the following operations has been abandoned?

    (A) gastric bypass
    (B) jejunoileal bypass
    (C) gastric partitioning
    (D) gastric stapling
    (E) vertical banded gastroplasty

    (2:1137–1139, 1164)

29. The following statements concern the composition of frequently used intravenous solutions. Which is NOT correct?

    (A) isotonic 0.9% NaCl contains 154 mEq/L of Na, Cl, and NaCl
    (B) 5% dextrose in 0.45% NaCl contains 50 g/L of glucose and 77 mEq/L of Na and Cl
    (C) lactated Ringer's solution contains Na 130 mEq/L, Cl 109 mEq/L, and HCO_3 28 mEq/L

(D) all of the solutions, isotonic NaCl, lactated Ringer's solution, and 5% dextrose in 0.45% NaCl, contain no potassium
(E) 3% NaCl contains 513 mEq/L of NaCl

(1:18)

30. In only one of the following clinical situations is a radical mastectomy clearly indicated.

(A) carcinoma of the breast with palpable nodes in the ipsilateral axilla
(B) carcinoma of the breast fixed to the pectoral muscle
(C) carcinoma in a lactating breast
(D) carcinoma develops in the other breast 5 years after radical mastectomy
(E) carcinoma in a male breast with a palpable axillary lymph node

(3:563)

31. The occurrence of polyposis coli, plus osteomas or exostoses, multiple epidermoid or sebaceous cysts, desmoid tumors often in abdominal incisions, and mesenteric fibromatosis makes up

(A) Gardner's syndrome
(B) Petersen's syndrome
(C) Peutz-Jegher's syndrome
(D) Meigs' syndrome
(E) Mallory-Weiss syndrome

(2:1194)

32. In which of the following fractures in an adult is operation NOT indicated?

(A) comminuted fracture of the head of the radius
(B) transverse fracture of the patella
(C) fracture of the medial humeral epicondyle
(D) fracture of the middle third of the clavicle with overriding
(E) fracture of the olecranon

(2:1964)

33. Wound dehiscence is rare under the age of 30, but in patients over 60, about 5% who have a laparotomy suffer from this complication. Which of the following statements is INCORRECT?

(A) the most important factor is the adequacy of the closure
(B) dehiscence is often the result of too few stitches placed too close to the wound margins
(C) increased intraabdominal pressure increases the risk of dehiscence
(D) transverse incisions have a lower incidence of dehiscence than have vertical incisions

(E) the use of catgut or polyglycolic acid sutures is associated with an increased incidence of wound dehiscence *(1:24)*

34. Regardless of the anatomic site of the tumor, pain is the most common initial complaint of a patient with carcinoma of the pancreas. The characteristics of this pain include all of the following EXCEPT

(A) the pain is vague and located in the epigastrium, with radiation to the back
(B) the pain is improved if the patient lies down
(C) the pain is improved if the patient bends forward
(D) the pain may not be improved with the administration of morphine
(E) frequently the cause of the abdominal pain is not diagnosed until the disease is far advanced *(3:1194)*

35. A woman aged 60 complains that she tires easily and feels weak. She is found to be anemic. Which of the following studies should be performed whenever possible?

(A) upper gastrointestinal series
(B) barium enema and colonoscopy
(C) sigmoidoscopy
(D) gastroscopy and duodenoscopy
(E) estimation of the serum carcinoembryonic antigen *(1:598)*

36. The congenital anomaly most commonly associated with an imperforate anus is

(A) tracheoesophageal fistula
(B) congenital heart disease
(C) talipes equinovarus
(D) malrotation of the intestine
(E) genitourinary abnormality *(6:1139)*

37. Hypoparathyroidism occurs as a complication of thyroidectomy, especially when performed for carcinoma or recurrent goiter. One of the following statements concerning this problem is INCORRECT.

    (A) the serum calcium is low, and the serum phosphorus is high
    (B) latent tetany is indicated by paresthesias and positive Chvostek and Trousseau signs
    (C) patients with the worst prognosis are those who develop symptoms after a long delay
    (D) acute hypoparathyroid tetany can be controlled by calcium chloride 10 to 20 ml of a 10% solution given intravenously
    (E) the management of chronic hypoparathyroidism is difficult because the difference between the controlling and intoxicating dose of vitamin D is small

    (1:255-256)

38. Controversy has surrounded the management of pancreatic pseudocysts. At the present time, one of the following methods of treatment is NOT justified.

    (A) operate if there is no evidence of resolution on a sonogram after 6 weeks
    (B) observe and manage conservatively
    (C) operate if the cyst becomes secondarily infected
    (D) perform internal drainage when possible
    (E) hemorrhage is an indication for operation

    (3:1189)

39. During an operation, the ureter sustains a transverse laceration involving 75% of its circumference at a distance of about 5 cm from the ureterovesical junction. The correct treatment would be

    (A) primary suture over a ureteric catheter
    (B) drainage
    (C) ligature proximal to the ureteric injury
    (D) ureterosigmoidostomy
    (E) end-to-side anastomosis to the bladder

    (2:1722)

40. Acute renal failure after surgery most often develops when one or more of the following are present.

    (A) preexisting renal disease
    (B) hypotension for more than 30 minutes
    (C) multiple blood transfusions
    (D) use of aminoglycoside antibiotics
    (E) hypertension for 1 hour

    (1:34)

41. A size 24 French urethral catheter

    (A) is 24 mm in external circumference
    (B) is 24 mm in diameter
    (C) has a length of 24 cm
    (D) allows a flow of 24 ml of urine/min
    (E) has an internal circumference of 24 mm

    (2:1687)

42. Which of the following testicular tumors is the most radiosensitive?

    (A) seminoma
    (B) choriocarcinoma
    (C) teratoma
    (D) carcinoma
    (E) interstitial cell tumor

    (2:1720)

43. A 1 cm calculus in the upper third of the ureter with infection of the urine and nonfunction of the kidney on an intravenous pyelogram is best treated by

    (A) antibiotics
    (B) nephrectomy
    (C) ureteral transvesical cystoscopic manipulation
    (D) ureteral catheter
    (E) ureterolithotomy

    (2:1699)

44. A young, previously healthy male is noted to have an abscess in the liver after a visit to the Sudan. A serologic test for antibody to *Entamoeba histolytica* is positive. Which of the following is NOT appropriate?

    (A) commence treatment with metronidazole
    (B) insert a percutaneous catheter and aspirate the abscess, sending pus for culture
    (C) if no secondary infection is present, treat also with chloroquine, emetine, and diiodohydroxyguinoline for possible associated systemic disease
    (D) drain the abscess widely
    (E) use follow-up sonograms to study size of the abscess

    (3:1075)

45. A 60-year-old man has a hard nodule on the right lobe of the prostate. Acid phosphatase levels are normal. Biopsy is performed and reveals adenocarcinoma of the prostate. A chest x-ray and full skeletal x-ray survey are negative. The preferred treatment would be

(A) suprapubic prostatectomy
(B) orchidectomy and estrogen therapy
(C) radical perineal prostatectomy
(D) transurethral resection of the prostate
(E) orchidectomy alone   *(2:1717)*

46. Which of the following is NOT a frequent symptom of internal hemorrhoids?

(A) bright red blood unmixed with stool
(B) severe pain
(C) prolapse with defecation
(D) pruritus
(E) discharge of mucus   *(1:633)*

47. A 50-year-old male has noticed the recent onset of a left varicocele, which has developed rather rapidly. With which of the following is this lesion likely to be associated?

(A) carcinoma of the left testicle
(B) portal hypertension
(C) carcinoma of the left kidney
(D) congestive cardiac failure
(E) retroperitoneal fibrosis   *(2:1685)*

48. The local degree of platelet activation and thrombus formation depends in part on a balance between the opposing actions of thromboxane A2 and which of the following substances?

(A) prostacyclin
(B) cholesterol
(C) prostaglandin E_2
(D) triglycerides
(E) all of the above   *(4:298)*

49. Pyuria without bacilluria and associated with gross hematuria is most commonly due to

(A) bladder stone
(B) urethritis
(C) perinephric abscess
(D) tuberculosis of the kidney
(E) carcinoma of the renal pelvis   *(1:848)*

Questions 50 through 52

A 2-day-old infant has had progressive vomiting since birth. No meconium has been passed, and there is a sausage-shaped mass in the right lower quadrant.

50. The most likely diagnosis is

(A) intussusception
(B) reduplication of the gut
(C) malrotation of the intestine

(D) meconium ileus
(E) acute appendicitis   *(1:1113-1114)*

51. In the patient described in the preceding question, which of the following tests would you NOT advise?

(A) tests for cystic fibrosis
(B) chest x-ray
(C) upper gastrointestinal series
(D) diagnostic enema
(E) abdominal plain x-ray   *(1:1113-1114)*

52. Which of the following would be the best form of therapy for the patient described in the preceding two questions?

(A) prepare for 48 hours with proper conservative therapy and then operate
(B) hydrate and treat with enemas of acetylcysteine or gastrografin
(C) treat with long tube and instillation of pancreatin
(D) treat with laxatives
(E) none of the above   *(1:1113-1114)*

53. An aneurysm of the subclavian artery associated with thoracic outlet compression most frequently produces major symptoms because of

(A) thrombosis
(B) rupture
(C) peripheral vascular spasm
(D) pressure on adjacent nerves and veins
(E) peripheral embolism   *(5:338)*

Questions 54 through 56

A 45-year-old farm worker from southern California has an ulcerated lesion 1 × 1.5 cm on the right lateral portion of the lower lip. He has poor oral hygiene. Firm nodes are palpable in the right submental triangle. The patient also has a peripheral coin lesion in the right lung, which shows some calcification and a central area of cavitation. The patient had gonorrhea at age 20.

54. The treatment would be

(A) wide excision and plastic closure
(B) wide excision and right radical neck dissection
(C) wide excision and thoracotomy with sequential resection of pulmonary lesion
(D) x-ray therapy
(E) dependent on biopsy of the lip lesion
                                          (2:565, 685)

55. The most likely diagnosis of the lip lesion described in the preceding question is

(A) squamous cell carcinoma
(B) basal cell carcinoma
(C) coccidioidomycosis
(D) syphilis
(E) tuberculosis   *(2:565)*

56. The lip lesion in the patient described in the preceding two questions has been adequately treated. The best diagnostic test for the lung lesion is

(A) skin test for coccidioidomycosis
(B) tomograms of the lung lesion
(C) Wasserman reaction
(D) bronchogram
(E) skin test for histoplasmosis   *(2:685)*

57. Which of the following cranial nerves transmits taste sensation from the anterior two thirds of the tongue?

(A) trigeminal nerve (fifth)
(B) facial nerve (seventh)
(C) glossopharyngeal nerve (ninth)
(D) vagus nerve (tenth)
(E) hypoglossal nerve (twelfth)   *(15:1174)*

58. A structure that lies anterior to the anterior scalene muscle is the

(A) subclavian artery
(B) subclavian vein
(C) cervical rib
(D) brachial plexus
(E) cervical sympathetic chain   *(5:26)*

59. The structures under the inguinal ligament from medial to lateral are

(A) lacunar ligament
femoral canal
femoral artery
femoral vein
femoral nerve
(B) lacunar ligament
femoral canal
femoral vein
femoral artery
femoral nerve
(C) lacunar ligament
femoral canal
femoral vein
femoral nerve
femoral artery

(D) femoral canal
femoral vein
femoral artery
femoral nerve
lacunar ligament
(E) femoral canal
lacunar ligament
femoral vein
femoral nerve
femoral artery   *(15:762)*

60. In a patient with massive venous thrombosis of the lower extremity who has thrown two pulmonary emboli, which of the following would not be indicated?

(A) interruption of the inferior vena cava
(B) fibrinolytic agents
(C) anticoagulant drugs
(D) ligature of the ankle-perforating veins
(E) elevation of the lower limb   *(4:1357-1383)*

61. The best treatment of a small carotid body tumor in a patient aged 45 is

(A) radiotherapy
(B) resection with ligature of the carotid artery
(C) resection with preservation of the carotid artery
(D) resection with graft replacement of the carotid artery
(E) no treatment   *(3:1825)*

62. A patient has an arteriovenous fistula between the superficial femoral artery and vein. Which one of the following does NOT occur?

(A) increased oxygen content of the venous blood proximal and distal to the fistula
(B) the distal limb is not ischemic
(C) pulse rate rises on compression of the proximal artery close to or at the site of the fistula
(D) an aneurysm will form if the fistula perforates and forms a false sac
(E) the pulse pressure is raised   *(2:933)*

63. A patient with stenosis of one renal artery will often have

(A) glomerular fibrosis
(B) arterial hypertension
(C) elevated blood urea nitrogen
(D) hematuria
(E) pyuria   *(2:1007-1011)*

64. Which of the following operations should NOT be performed on a patient with an arteriovenous fistula of a main artery in an extremity because gangrene may follow?

    (A) repair of the artery and the vein
    (B) ligature of the artery proximal to the fistula
    (C) quadruple ligature of the artery and vein proximal and distal to the fistula
    (D) ligature of the artery and vein proximal to the fistula
    (E) repair of the arterial defect through the vein with subsequent ligature of the vein
    (4:873)

65. In traumatic arteriovenous fistula, all the following are present EXCEPT

    (A) hyperemia in region of fistula
    (B) elevated pulse rate
    (C) normal diastolic pressure
    (D) venous engorgement regionally
    (E) increased cardiac output   *(4:862)*

66. In a patient with reversal of the blood flow in a vertebral artery, the obstruction is most commonly found in the

    (A) internal carotid artery
    (B) common carotid artery
    (C) opposite vertebral artery
    (D) proximal subclavian artery
    (E) distal subclavian artery   *(4:1200)*

67. A middle-aged woman has a venous stasis ulcer just above the medial malleolus of the ankle joint. Which of the following most frequently does more harm than good?

    (A) bedrest and elevation of the limb
    (B) application of topical antibiotics to the ulcer
    (C) ligature of the ankle-perforating veins
    (D) application of an Unna boot
    (E) application of a pad and compression bandage   *(4:1397-1399)*

68. A Syme's amputation is performed with bone section through the

    (A) metatarsal bones
    (B) distal tarsal bones
    (C) proximal tarsal bones
    (D) ankle joint
    (E) tibia and fibula just proximal to the ankle joint   *(1:706)*

69. The abdominal aorta may be exposed by a transperitoneal or an extraperitoneal incision. Which of the following is a CONTRAINDICATION to the extraperitoneal approach?

    (A) chronic obstructive pulmonary disease
    (B) obesity
    (C) disease of the right common iliac artery
    (D) multiple previous abdominal operations
    (E) absence of an experienced assistant   *(7:87)*

70. Which of the following antimicrobial drugs is best administered orally?

    (A) cefamandole
    (B) cefazolin
    (C) cephalothin
    (D) amikacin
    (E) ciprofloxacin HCl   *(8:41, 45-46)*

71. All of the following may be present subsequent to embolic obstruction of the femoral artery EXCEPT

    (A) pallor of the extremity
    (B) ankle edema
    (C) absence of the distal pulses
    (D) paralysis of the leg and foot
    (E) strong external iliac pulse   *(4:450-451)*

72. Lasers are becoming an increasingly important tool for surgeons. For years, argon lasers have been used by ophthalmologists. Which of the following statements about lasers is UNTRUE?

    (A) the laser boils intracellular water, exploding the cells in its path
    (B) the CO_2 laser provides a good cutting beam
    (C) the Nd:YAG laser provides destructive coagulation of tissues
    (D) the letters Nd:YAG stand for neodymium:yttrium-argon-garnet
    (E) a contaminated wound can be coverted to a clean wound with proper application of the laser beam to the wound surface *(3:256)*

73. A portacaval shunt in a patient with asymptomatic esophageal varices will

    (A) increase the risk of variceal hemorrhage
    (B) not increase the life expectancy
    (C) decrease the incidence of encephalopathy
    (D) increase ascites
    (E) accelerate the cirrhosis of the liver *(12:132)*

74. The nerve most likely to be injured by retraction or dissection during the operation of carotid thromboendarterectomy is the

(A) glossopharyngeal
(B) vagus
(C) spinal accessory
(D) hypoglossal
(E) superior laryngeal   *(4:1251)*

75. The characteristics of the Peutz-Jeghers syndrome include all EXCEPT

(A) pigmentation of the mucosa of the mouth and lips
(B) polyposis of the intestines
(C) pigmentation of palms of the hands and soles of feet
(D) the intestinal lesions are precancerous
(E) is inherited as a mendelian dominant   *(1:583)*

76. The indications for colectomy in a patient with ulcerative colitis include

(A) proved or suspected perforation
(B) toxic megacolon unresponsive to treatment
(C) uncontrolled arthritis and skin lesions
(D) long-standing colitis with polyps
(E) all of the above   *(1:621)*

77. In acute appendicitis, which of the following physical signs is the most diagnostic?

(A) hypoactive bowel sounds
(B) rebound tenderness
(C) rectal tenderness
(D) palpable mass
(E) localized tenderness   *(1:556)*

78. All of the following statements concerning infection with the parasite *Entamoeba histolytica* (amebiasis) are correct EXCEPT

(A) 10% of the world population is infected with this parasite
(B) the trophozoites often inhabit the colon where they subsist on bacteria, usually without causing symptoms
(C) amebic dysentry develops when the amebas invade the wall of the colon, undermining the mucosa and producing ulcers
(D) localized intestinal disease may cause a stricture or an ameboma

(E) diffuse amebic hepatitis precedes the development of an amebic liver abscess   *(1:117)*

Questions 79 and 80

A 55-year-old man had a hernia repair under general anesthesia. On the next day, he is noted to be dyspneic and have a fever of 101°F. Examination reveals decreased breath sounds over the right chest.

79. The most likely diagnosis is

(A) pneumonia
(B) pneumothorax
(C) atelectasis
(D) pleural effusion
(E) pulmonary embolism   *(2:461–463)*

80. The best treatment of the patient described in the preceding question would be to

(A) start antibiotics
(B) do endotracheal suction
(C) start anticoagulants
(D) wrap and elevate the legs
(E) aspirate the chest   *(2:461–463)*

81. A patient with renal failure who is well controlled by renal dialysis is probably in anesthesia risk category

(A) I
(B) II
(C) III
(D) IV
(E) V   *(3:168)*

82. The triad of gastrointestinal bleeding, right upper quadrant pain, and jaundice suggests a diagnosis of

(A) hepatoma
(B) hemobilia
(C) aortoenteric fistula
(D) choledochal cyst
(E) duodenal diverticulum   *(3:1094)*

83. Lymphocytic gastric submucosal infiltration associated with benign gastric ulcer is known as

(A) Ménétrier's disease
(B) pseudolymphoma
(C) hypertrophic gastropathy
(D) atrophic gastritis
(E) granulomatous gastritis   *(3:857–858)*

84. The dorsalis pedis artery arises from the

    (A) femoral artery
    (B) popliteal artery
    (C) anterior tibial artery
    (D) posterior tibial artery
    (E) peroneal artery   *(15:775)*

85. The 11th (spinal accessory) cranial nerve inner-
    vates which of the following muscles?

    (A) trapezius and deltoid
    (B) trapezius and sternomastoid
    (C) serratus anterior
    (D) omohyoid
    (E) strap muscles (infrahyoid muscles) *(15:1189)*

86. The superior parathyroid glands are derived from

    (A) the thyroglossal duct
    (B) the third branchial pouch
    (C) the fourth branchial pouch
    (D) the second branchial cleft
    (E) Rathke's pouch   *(2:1578)*

87. The most accurate diagnostic indicator of gas-
    troesophageal reflux is

    (A) a pressure of 0 to 5 mm Hg at the lower
        esophageal high pressure zone
    (B) a pressure below 20 mm Hg at the high
        pressure zone
    (C) 24-hour pH electrode monitoring
    (D) esophagoscopy
    (E) acid perfusion (Bernstein test)   *(3:705)*

Questions 88 and 89

A 25-year-old man suffers a major burn of the lower
part of the body. It is mostly second degree and covers
about 30% of the body surface. The early response to
treatment is satisfactory, but after 24 hours, the patient
is noticed to have tachypnea, and an increased effort
is required for him to breathe. Arterial blood gas measurements show the Po₂ to be 58 mm Hg. The chest
x-ray shows diffuse pulmonary infiltrates, and the heart
is not enlarged.

88. The probable cause of this problem is

    (A) atelectasis
    (B) pulmonary edema
    (C) pneumonia
    (D) respiratory distress syndrome
    (E) aspiration pneumonia   *(2:131)*

89. The correct treatment for the patient described
    is

    (A) immediate tracheostomy
    (B) large doses of antibiotics
    (C) diuretics
    (D) immediate intubation and positive
        pressure ventilation
    (E) tracheal suction through a bronchoscope,
        if necessary   *(2:136)*

Questions 90 and 91

A 43-year-old man was asymptomatic before vomiting
bright red blood and the passage of tarry stools. Examination reveals a blood pressure of 60/40 and a
hemoglobin of 8 g. He is transfused with 2000 ml of
whole blood. Twelve hours later, he vomits large quantities of bright red blood, and his blood pressure is 60/
40 with a hemoglobin of 7 g.

90. The most likely diagnosis is

    (A) duodenal ulcer
    (B) gastric ulcer
    (C) esophageal varices
    (D) acute gastritis
    (E) carcinoma of the stomach   *(2:1125)*

91. In the patient described, you should recommend

    (A) immediate operation, with blood
        transfusion
    (B) elective surgery after control of the shock
    (C) transfusion and an upper gastrointestinal
        series when stable
    (D) transfusion and esophagoscopy when
        stable
    (E) intragastric milk and antacids   *(2:1128)*

**DIRECTIONS (Questions 92 through 158): Each
question consists of an introduction followed by
five statements. Mark T (true) or F (false) after
each statement.**

92. The pathophysiologic consequences of severely
    and acutely elevated intracranial pressure are

    (A) bradycardia
    (B) fall in systolic blood pressure
    (C) fall in respiratory rate
    (D) oliguria
    (E) abducens nerve paralysis   *(1:751–752)*

93. Any patient sustaining an injury above the clavicle or a head injury resulting in an unconscious state should be suspected of having an associated cervical spinal column injury. The following statements concern this problem.

    (A) if the patient has pain, tenderness, or decreased motion of the neck, the cervical spine should be immobilized at once
    (B) many fractures of the C3 to C7 spinal segment are caused by automobile accidents or sports injuries
    (C) in general, the easier the reduction of a cervical spinal dislocation, the more stable will be the reduction
    (D) if the x-ray does not show C7, the shoulders should be pulled towards the head
    (E) a cervical spinal injury requires immobilization of the entire patient with a semirigid cervical collar and backboard before and during transfer to a definitive care center   (3:1431-1435)

94. Clinical manifestations of tentorial herniation may include

    (A) ipsilateral (side of the lesion producing herniation) mydriasis
    (B) contralateral hemiparesis
    (C) decerebrate rigidity
    (D) ipsilateral hemiparesis
    (E) contralateral hemianopsia   (1:741)

95. The following statements concern extradural hemorrhage due to a fracture of the temporal bone.

    (A) typical history: minor head injury, unconsciousness, lucid interval, then headache, nausea, and vomiting, with increasing unconsciousness
    (B) as the situation progresses, the pulse rate rises and the blood pressure falls
    (C) the pupil usually becomes dilated and fixed on the side opposite the head injury
    (D) if an extradural hemorrhage is suspected, a trephine hole should be placed over the temporal bone as soon as possible
    (E) extradural hemorrhage most commonly follows a linear fracture of the temporal bone   (3:1382-1387)

96. In the evaluation of the severity of a head injury

    (A) the longer the period of retrograde amnesia, the more severe the cerebral injury is likely to be
    (B) if there is no retrograde amnesia, the degree of cerebral injury is likely to be slight, even if there is marked damage to the skull
    (C) lumbar puncture has no role in the diagnosis of an obvious head injury
    (D) absence of retrograde amnesia means that extradural or subdural hematomas are unlikely to develop
    (E) eye opening is misleading   (1:744-747)

97. Subarachnoid hemorrhage may be due to an aneurysm, arteriovenous malformation, or sometimes another cause. The following statements are about this condition.

    (A) the onset is often explosive: severe headache, nausea, vomiting, and perhaps seizures or unconsciousness
    (B) the onset rarely occurs during sleep
    (C) cerebral arterial spasm frequently develops
    (D) lumbar puncture is dangerous in these patients and should not be performed
    (E) after transfer to a neurosurgical center, the diagnosis should be confirmed by cerebral angiography   (3:1375-1378)

98. The following statements are about fat embolism.

    (A) most patients are symptomatic within 24 hours of the trauma that produced fat embolism
    (B) it occurs with burn trauma as well as with fractures of the long bones
    (C) the main symptoms relate to pulmonary pathology
    (D) in a patient with extensive trauma, an elevated serum lipase level in the first 48 hours is probably due to pancreatitis rather than to fat embolism
    (E) intravenous alcohol is the treatment of choice   (2:470-471)

99. The clinical diagnosis of fat embolism is suggested by

    (A) delirium
    (B) tachycardia
    (C) petechiae
    (D) a sudden rise in the hematocrit
    (E) respiratory distress syndrome   (2:470-471)

100. Aortic valvular stenosis characteristically produces

(A) systemic arterial hypertension
(B) left ventricular hypertrophy
(C) cyanosis
(D) a small pulse pressure
(E) a diastolic murmur   *(2:836)*

101. Pulmonary osteoarthropathy often is associated with

(A) chronic emphysema
(B) pulmonary tuberculosis
(C) pulmonary malignant tumors
(D) acute pulmonary abscess
(E) rheumatoid arthritis   *(2:2037)*

102. The following statements concern choledochal cyst.

(A) the cyst is often palpable in the upper abdomen
(B) a HIDA scan provides a cholangiogram demonstrating the cyst
(C) the present treatment is cystectomy and anastomosis of the proximal hepatic ducts to a Roux loop of jejunum
(D) the liver is usually normal in these patients
(E) in most older children, the classic triad of jaundice, abdominal pain, and cyst exists   *(3:1286)*

103. The following statements refer to characteristics of pheochromocytoma.

(A) pheochromocytomas are familial
(B) extraadrenal tumors secrete more epinephrine than norepinephrine
(C) tumors are more likely to be multiple or bilateral in children than in adults
(D) multiple neurofibromatosis occurs in about 75% of patients
(E) they usually cause sustained hypertension in the adult   *(2:1520-1528)*

104. Following appendectomy, the patient develops a wound infection, and *Clostridium perfringens* is cultured from the pus. The patient has no clinical signs of clostridial myonecrosis (gas gangrene). Treatment should consist of

(A) specific antitoxin
(B) antibiotics
(C) hyperbaric oxygen
(D) open drainage and debridement of dead tissue
(E) observation only   *(1:110)*

105. The treatment of a patient with tetanus includes

(A) excision and debridement of the wound
(B) control of convulsions
(C) antibiotics
(D) large doses of tetanus toxoid
(E) human tetanus immune globulin *(1:112-113)*

106. Acute cholecystitis is diagnosed in an otherwise healthy woman aged 40. The following statements concern her management.

(A) the majority of such cases resolve without operation
(B) operative cholangiography should be performed when it is safe to do so
(C) when technically possible, a cholecystectomy should be performed
(D) cholecystostomy is an acceptable alternative to cholocystectomy in elderly, poor-risk patients
(E) on practical grounds, early operation avoids a second hospitalization for a cholecystectomy   *(3:1142)*

107. A glomus tumor

(A) is nearly always painful
(B) occurs only on the hand
(C) changes color with temperature
(D) is comprised of blood vessels and nerves
(E) is treated by meticulous dissection and total excision   *(2:513)*

108. A 60-year-old man has suffered three episodes of left spontaneous pneumothorax during the past year. His general health is good, but he has had a chronic cough for years. The left lung is 60% collapsed, and no other pulmonary lesion is seen on the chest films.

(A) tuberculosis is the most probable cause of the spontaneous pneumothorax
(B) spontaneous pneumothorax occurs most commonly in men considerably younger than this patient
(C) catheter thoracentesis or closed tube drainage should be instituted in the eighth interspace in the posterior axillary line
(D) definitive treatment will likely require thoracotomy
(E) this patient probably has generalized emphysema   *(1:291-293)*

109. A severe form of the carpal tunnel syndrome involving the median nerve causes atrophy of the

    (A) dorsal interosseous muscles
    (B) volar interosseous muscles
    (C) muscles of the hypothenar eminence
    (D) muscles of the thenar eminence
    (E) the little finger   (1:1070)

110. The following statements concern Meckel's diverticulum.

    (A) it is a cause of massive rectal bleeding in pediatric patients
    (B) the rectal bleeding is characteristically painless
    (C) a technetium-99 radionuclide scan is a valuable diagnostic study
    (D) the mortality of operation in a patient with complications is low
    (E) persistent loss of small amounts of blood is a frequent finding.   (3:947-948, 1282)

111. In a 15-year-old child who has a large, symptomatic pulmonary arteriovenous fistula, the following would be expected.

    (A) polycythemia
    (B) pulmonary artery hypertension
    (C) cyanosis
    (D) opacification of the lesion on archaortography
    (E) low pulmonary venous pressure   (1:382)

112. Following trauma

    (A) ACTH release usually is suppressed
    (B) hormonal response depends on whether or not the afferent nerve supply to the traumatized area is intact
    (C) ACTH release is dependent on the presence of intact adrenal glands
    (D) the ACTH level usually is increased
    (E) the cortisol level usually is increased   (2:1-9)

113. Hemorrhage and hypovolemia stimulate the secretion of

    (A) renin
    (B) aldosterone
    (C) antidiuretic hormone
    (D) growth hormone
    (E) glucagon   (2:14-16)

114. The following are true of ulcerative colitis.

    (A) the rectum often is spared

    (B) malignancy occurs more frequently than in the general population
    (C) malignancies are more likely to occur on the left side
    (D) 15% of ulcerative colitis-related malignancies are multicentric
    (E) the incidence of malignancy is related to both the extent and the duration of disease   (3:1015)

115. Necrotizing fasciitis is an uncommon but important clinical entity. If not promptly recognized and treated, the mortality can be very high. The following statements are about this entity.

    (A) there is extensive necrosis of the superficial fascia, with widespread undermining of the surrounding tissues
    (B) in about 90% of patients, the bacteria are beta-hemolytic streptococci or coagulase-positive staphylococci or both. In 10%, the bacteria are gram-negative enteric pathogens
    (C) cellutitis and edema with extreme systemic toxicity occur
    (D) treatment consists of radical debridement of the involved fascia plus antibiotics, such as an aminoglycoside, clindamycin, and ampicillin
    (E) excision of the fascia must be carried out promptly   (2:181)

116. These statements relate to thyroglossal duct cyst.

    (A) the cyst may become infected
    (B) it may represent the patient's only thyroid tissue
    (C) a thyroid scan will demonstrate the presence or absence of thyroid tissue in the normal location
    (D) surgical excision requires removal of the cyst and the duct remnant to the foramen caecum of the tongue
    (E) it is necessary to remove the center of the hyoid bone as part of the excision   (3:1346)

117. The following statements are in regard to osmolality of a solution.

    (A) 1 mmol of sodium chloride constitutes 1 mOsm
    (B) 1 mmol of sodium sulfate (Na_2SO_4) constitutes 3 mOsm
    (C) 1 mmol of calcium chloride ($CaCl_2$) constitutes 2 mOsm

(D) 1 mmol of glucose constitutes 1 mOsm

(E) 1 mmol of urea constitutes 1 mOsm

(2:47-48)

118. The following statements concern imperforate anus.

(A) in about half the patients, there are other congenital abnormalities

(B) it is important to determine if the blind rectal pouch is located above or below the puborectalis muscle

(C) a fistula between the rectum and urinary tract is common in females

(D) the most important element in definitive repair is the accurate placement of the rectum through the puborectalis sling of the levator ani complex

(E) for boys with a high defect or a urinary tract fistula, best results are obtained with a divided colostomy followed by definitive repair at the age of 6 months *(3:1275-1278)*

119. In high-output renal failure

(A) there is usually a period of oliguria initially

(B) because of the large volume of urine excreted, it frequently is necessary to give large amounts of potassium salts

(C) water restriction results in a prompt significant decrease in urine output

(D) the renal response to vasopressin is abnormal

(E) failure to recognize the problem may lead to death from hyperkalemia, hypernatremia, or acidosis *(2:67)*

120. The following statements are about elemental diets.

(A) they contain all fat-soluble vitamins except vitamin K

(B) the diets with very high nitrogen content are more palatable than the lower nitrogen preparations

(C) they contain no bulk

(D) because they are unpalatable, each total dose of 200 ml of the standard solution should be swallowed as quickly as possible

(E) water may be added to compensate for excessive pure water losses *(2:74)*

121. Instances in which parenteral hyperalimentation is indicated include

(A) an adult who remains decerebrate 8 weeks after an accident

(B) a patient with excessive metabolic requirements following severe injury

(C) as preparation of the bowel for left colectomy for carcinoma

(D) prolonged paralytic ileus following multiple operations for a pancreatic abscess

(E) preoperative treatment of severe relapsing pancreatitis *(2:74-78)*

122. The following are indications for exploration of penetrating wounds of the neck and thoracic inlet.

(A) thoracic wounds whose trajectory traverses the superior mediastinum or thoracic inlet

(B) radiologic evidence of a widened mediastinum

(C) a large hematoma

(D) any wound above the clavicle or manubrium that penetrates the platysma muscle

(E) a stab wound of the esophagus *(2:221-223)*

123. The following symptoms and signs are associated with ischemia of an extremity following the casting of a fracture.

(A) motor paralysis

(B) pallor

(C) severe pain

(D) sensory paralysis

(E) extreme swelling *(2:1958)*

124. Pyogenic osteomyelitis of the vertebral column

(A) causes severe back pain that is not relieved by rest

(B) is most common during adolescence and in young adulthood

(C) does not usually cause marked collapse of the vertebral bodies

(D) is most common in the cervical region

(E) is most often due to *Staphylococcus aureus* infection *(2:1845-1846)*

125. Peritoneal lavage is used as a diagnostic procedure in an adult who has sustained blunt abdominal trauma. A liter of Ringer's lactate solution is infused into the peritoneal cavity. In the returned fluid a positive test is indicated by

    (A) bile in the fluid
    (B) greater than 25,000 RBC/mm³
    (C) greater than 500 WBC/mm³
    (D) bacteria in the fluid
    (E) fluid amylase of 25 units   *(2:230–231)*

126. A young adult has sustained blunt trauma to the abdomen. At operation, the pancreas is found to be completely transected, but the spleen and duodenum are intact. The following procedures would be considered good surgical treatment.

    (A) distal pancreatectomy; oversewing the proximal severed end
    (B) oversewing the distal severed end of the pancreas and pancreaticojejunostomy to the proximal end
    (C) pancreaticojejunostomy to both proximal and distal severed ends
    (D) thorough drainage of the area only
    (E) total pancreatectomy   *(2:251–253)*

127. The following statements concern a patient who has been burned.

    (A) a second degree burn is erythematous, weeping, painful, and blistered
    (B) the skin in a third degree burn may regenerate from epithelial cells surrounding the hair follicles and sweat glands
    (C) if the rule of nines is used to estimate the percentage of the body surface involved by a burn, the right lower extremity represents 9%
    (D) tetanus prophylaxis is mandatory for burn patients except those actively immunized within the preceding 12 months
    (E) a circumferential third degree burn may cause ischemia of an extremity, and escharotomy is then required   *(2:271)*

128. At present, the following procedures is/are thought to decrease the incidence of tumor spread at the time of surgery.

    (A) the use of 0.5% formaldehyde to prevent local recurrence from carcinoma of the cervix
    (B) the use of plastic drapes to protect the edges of the incision
    (C) electric cauterization of the cut surface of a tumor entered during the course of the operation
    (D) irrigation of the wound with sodium hypochlorite
    (E) the intravenous administration of 5-fluorouracil   *(2:338–339)*

129. The following statements are about soft tissue tumors.

    (A) if the tumor can be easily shelled out, it is probably benign
    (B) sarcomas lying within muscle groups require the removal of all muscle bundles from their origin to their insertion within that fascial compartment
    (C) it is necessary to remove the fascia but not necessary to remove muscle tissue in the immediate region of a subcutaneous sarcoma in the thigh
    (D) soft tissue sarcomas have a compressed zone of neoplastic cells, which form a pseudocapsule
    (E) the nodular melanoma has a better prognosis than does a lentigo maligna   *(2:339)*

130. The cure rate for epidermoid carcinoma of the following sites is approximately equal using either radiation therapy or surgery.

    (A) lip
    (B) lung
    (C) anus
    (D) salivary gland
    (E) stomach   *(2:345)*

131. The following statements concern acute appendicitis:

    (A) deaths from appendicitis are confined almost entirely to patients with perforation
    (B) pain usually is the first symptom
    (C) the standard laboratory determinations are of great value
    (D) anorexia is an important symptom
    (E) rectal or pelvic examinations are essential   *(3:969–971)*

132. Secondary hyperparathyroidism has become much more common since the initiation and wide use of maintenance hemodialysis in patients with renal disease. The following statements concern their problem.

(A) secondary hyperparathyroidism is commonly associated with renal osteodystrophy
(B) persistent and symptomatic hypercalcemia is an indication for parathyroidectomy if a renal transplant is being considered
(C) about 25% of patients with renal osteodystrophy have parathyroid hyperplasia
(D) total parathyroidectomy combined with autografting of some parathyroid tissue to the muscles of the forearm is a valid procedure
(E) secondary hyperparathyroidism may cause some pain and itching   (3:629)

133. The relative incidence of gastric to duodenal ulcer is increasing in the USA. The following statements concern gastric ulcer.

(A) most patients with duodenal ulcer do well with medical management. Patients with gastric ulcer have a higher rate of recurrence and of more serious complications
(B) gastroscopy is more accurate than radiology in the diagnosis of gastric ulcer and additionally affords an opportunity for biopsy
(C) the risk of developing carcinoma in the gastric remnant after gastric resection for peptic ulcer is the same as that for the unoperated stomach
(D) malignancy is a possibility for all gastric ulcers
(E) it is proper to treat patients with a gastric ulcer not having the characteristics of malignancy with a rigidly prescribed 6-week test of healing by medical means
                         (3:830–832,883)

134. A healthy 17-year-old male is bitten on the leg by a snake. He has the snake in a brown paper bag—a copperhead. He consults you ½ hour after the event.

(A) apply a tourniquet proximal to the bite, tight enough to obstruct both the venous and arterial flow
(B) apply a tourniquet proximal to the bite to occlude the venous and lymphatic return but not the arterial flow
(C) surgically excise the bitten area
(D) give broad-spectrum antibiotics
(E) prepare to do a fasciotomy, if necessary
                         (3:286)

135. The following statements concern epidermoid carcinoma of the esophagus.

(A) dysphagia is the first, most important, and most constant symptom
(B) esophagoscopy should be performed on all patients in whom the diagnosis is suspected
(C) in the USA, the operability rate is reported to be about 33%
(D) in China, the 5-year survival rate after resection is reported to be about 33%
(E) the lymphatic drainage of the esophagus is not segmental   (3:737–746)

136. A patient after multiple injuries caused by trauma is diagnosed as suffering from the adult respiratory distress syndrome. The following statements concerning the treatment are either true or false.

(A) continuous positive pressure ventilation is rarely required
(B) steroids in large doses are of value
(C) diuretics help by reducing excess body water
(D) heparin may be required if disseminated intravascular coagulation is suspected
(E) antibiotics rarely are indicated   (3:39, 61.

137. The following statements concern the anatomy and physiology of the rectum and anal canal.

(A) the distal part of the anal canal is lined for about 2 cm with squamous epithelium that does not secrete mucus
(B) the rectum is lined by mucus-secreting columnar epithelium
(C) the mucus-secreting columnar epithelium is almost devoid of somatic receptor nerve endings
(D) the squamous epithelium contains sensory receptor nerve endings of a specialized type
(E) the terminal part of the circular muscle of the rectum is greatly enlarged to form the internal sphincter. The visceral tone of this sphincter is most important in maintaining a closed anal canal
                         (3:1035–1038)

138. The following five statements concern the prophylaxis of tetanus in patients with a wound.

 (A) the wound was made with a knife 2 hours earlier. The patient has been fully immunized and the last dose given within 5 years. No booster dose of toxoid is indicated
 (B) the patient has a leg wound due to crushing by a tractor, and the immunization history is not known. Give both 0.5 ml adsorbed toxoid and at least 250 units of tetanus immune globulin
 (C) tetanus antitoxin of animal origin is rarely given because of the danger of anaphylaxis
 (D) tetanus is the result of local infection; therefore, proper initial wound care is of paramount importance
 (E) when giving 0.5 ml of adsorbed toxoid and tetanus immune globlin, separate needles and syringes are required   *(3:328)*

139. A 30-year-old female has a slowly enlarging painless oval mass on the medial side of the upper thigh. It is 8 cm by 6 cm in size. The clinical diagnosis is a soft tissue sarcoma.

 (A) biopsy is essential
 (B) if possible the mass should be excised with a wide margin
 (C) simple enucleation increases the chances for spread and decreases the possibility of cure
 (D) high-dose precision radiation therapy (6000 to 7000 rads) is a valuable therapeutic tool
 (E) these tumors are encapsulated   *(3:526)*

140. The following statements concern infection in the anorectal region.

 (A) abscesses in this area should be drained as soon as they are diagnosed
 (B) a fistula in ano may be intersphincteric, transsphincteric, suprasphincteric, or extrasphincteric. In each case, the sphincters referred to are the external sphincter muscles
 (C) by definition, a fistula is an abnormal communication between two epithelial surfaces
 (D) treatment is to drain the primary source and to lay the whole track open
 (E) complete division of the sphincter muscle mass renders the patient incontinent
      (3:1049)

141. The subphrenic spaces are an important site of intraabdominal infection. The following are statements concerning subphrenic abscess.

 (A) there may be an associated sterile pleural effusion on the involved side
 (B) an air–fluid level can be demonstrated in less than 5% of patients
 (C) pain at the tip of the shoulder and hiccups may reflect diaphragmatic irritation
 (D) a large collection of pus may accumulate with few symptoms or signs
 (E) ultrasound is a helpful diagnostic test
      (2:1413)

142. Cyclosporine selectively inhibits activated T lymphocytes and prevents these T cells from manufacturing or releasing interleukin 2. The following statements refer to cyclosporine.

 (A) cyclosporine induces immunosuppression without myelosuppression
 (B) cyclosporine is given intravenously
 (C) cyclosporine is nephrotoxic
 (D) the administration of steroids with cyclosporine permits a smaller dose of cyclosporine and less nephrotoxicity
 (E) kidney transplantation has benefited from the use of cyclosporine, but patient management has become more complex
      (3:443)

143. The following statements concern acute traumatic rupture of the diaphragm.

 (A) it follows severe crush injuries to the thorax or abdomen
 (B) the injury may be misdiagnosed as a hemothorax
 (C) CT scans and liver scans are useful diagnostic tools
 (D) treatment is supportive; early operation is rarely required
 (E) herniation of the liver through the right diaphragm is rare but may occur   *(3:364)*

144. Ulcerative colitis is a diffuse inflammatory disease of the mucous lining of the colon and rectum. The following statements concern this condition.

 (A) the etiology remains unknown
 (B) the most frequent symptoms are diarrhea, abdominal pain, and rectal bleeding, in that order

(C) total removal of the colon and rectum
cures ulcerative colitis
(D) fistula in ano is more common than in
other forms of inflammatory bowel disease
(E) psychologic factors have long been
thought to play a critical role in
exacerbations of this disease   *(3:1012-1017)*

145. The following statements concern carcinoma of
the breast. Which are true and which are false?

(A) Paget's disease of the nipple is always
associated with an underlying carcinoma
often undetected by palpation
(B) xeroradiography and mammography are
equivalent diagnostic procedures
(C) the accuracy of diagnosis of breast cancer
on physical examination is only 70% in
the most experienced hands
(D) the mortality rate from breast cancer is
the same in Japan and the USA
(E) breast cancer is most commonly found in
the upper and inner quadrant of the
breast   *(3:542-553)*

146. The following complications of ulcerative colitis
require urgent operation.

(A) massive bleeding
(B) fulminant unresponsive colitis
(C) stricture and obstruction
(D) toxic megacolon
(E) carcinoma   *(3:1017)*

147. Carcinoma of the colon and rectum is a leading
cause of death and disability in the USA. The
following statements concern this problem.

(A) any change in bowel habit in a person
over 40 demands investigation
(B) hemorrhoids should not be accepted as
the cause of a patient's symptoms until
complete study has excluded the presence
of other disease
(C) removal of a resectable primary lesion is
not indicated in the presence of
metastases
(D) chemotherapy still suffers from the lack of
an ideal drug
(E) surgical excision is the usual curative
therapy for colonic cancer   *(3:1004-1009)*

148. The following statements concern gastroesophageal reflux.

(A) heartburn and regurgitation are relieved
by lying flat in bed

(B) bleeding from gastroesophageal reflux
usually presents as chronic anemia
(C) in advanced cases, stricture leads to
mechanical obstruction
(D) the chest pain associated with
gastroesophageal reflux generally is
described as heartburn
(E) in a few patients, severe acute esophagitis
may cause massive upper gastrointestinal
hemorrhage   *(3:758-760)*

149. Primary peritonitis is uncommon. The following
statements concern this condition.

(A) primary peritonitis refers to inflammation
of the peritoneal cavity without a
documented source of contamination
(B) children with the nephrotic syndrome and
systemic lupus erythematosus are
particularly susceptible
(C) in recent years, the bacterial flora has
changed from gram-negative to gram-
positive organisms
(D) these patients have acute abdominal
tenderness, fever, and leukocytosis
(E) the diagnosis may only be established at
laparotomy   *(3:783)*

150. The following statements concern villous adenomas of the rectum.

(A) they are soft, velvety, sessile projections
usually covered with thick mucus
(B) they are easily felt on digital examination
of the rectum
(C) villous adenomas have a high malignant
potential
(D) occasionally these patients have mucus
discharge of 1 to 3 L per day containing
25 to 35 mEq K and 100 to 150 mEq
Na/L
(E) if invasive cancer is present, the prognosis
is better than it is with ordinary colon or
rectal carcinoma   *(3:1003-1005)*

151. The following statements concern a relatively rare problem, retroperitoneal fibrosis.

    (A) an association with the ingestion of methysergide has been reported
    (B) the structures involved include the ureters, vena cava, aorta, and duodenum
    (C) it is more common in women than men
    (D) an intravenous pyelogram is the most definitive diagnostic test
    (E) the process is similar to that seen in mediastinal fibrosis and Riedel's thyroiditis   (3:787)

152. The following statements are about the stimulation or the inhibition of gastric secretion.

    (A) fat in the duodenum in an absorbable form is an effective inhibitor of postprandial gastric secretion
    (B) the gastric phase of secretion is stimulated by food in the stomach; the humoral mediator for this is the hormone gastrin
    (C) vagus nerve stimulation releases acetylcholine from the vagal nerve endings in the mucosa of the fundus, which stimulates acid secretion by the parietal cells and the release of pepsinogen by the chief cells
    (D) since pepsin is active only in an acid environment, a peptic ulcer cannot occur in the absence of acid
    (E) the contribution of the intestinal phase to total gastric secretory output is difficult to estimate and apparently is not significant   (3:815-820)

153. The following statements concern acute appendicitis.

    (A) the sequence of symptoms usually begins with diffuse abdominal pain felt most prominently in the epigastrium or around the umbilicus, followed by anorexia and some nausea
    (B) after a variable time, the pain shifts to the right lower quadrant and becomes localized
    (C) a high fever over 39°C is usual
    (D) if vomiting precedes the onset of abdominal pain, the diagnosis should be questioned
    (E) a patient with an abnormally located appendix is likely to have an atypical history, particularly of pain   (3:969-972)

154. The following statements concern follicular adenoma of the thyroid gland.

    (A) adenomas of the thyroid may develop after irradiation of the neck
    (B) excision of the whole adenoma is sound practice
    (C) after excision of a follicular adenoma, permanent thyroid hormone replacement is necessary to reduce the incidence of recurrence
    (D) needle biopsy is valuable as a method of distinguishing a follicular adenoma from a follicular adenocarcinoma
    (E) ultrasound using present techniques can differentiate among solid adenomas, carcinomas, and nontoxic thyroid nodules   (3:601)

155. A marginal or gastrojejunal ulcer may occur after a partial gastrectomy or gastrojejunostomy. The following statements are related to this problem.

    (A) the reason for the original operation was duodenal ulcer in at least 9 of 10 patients
    (B) fiberoptic endoscopy is the best diagnostic study
    (C) a gastrojejunocolic fistula may form
    (D) today, treatment with cimetidine and antacids is effective
    (E) pain is the most common symptom (3:844)

156. Multiple endocrine neoplasia type II (MEN II), although rare, is being recognized increasingly in the families of patients with medullary carcinoma of the thyroid.

    (A) the syndrome consists of a triad of inherited neoplasms: medullary carcinoma of the thyroid, pheochromocytoma, and parathyroid hyperplasia
    (B) pheochromocytomas in patients with MEN II frequently are bilateral
    (C) the surgical treatment of medullary carcinoma of the thyroid is subtotal thyroidectomy
    (D) metastasis from medullary carcinoma of the thyroid responds well to radiotherapy
    (E) thyrocalcitonim levels in the plasma are elevated in virtually all patients with medullary carcinoma of the thyroid   (3:612-617)

157. Traumatic rupture of the duodenum is not common because the duodenum is deep in the ab-

dominal cavity and well protected. The following statements are related to this injury.

(A) most injuries are due to penetrating wounds
(B) associated injuries to the pancreas, liver, and inferior vena cava are a major factor in the prognosis
(C) the diagnosis of retroperitoneal rupture due to blunt trauma may be difficult even at laparotomy
(D) retroperitoneal hematomas adjacent to the duodenum should not be opened unless a diagnosis of duodenal rupture has been previously established
(E) plain x-ray films may show free air in the peritoneum or streaks of air in the retroperitoneum around the duodenum

(3:847)

158. The following statements concern the etiology, diagnosis, and treatment of pharyngoesophageal diverticulum (Zenker's diverticulum).

(A) these are true diverticula consisting of all layers of the wall of the esophagus
(B) they usually occur in older patients
(C) dysphagia is the main symptom and esophageal carcinoma the main differential diagnosis
(D) a two-stage resection is preferred because it is safer
(E) the diverticulum is usually located on the right side of the neck

(3:726)

DIRECTIONS (Questions 159 through 180): Each of the numbered items or incomplete statements in this section is followed by answers or by completions of the statement. Select the ONE lettered answer or completion that is BEST in each case.

159. Of the following statements referring to the Heimlich maneuver, which is INCORRECT?

(A) the Heimlich maneuver consists of placing your arms around the choking person from behind; one fist is grasped in the other hand and both hands are then briskly brought into the subxiphoid area to apply pressure to the diaphragm
(B) a frequent indication is a bolus of meat caught between the vocal cords
(C) laryngospasm and the bolus make the patient mute
(D) a first step is to strike an adult on the back or to turn a child upside down

(E) if the Heimlich maneuver fails, an alternative airway must be established immediately with a tracheotomy

(3:1322)

160. The complications of diverticulitis of the colon include all of the following EXCEPT

(A) carcinoma of the colon
(B) perforation and general peritonitis
(C) perforation and local abscess
(D) intestinal obstruction
(E) colovesical fistula

(3:997-999)

161. The advantages of a rigid dressing to a major lower limb amputation stump, such as a plaster cast without an attached prosthesis, include all of the following EXCEPT

(A) immobilization of the tissues near the wound
(B) control of edema and swelling
(C) prevention of joint contractures
(D) accelerated maturity of the stump
(E) protection from trauma to the wound

(4:1495-1496)

162. The common and superficial femoral arteries have been injured and even stripped during the operation of long saphenous vein ligature and stripping. The best way to avoid these iatrogenic disasters is to

(A) dissect the structures in the groin accurately
(B) note the color of the veins and arteries
(C) mark the varices before the operation
(D) pass the stripper from the groin to the ankle
(E) pass the stripper from the ankle to the groin

(5:39)

163. The complement system carries out all of the following functions EXCEPT

(A) damages bacterial cell walls
(B) injects lytic enzymes into bacterial cells
(C) releases chemotatic substances
(D) produces immune adherence
(E) prepares bacteria for phagocytosis

(3:260)

164. The gastrointestinal hormone gastrin has both gastric and extragastric biologic actions. Which of the following functions are NOT due to gastrin?

(A) gastric acid secretion
(B) gastric pepsin secretion
(C) contraction of the lower esophageal sphincter
(D) relaxation of the gallbladder
(E) increased gastric mucosal blood flow

(20:135-147)

165. At which of the following locations do traumatic aneurysms of the aorta occur?

(A) the ascending aorta
(B) the aortic arch
(C) the thoracic aorta distal to the left subclavion artery at the ligamentum arteriosum
(D) the aorta adjacent to the diaphragm
(E) the infrarenal abdominal aorta

(3:1812)

166. In a young adult male, the central venous pressure is decreased and the pulmonary capillary wedge pressure is decreased. He is hypotensive. The most likely problem is

(A) hypovolemia
(B) pulmonary hypertension
(C) right ventricular failure
(D) hypervolemia
(E) pulmonary embolism

(5:234)

167. Damage to all of the following cranial nerves has been reported following exposure of the bifurcation of the common carotid artery. Which of the following nerves is most frequently injured in this way?

(A) the facial nerve (VII)
(B) the glossopharyngeal nerve (IX)
(C) the vagus nerve (X)
(D) the spinal accessory nerve (XI)
(E) the hypoglossal nerve (XII)   *(4:1304-1305)*

168. The majority of surgical wound infections are caused by

(A) staphylococci
(B) streptococci
(C) *Escherichia coli*
(D) *Pseudomonas aeruginosa*
(E) *Proteus*

(3:273)

169. In 1929, Mallory and Weiss described four alcoholic patients who bled from a longitudinal tear in the esophagogastric mucosa. Of the five statements concerning this syndrome, only one is correct. Which one is it?

(A) 90 to 100% of these patients are moderate or severe alcoholics
(B) in 50% of these patients, vomiting precipitates the problem
(C) nearly all patients with the Mallory-Weiss syndrome stop bleeding spontaneously
(D) vagotomy is the recommended treatment
(E) most patients can be treated at home without admission to a hospital   *(3:846)*

170. Since the rectum is adjacent to the cervix and body of the uterus, radiation to these structures may injure the rectum. Only one of the following statements concerning radiation proctitis is correct.

(A) simple supportive therapy—low-residue diet, stool softeners, sedation, and antispasmodics—is rarely effective
(B) a defunctioning proximal colostomy is often required
(C) most patients receiving radiation at these sites develop transient and self-limiting diarrhea
(D) a rectovaginal fistula from radiation injury often heals spontaneously
(E) oral steroids, sulfasalazine, and steroid enemas are not indicated   *(3:1042)*

171. A major factor in returning blood from the lower limbs to the heart, particularly when an individual is standing erect, is the calf muscle pump. Which of the following is NOT a function of this muscle pump?

(A) reduction of venous pressure in the dependent lower limb
(B) reduction of venous blood pressure in an exercising limb
(C) improvement of arterial blood flow to the exercising muscles of the limb
(D) increase in the return of venous blood to the right heart
(E) reduction of intestitial fluid in the leg and foot   *(4:152-154)*

172. The most serious threat to life when an echinococcal cyst ruptures is

(A) hemorrhage
(B) peritoneal seeding of daughter cysts
(C) sepsis

(D) anaphylaxis
(E) hepatorenal syndrome   *(3:1089)*

173. The treatment of a recent caustic burn of the esophagus consists of each of the following EXCEPT

(A) the most important step is immediate verification of the etiologic agent
(B) if possible, obtain the container that held the caustic agent
(C) induce vomiting and institute gastric lavage as soon as possible
(D) esophagoscopy is useful to define the depth of the burn but must be terminated at the proximal point of injury
(E) patients with signs of dysphagia, stridor, or hoarseness should be treated immediately with steroids and antibiotics
          (3:767–772)

174. Retrograde ejaculation in the male patient may follow injury to which of the following nerves?

(A) the second lumbar sympathetic ganglion
(B) more than 5 inches of the lumbar sympathetic chain
(C) the preaortic and preiliac plexus of autonomic nerves
(D) the genitofemoral nerve
(E) the ilioinguinal nerve   *(10:479)*

175. Wound hematoma is a common complication. Which of the following statements concerning wound hematoma is INCORRECT?

(A) hematomas occurring after thyroid or carotid surgery are particularly dangerous
(B) hematomas after thyroid or carotid surgery should be observed carefully
(C) most hematomas are due to imperfect hemostasis
(D) the risk of hematoma is higher in patients who have been given anticoagulants
(E) hematoma found days after surgery may be evacuated by gentle compression of the wound edges   *(1:23)*

176. The following statements concern reconstruction operations on the breast. Select the statement that is the most accurate.

(A) general anesthesia is preferred in both augmentation and reduction mammaplasty
(B) carcinoma is found in about 6% of specimens after subcutaneous mastectomy

(C) if a hematoma occurs, the management is a compression dressing
(D) even with antibiotic coverage, infection is not uncommon
(E) the blood supply of the nipple is best preserved by keeping a small segment of breast tissue to protect this region during subcutaneous mastectomy   *(3:557)*

177. Morbid obesity has been defined by the National Institutes of Health as 45 kg overweight or 200% or more of desirable weight according to Metropolitan Life Insurance Standards. One of the following statements is INCORRECT.

(A) morbid obesity exerts profound effects through excessive production of estrogen by the large volume of fat cells
(B) complications are fewer and less severe with gastric bypass than with intestinal bypass
(C) after weight loss, hypertension usually improves and many patients become normotensive
(D) weight loss after operation is not associated with a fall in the serum cholesterol or triglycerides
(E) the most dramatic results of a successful gastric bypass operation are on the patient's personal and emotional state
          (3:936–944)

178. The blind loop syndrome may follow surgery and also is associated with other situations, such as stricture of the small intestine, bowel stasis, small bowel diverticula, and scleroderma. One of the following statements concerning this problem is INCORRECT.

(A) the syndrome is always due to small bowel stasis and subsequent infection
(B) the syndrome is usually associated with constipation
(C) the hematologic problems associated with this syndrome revolve around vitamin B_{12} and folic acid deficiency
(D) treatment should include surgical correction of the cause of the intestinal stasis if possible
(E) the diagnosis can be confined by a pernicious anemia-like urinary excretion of vitamin B_{12} *(3:959)*

179. Which of the following statements concerning anal fissure is INCORRECT?

(A) it is a linear ulcer situated to either side of the midline posteriorly

(B) because it involves the highly sensitive squamous epithelium, it is often painful

(C) the pain persists for several hours after defecation

(D) there may be a skin tag at the base of the fistula that is known as the "sentinel pile"

(E) spotting with bright red blood occurs

(3:1649)

180. The incidence of overwhelming postsplenectomy sepsis has focused attention on the immunologic function of the spleen. The condition

(A) is seen 4 times as often in the splenectomized population as in the general population

(B) is most likely to occur several years after splenectomy

(C) occurs with nausea, vomiting, headache, confusion, shock, and coma

(D) carries the highest risk for elderly patients

(E) is usually due to staphylococcus infection

(3:1228)

Answers and Explanations

1. **(D)** In the newborn infant, for whom the risk of incarceration is high, repair is advisable before the child is discharged from hospital.

2. **(C)** Traumatic rupture of the thoracic aorta does not involve the pericardium, although a cardiac contusion can occur as a separate event.

3. **(C)** Rectal stricture is common in patients with lymphogranuloma venereum. It may resemble carcinoma of the rectum. It is not a precancerous lesion. The cancer, if present, has occurred incidentally. However, in each case malignancy should be ruled out by a biopsy.

4. **(B)** In general, if an inoperable carcinoma of the head of the pancreas is found at operation, it is best to perform both a cholecystojejunostomy and a gastroenterostomy.

5. **(B)** Rapid rewarming of the frozen part is the single most effective maneuver for preserving potentially viable tissue. Slow rewarming is not as effective in maintaining tissue viability and results in more extensive microvascular damage. Also, 36°F is the temperature of many domestic refrigerators.

6. **(A)** Hypothyroidism does not raise the serum calcium; hyperthyroidism does.

7. **(A)** Allen's test is useful in determining the state of the palmar arch arterial circulation. It should be performed before either the radial or ulnar artery is interrupted or cannulated.

8. **(A)** Medical treatment is not an alternative to surgery. A trial of medical management is nearly always fatal in patients with acute suppurative cholangitis.

9. **(B)** Other congenital abnormalities are frequent. Congenital heart abnormalities are present in 20 to 25% and imperforate anus in 10% of infants with a TEF.

10. **(A)** A lead point is seen in adults; it is rare in children. Red currant jelly stools are common. A sausage-shaped mass is palpable in most patients. Barium enema reduction is safe if a surgeon has seen the patient and proper precautions are taken.

11. **(C)** The treatment of appendicitis during pregnancy is immediate operation. Because of the extreme seriousness of perforation in a pregnant patient, it is better to remove a normal appendix than risk the consequences.

12. **(B)** Hemodynamic measurements on patients in shock caused by sepsis frequently reveal a high cardiac index and low peripheral resistance.

13. **(A)** When possible, the gastrointestinal tract should be used to provide nutrition. When the voluntary intake falls below requirements, feeding by a small nasogastric tube and constant infusion pump may be used. Intravenous feeding should be used only if these measures prove to be inadequate.

14. **(C)** The disc herniates in a posterior and lateral direction, not anterior and lateral.

15. **(D)** In patients with proximal small bowel obstruction, biliary colic or renal colic vomiting occurs soon after the onset of pain.

16. **(A)** In the early stages, hyperthyroidism is often present. In the established case, hypothyroidism is the most common presenting problem.

17. **(C)** The history of vomiting and retching with hematemesis and melena followed by the sudden onset of epigastric flank and back pain is characteristic of spontaneous perforation of the esophagus. Of special interest is the finding of marked or boardlike abdominal rigidity with no tenderness, no rebound, and audible peristaltic sounds. These findings occur only in retroperitoneal inflammation of sudden onset and in tetanus. Here, the perforation of the distal esophagus led to spreading inflammation in the upper retroperitoneal space. The spread was not upward into the mediastinum—hence no mediastinal emphysema, no pleural effusion, no chest pain, no cervical emphysema, and no dyspnea.

18. **(A)** A pneumothorax may be demonstrated on the chest film, but the tear in the esophagus can be best demonstrated during a swallow of a water-soluble contrast medium.

19. **(B)** Immediate repair through a left thoracotomy incision with drainage and antibiotics is mandatory in such a patient.

20. **(C)** Adhesions with symptoms of mild to severe intestinal obstruction may occur many years after any abdominal operation. They are the most common cause of mechanical intestinal obstruction.

21. **(B)** Upright abdominal films may show a ladderlike pattern of dilated small bowel loops with air–fluid levels. Such features may be minimal or absent in early obstruction.

22. **(B)** This patient has suffered from repeated attacks of increasing severity. This particular attack has subsided. It is, therefore, a good time to attempt correction of this problem before strangulation obstruction develops.

23. **(D)** Esophageal dysfunction occurs commonly in patients with scleroderma.

24. **(A)** Bile is not present in the vomitus because the obstruction is proximal to the ampulla of Vater.

25. **(B)** The application of heat to an ischemic extremity may produce significant thermal damage to the skin and subcutaneous tissues and should be avoided.

26. **(A)** Although a paraesophageal hernia may occur in combination with a sliding hiatus hernia, in its pure form, a paraesophageal hernia is not associated with reflux esophagitis.

27. **(D)** It was originally thought that the CEA level in the serum was specific for carcinoma of the colon and pancreas. This proved to be incorrect. Today the CEA level is used for follow-up study of patients after the resection of a carcinoma of the large intestine. A rise indicates a recurrence often before it is clinically detectable.

28. **(B)** Jejunoileal bypass produces significant weight loss, but the procedure has been abandoned because of the serious long-term complications, including hepatic steatosis, cirrhosis, gallstones, avitaminosis, hair loss, blind loop syndrome, hypocalcemia, and hypokalemia.

29. **(D)** Lactated Ringer's solution contains 4 mEg/L of potassium; 0.9% NaCl and 5% dextrose in 0.45% NaCl contain no potassium.

30. **(E)** In the male breast, carcinoma is relatively slow growing and excellent survival data have been achieved with radical mastectomy.

31. **(A)** Gardner's syndrome is a familial condition with the components listed. The polyps are true neoplasms and malignant change is common. The treatment of the intestinal polyposis is the same as that for other forms of familial polyposis coli.

32. **(D)** Fractures of the clavicle unite even with overriding. Open reduction is rarely required.

33. **(D)** There is no evidence that the kind of incision is related to the incidence of wound dehiscence. However, long paramedian incisions that denervate much of the rectus abdominis muscle are an exception.

34. **(B)** The pain characteristically is made worse by lying down and improves when the patient stands up or bends forward.

35. **(B)** This patient may have carcinoma of the ascending colon. A barium enema is still the most widely used method of diagnosing carcinoma of the right colon, although colonoscopy is also helpful if an expert colonoscopist is available.

36. **(E)** A variety of congenital abnormalities may be associated with an imperforate anus, but genito urinary ones are noted in 30 percent of patients.

37. **(C)** In general, the more rapid the onset of symptoms and signs of hypoparathyroidism, the worse the prognosis.

38. **(B)** In view of prospective data regarding the natural history of untreated pseudocysts, nonoperative prolonged observation can no longer be justified.

39. **(A)** If a ureteric injury of this type is recognized, the correct treatment is primary suture over an indwelling ureteric catheter.

40. **(E)** Postoperative acute renal failure is not associated with high blood pressure. It is more common in patients aged over 60, after operations near to the renal arteries, in septic patients, and when hemolysis develops.

41. **(A)** Instruments for passage through the urethra usually are numbered according to the French system, the number being the outside circumference in millimeters. A size 24 French catheter, therefore, has an outside circumference of 24 mm.

42. **(A)** A seminoma of the testis is a very radiosensitive tumor.

43. **(E)** A nonfunctioning kidney on an intravenous pyelogram is an indication for ureterolithotomy, or lithotripsy can be tried if it is available.

44. **(D)** Open drainage of an amebic abscess should be reserved for the relatively few with secondary infection.

45. **(C)** This is the only type of prostatic carcinoma that is surgically curable. The procedure is a radical perineal prostatectomy or radiation therapy.

46. **(B)** It is important to remember that severe pain is not associated with internal hemorrhoids but occurs with thrombosed external hemorrhoids.

47. **(C)** The acute onset of a left varicocele after the age of 40 years suggests left renal vein occlusion secondary to a renal carcinoma.

48. **(A)** Prostacyclin is a vasodilator and the most potent known inhibitor of platelet aggregation.

49. **(D)** Tuberculosis of the kidney often causes pyuria that is sterile and attacks of hematuria.

50. **(D)** Meconium ileus accounts for about 20% of cases of intestinal obstruction in the newborn. The distal ileum is obstructed by inspissated meconium.

51. **(C)** An upper gastrointestinal series may be harmful to a patient with meconium ileus. A barium enema may be of value to exclude colonic atresia and megacolon.

52. **(B)** Until recently, the best treatment was to hydrate and operate immediately, but recently, success has been reported with the nonoperative treatment of acetylcysteine or Gastrografin enemas.

53. **(E)** The subclavian aneurysm associated with the thoracic outlet compression syndrome often becomes apparent because of peripheral embolism, the patient not having recognized the problem before.

54. **(E)** It is probable that this patient has a carcinoma of the lip. A biopsy should precede treatment. The pulmonary lesion might be coccidioidomycosis.

55. **(A)** Carcinoma of the lip is associated with poor dental hygiene. Coccidioidomycosis does not cause ulcers of the lips.

56. **(A)** Skin tests demonstrate that many people in endemic areas have coccidioidomycosis, but in the majority, it is asymptomatic.

57. **(B)** The chorda tympani branch of the facial (seventh) cranial nerve, which runs in the sheath of the lingual nerve, transmits the sensation of taste from the anterior two thirds of the tongue.

58. **(B)** The anterior scalene muscle lies between the subclavian vein in front and the subclavian artery behind.

59. **(B)** The lacunar or reflected inguinal ligament is medial to the femoral canal. The femoral canal, the femoral vein, artery, and nerve are lateral.

60. **(D)** In a patient of this type, the important thing is to prevent further pulmonary emboli. Postphlebitic symptoms can be treated later.

61. **(C)** Carotid body tumors are rare. They grow slowly. Malignant change is rare. When large, they produce nerve paralysis, dysphagia, and pain. Early removal is recommended because it is easier to preserve the carotid artery if the tumor is small.

62. **(C)** Obliteration of the fistula by digital pressure slows the pulse rate. The bradycardia phenomenon was described by Nicoladoni in 1875.

63. **(B)** Reduction or dampening of the arterial pulse pressure in the renal artery beyond a stenosis is thought to be the stimulus that initiates the renal pressor mechanism.

64. **(B)** Ligature of the artery proximal to an arteriovenous fistula without ligature of the accompanying vein allows the collateral circulation to return to the heart through the fistula and the vein. Peripheral gangrene often follows.

65. **(C)** The diastolic blood pressure is reduced in patients with an arteriovenous fistula. This is part of the increased pulse pressure that develops in these patients.

66. **(D)** Thrombosis of the subclavian artery proximal to the origin of the vertebral artery produces the subclavian steal syndrome.

67. **(B)** Antibiotics applied directly to venous stasis ulcers of the leg may produce a local sensitivity reaction and make the ulcer worse.

68. **(E)** The malleoli of the tibia and fibula are resected to provide a continuous flat surface, and the bones are trimmed so that there are no pressure points.

69. **(E)** The extraperitoneal approach can be difficult if the assistant is inexperienced.

70. **(E)** Ciprofloxacin HCl cannot be dissolved to make an intravenous or intramuscular injection.

71. **(B)** Ankle edema is not associated with acute femoral arterial occlusion.

72. **(D)** The letters Nd:YAG stand for neodymium:yttrium-aluminum-garnet. The most frequently used lasers are the CO_2, argon, and Nd:YAG lasers.

73. **(B)** Controlled trials have shown that a prophylactic portacaval shunt in an asymptomatic patient with varices does not increase the life expectancy.

74. **(D)** The hypoglossal nerve crosses the internal and external carotid arteries close to their origin from the common carotid artery.

75. **(D)** The intestinal lesions are hamartomas, and, therefore, the malignant potential is very small.

76. **(E)** About 75% of patients with ulcerative colitis are treated medically. All of the listed items are indications for colectomy.

77. **(E)** Localized tenderness is the one essential physical finding that must be sought by precise one-finger palpation.

78. **(E)** The concept of ambeic hepatitis, implying diffuse liver involvement, is not supported by histologic evidence. The abscess usually is solitary, and the liver remote from the abscess is normal.

79. **(C)** Atelectasis is the most common postoperative complication. It usually develops in the first 24 to 48 hours after operation.

80. **(B)** The treatment consists of stimulating the patient to breathe deeply and to cough. Endotracheal suction helps this.

81. **(C)** A patient with a well-controlled major system disease is in risk category III. Patients with multiple-system, nonlife-threatening diseases and with limitations of daily activities also are in this class. Class I includes patients who are healthy but excludes the very young or very old, who would be in class II. Class II patients have single-system, controlled disease that is not incapacitating. Class IV patients have severe, debilitating, end-stage disease that poses danger of death due to organ failure. Stage V patients are preterminal.

82. **(B)** The classic triad of gastrointestinal bleeding, right upper quadrant pain, and jaundice should suggest a diagnosis of hemobilia. Because hemobilia is rare, it is important to keep in mind

because it may be correctable if recognized in time. Suspicion should be high if there has been trauma or biliary tract manipulation.

83. **(B)** Gastric lymphocytic submucosal infiltration is usually a response to benign gastric ulcer and is known as pseudolymphoma. Differentiation from follicular lymphoma can be difficult, and errors occur in both directions. Ménétrier's disease is mucous cell hypertrophy, hypertrophic gastropathy involves all mucosal cells, granulomatous gastritis is a manifestation of sarcoid or Crohn's disease, and atrophic gastritis is self-explanatory.

84. **(C)** The dorsalis pedis artery is the continuation of the anterior tibial artery.

85. **(B)** The spinal accessory nerve supplies the trapezius and sternomastoid muscles.

86. **(C)** The superior parathyroid glands develop from the fourth branchial pouch.

87. **(C)** The normal range of pressure in the lower esophageal high pressure zone, the functional sphincter, is 10 to 20 mm Hg, but variation from this pressure is poorly correlated with reflux. Patients with very low pressures, 0 to 5 mm Hg, are more likely to have reflux, but patients may have reflux with high pressures and no reflux with low pressure. Esophagoscopy with biopsy is a confirmatory test of the damage done by chronic reflux but is not a direct measure of active reflux. Infusion of 0.1 N HCl (Bernstein test) may reproduce reflux symptoms and aid in differential diagnosis but is again indirect evidence. Barium swallow has proven unreliable. Twenty-four hour monitoring with an indwelling pH electrode is the most accurate diagnostic study.

88. **(D)** The respiratory distress syndrome was at first thought to follow use of the pump oxygenator. It is now known to follow many severe situations, including major trauma and burns.

89. **(D)** Prompt intubation and positive pressure ventilation can nurse the respiratory distress syndrome, which is often fatal if not treated in this way.

90. **(A)** Duodenal ulcer can cause major hemorrhage without a history of preceding ulcer pain.

91. **(A)** Major rebleeding in hospital is attended by a mortality of 25%. A policy of early surgery is recommended to improve these results.

92. **(A) (T), (B) (F), (C) (T), (D) (F), (E) (T)** The consequences are a rise in systolic blood pressure, bradycardia, and a fall in respiratory rate, with a VI nerve paralysis.

93. **(A) (T), (B) (T), (C) (F), (D) (F), (E) (T)** An easily reduced cervical spine dislocation is usually unstable. The shoulders should be pulled down toward the feet to see C7.

94. **(A) (T), (B) (T), (C) (T), (D) (T), (E) (T)** Compression of nerve III can produce ipsilateral mydriasis, and compression of the midbrain results in decerebrate rigidity. Compression of the ipsilateral cerebral peduncle causes hemiparesis. The contralateral cerebral peduncle may be compressed to produce a false localizing sign, ipsilateral hemiparesis. Contralateral hemianopsia, due to posterior cerebral artery compression, can be another false localizing sign.

95. **(A) (T), (B) (F), (C) (F), (D) (T), (E) (T)** As the situation progresses, the pulse slows and the blood pressure rises. The pupil usually becomes dilated and fixed on the same side as the injury.

96. **(A) (T), (B) (T), (C) (T), (D) (F), (E) (F)** The period of retrograde amnesia is a good guide to the degree of cerebral injury but it in no way is a guide to the development of extradural or subdural hematomas. Lumbar puncture is not useful and can be very dangerous.

97. **(A) (T), (B) (T), (C) (T), (D) (F), (E) (T)** The diagnosis of subarachnoid hemorrhage should be verified by CT scan or lumbar puncture if the scan is negative.

98. **(A) (T), (B) (T), (C) (T), (D) (T), (E) (F)** Sixty percent of patients are symptomatic within 24 hours of the trauma. In fat embolism, the serum lipase level usually begins to rise on the third day and reaches a maximum 7 to 8 days after injury. The lipase level is increased by heparin therapy. The use of intravenous alcohol is debatable.

99. **(A) (T), (B) (T), (C) (T), (D) (F), (E) (T)**
Cardiac, cerebral, and pulmonary symptoms occur. Tachypnea and tachycardia are characteristic. Dyspnea, cyanosis, and blood-tinged tracheobronchial secretions suggest the diagnosis. If the fat emboli pass through the pulmonary filter and lodge in the cerebral vessels, symptoms may be confusion, acute psychoses, or coma. A sudden fall in the hematocrit can occur with hemorrhage into the pulmonary tissue.

100. **(A) (F), (B) (T), (C) (F), (D) (T), (E) (F)**
The systolic systemic blood pressure is low or normal. A very small pulse pressure indicates severe stenosis. There is progressive concentric ventricular hypertrophy, but little cardiac dilatation. The patient is not cyanotic, and the murmur is systolic.

101. **(A) (T), (B) (T), (C) (T), (D) (F), (E) (F)**
The cause of hypertrophic pulmonary osteoarthropathy is unknown. It would not be expected to occur with acute infections of the lung or rheumatoid arthritis.

102. **(A) (T), (B) (T), (C) (T), (D) (F), (E) (F)**
Many of these infants and children also suffer from cirrhosis of the liver. The classic triad of jaundice, abdominal pain, and cystic mass is found in less than 20% of patients.

103. **(A) (T), (B) (F), (C) (T), (D) (F), (E) (T)**
Extraadrenal tumors lack the methylating enzyme needed to convert norepinephrine to epinephrine. Multiple neurofibromatosis occurs in about 5% of patients.

104. **(A) (F), (B) (T), (C) (F), (D) (T), (E) (F)**
Antitoxin is not of value therapeutically or prophylactically. This simple contamination might be treated adequately with only open drainage (and debridement if necrotic tissue is present), but antibiotics are a protection against the development of clostridial myositis and myonecrosis.

105. **(A) (T), (B) (T), (C) (T), (D) (F), (E) (T)**
Tetanus toxoid is a preventive measure, not a treatment. When the diagnosis of tetanus is first made, the patient is given 3000 to 6000 units of human tetanus immune globulin to fix the toxin. It may be necessary to repeat this.

106. **(A) (T), (B) (T), (C) (T), (D) (T), (E) (T)**
Cholecystostomy is good treatment for an elderly, poor-risk patient.

107. **(A) (T), (B) (F), (C) (T), (D) (T), (E) (T)**
Exquisite pain with slight pressure is characteristic of subungual glomus tumors. They consist of blood vessels and nerves of an arteriovenous shunt and usually develop in the extremities, particularly the hands and feet.

108. **(A) (F), (B) (T), (C) (F), (D) (T), (E) (T)**
Tuberculosis is now an uncommon cause of spontaneous pneumothorax. When it is the cause, pulmonary lesions usually are seen on the chest film. Spontaneous pneumothorax occurs most commonly in men between the ages of 15 and 35. Persistent air leaks and recurrent pneumothorax are usually treated by thoracotomy to excise apical blebs and to cause adhesion of the visceral pleura to the chest wall. For evacuation of the air, the catheter or tube is placed in the second anterior intercostal space.

109. **(A) (F), (B) (F), (C) (F), (D) (T), (E) (F)**
This syndrome is produced by compression of the median nerve between the volar carpal ligament and the tendons in the tunnel. The usual symptoms are aching and numbness over the median nerve distribution with sparing of the little finger. Severe compression causes thenar paralysis, with muscle atrophy.

110. **(A) (T), (B) (T), (C) (T), (D) (F), (E) (F)**
The mortality in patients with complications can be as high as 16%. Persistent loss of small quantities of blood is rarely due to a Meckel's diverticulum.

111. **(A) (T), (B) (F), (C) (T), (D) (F), (E) (T)**
Pulmonary artery blood shunts into the pulmonary veins, a right-to-left shunt. In late childhood, large lesions cause cyanosis, clubbing, and polycythemia. Pulmonary artery pressure is low. The lesion is demonstrated by injecting contrast medium into the right ventricle or pulmonary artery, not into the aortic arch.

112. **(A) (F), (B) (T), (C) (F), (D) (T), (E) (T)**
Following trauma to a normally innervated area of the body the ACTH and cortisol levels are increased. Paraplegic patients undergoing operative procedures to a denervated area do not respond with an increased ACTH level.

113. **(A) (T), (B) (T), (C) (T), (D) (T), (E) (T)**
Hemorrhage and hypovolemia also stimulate the secretion of epinephrine, norepinephrine, and cortisol.

114. **(A) (F), (B) (T), (C) (F), (D) (T), (E) (T)**
Ulcerative colitis almost invariably involves the rectum (90 to 95%). If the rectum is not involved, one should consider a diagnosis of Crohn's colitis. The incidence of malignancy, although not as high as previously thought, still is significantly higher than in the general population (10 to 20% chance within 20 years). Malignancies are evenly distributed throughout the colon, and 15% are multicentric. Malignancy is related to extent and duration of disease, although not necessarily to severity. Ulcerative proctitis, for example, is a more benign variant rarely associated with malignancy. On the other hand, childhood onset of ulcerative colitis results in a 3% incidence of carcinoma at 10 years and an additional 20% incidence with each succeeding decade.

115. **(A) (T), (B) (T), (C) (T), (D) (T), (E) (T)**
All the statements are true about this rare but frequently fatal disease.

116. **(A) (T), (B) (T), (C) (T), (D) (T), (E) (T)**
It is necessary in all cases to remove the center portion of the hyoid bone.

117. **(A) (F), (B) (T), (C) (F), (D) (T), (E) (T)**
Osmole and milliosmole refer to the number of osmotically active particles present in a solution. A millimole of sodium chloride, which dissociates nearly completely, constitutes a milliosmole of sodium and a milliosmole of chloride for a total of 2 mOsm. Na_2SO_4 and $CaCl_2$ each dissociate into three osmotically active particles. A millimole of an un-ionized molecule, such as glucose, provides only 1 mOsm.

118. **(A) (T), (B) (T), (C) (F), (D) (T), (E) (T)**
The presence of the vagina reduces the incidence of urinary tract fistulas in girls.

119. **(A) (F), (B) (F), (C) (F), (D) (T), (E) (T)**
High-output renal failure usually begins without a period of oliguria. Water restriction results in hypernatremia without a decrease in urine output. Even small doses of potassium salts administered intravenously can prove fatal in high-output failure. Usually, urea nitrogen continues to increase 8 to 12 days before it begins to decline, and during this time the blood/urine urea ratio is about 1 : 10. There is complete resistance to vasopression for 1 to 3 weeks after the blood urea nitrogen has declined.

120. **(A) (T), (B) (F), (C) (T), (D) (F), (E) (T)**
The high nitrogen diets are even more unpalatable than the lower nitrogen ones and are suitable only for tube feedings. Because they contain no bulk and leave little residue, they are indicated only when low residue is an advantage. If low residue is not an advantage, many cheaper, palatable nutritional supplements are preferable. Sipping 300 ml over a 1-hour period rather than gulping the solution down can sometimes prevent the unpleasant side effects of nausea, vomiting, and diarrhea.

121. **(A) (F), (B) (T), (C) (F), (D) (T), (E) (T)**
Intravenous hyperalimentation is contraindicated in patients for whom there is no hope of resuming a meaningful human existence. It is also contraindicated in patients whose nutritional status is not in jeopardy or can be supported more easily by oral alimentation. It is lifesaving in some patients with temporary excessive metabolic demands or with severe malabsorption problems as well as in others.

122. **(A) (T), (B) (T), (C) (T), (D) (T), (E) (T)**
All of the choices plus other obvious situations of life-threatening injury are indications for formal exploration of the injured area. Negative explorations are tolerated well, and an aggressive approach will detect some potentially fatal injuries in the apparently clinically negative neck wound.

123. **(A) (T), (B) (T), (C) (T), (D) (T), (E) (T)**
Most patients are made more comfortable by immobilization of the fracture, but if the cast has produced ischemia or if an arterial injury has not been corrected, pain continues to be severe and unrelenting. One may detect either sensory or motor paralysis or both. Glovelike anesthesia is an important early sign of ischemia. Pallor often is more easily detected in the upper extremity than in the lower extremity.

124. **(A) (T), (B) (T), (C) (T), (D) (F), (E) (T)**
The levels most commonly affected are the lumbar, thoracic, and cervical regions, in that order. Thoracic vertebral infection may lead one to suspect a dissecting aneurysm because of the severe, unremitting pain, which is aggravated by movement but is not relieved by rest. Severe

muscle spasm and marked tenderness over the spinous process may give one a clue to the diagnosis. Unlike tuberculosis of the spine, this type of infection usually does not result in marked collapse of the vertebral bodies.

125. (A) (T), (B) (F), (C) (T), (D) (T), (E) (F)
An RBC count in excess of 100,000/mm³ indicates a positive lavage. An elevated amylase and bacteria in the fluid are other indications of a positive lavage.

126. (A) (T), (B) (F), (C) (T), (D) (F), (E) (F)
Simple drainage is not adequate for this injury. The distal end must be removed, or it must be anastomosed in a fashion to permit internal drainage of the pancreatic juice from the distal end. Direct duct repair is not considered a preferred method but rather one that can be considered when the alternative is radical pancreatic resection in the critically ill patient. With distal pancreatic resection, splenectomy is performed to facilitate the operation.

127. (A) (T), (B) (F), (C) (F), (D) (T), (E) (T)
A third degree burn destroys all of the elements of the skin; therefore, regeneration from the deeper layers, such as hair follicles and sweat glands, is impossible. The rule of nines estimates each lower extremity as 18.

128. (A) (T), (B) (T), (C) (T), (D) (F), (E) (F)
Irrigation of the incision with various cytotoxic agents was popularized several years ago as a method of preventing recurrence, but its use has had little success.

129. (A) (F), (B) (T), (C) (F), (D) (T), (E) (F)
Far too often, a soft tissue sarcoma is incompletely removed because the internal portion can be so easily enucleated from the pseudocapsule. It is important that a wide margin of normal tissue, deep to the tumor as well as on the other sides, be excised, and this means excision of some subjacent muscle tissue.

130. (A) (T), (B) (F), (C) (T), (D) (F), (E) (F)
The cure rate for epidermoid carcinoma of a number of sites (e.g., skin, cervix, lip, larynx, anus) is approximately the same for both modes of treatment. Surgery gives the higher cure rate in stomach, lung, and salivary gland carcinomas.

131. (A) (T), (B) (T), (C) (F), (D) (T), (E) (T)
The customary determinations, particularly the leukocyte count, are of limited value.

132. (A) (T), (B) (T), (C) (F), (D) (T), (E) (T)
Virtually all patients with renal osteodystrophy have parathyroid hyperplasia.

133. (A) (T), (B) (T), (C) (F), (D) (T), (E) (T)
The risk of developing carcinoma in the gastric remnant after gastric resection for peptic ulcer appears to be substantially higher than the risk of spontaneous development of gastric carcinoma in the unoperated stomach.

134. (A) (F), (B) (T), (C) (T), (D) (T), (E) (T)
The tourniquet should obstruct the venous return not the arterial flow.

135. (A) (T), (B) (T), (C) (T), (D) (T), (E) (T)
All statements are true.

136. (A) (F), (B) (T), (C) (T), (D) (T), (E) (F)
Continuous positive pressure ventilation and antibiotics are both indicated.

137. (A) (T), (B) (T), (C) (T), (D) (T), (E) (T)
All statements are true.

138. (A) (T), (B) (T), (C) (T), (D) (T), (E) (T)
All statements are true.

139. (A) (T), (B) (T), (C) (T), (D) (T), (E) (F)
These tumors are not encapsulated; they possess a pseudocapsule.

140. (A) (T), (B) (T), (C) (T), (D) (F), (E) (T)
Division of all the sphincter muscle renders the patient incontinent. Therefore, in patients with fistulas of the extrasphincteric type, the whole track must not be laid open.

141. (A) (T), (B) (F), (C) (T), (D) (T), (E) (T)
An air–fluid level can be demonstrated in 25% of patients and establishes the diagnosis.

142. (A) (T), (B) (F), (C) (T), (D) (T), (E) (T)
Cyclosporine is virtually insoluble in water and, therefore, cannot be given intravenously. Although absorption through the gastrointestinal tract is slow and incomplete, it is given orally.

143. (A) (T), (B) (T), (C) (T), (D) (F), (E) (T)
Early operation is useful if the diagnosis is made and the condition of the patient permits.

144. (A) (T), (B) (T), (C) (T), (D) (F), (E) (T)
Fistula in ano is more common in Crohn's disease than in ulcerative colitis. It is now clear that patients with ulcerative colitis have no unusual predisposing factors when compared with matched controls.

145. (A) (T), (B) (T), (C) (T), (D) (F), (E) (F)
The mortality from breast cancer is lower in Japan than it is in the USA. The most common location is the upper and outer quadrant of the breast.

146. (A) (T), (B) (T), (C) (T), (D) (T), (E) (T)
All the complications listed require urgent colectomy, which incurs a higher morbidity and mortality than elective surgery (4 to 5% vs 1 to 2%). Toxic megacolon, especially when perforation has already occurred, as is frequently the case, is particularly deadly (17% mortality). Elective colectomy usually is chosen because of cancer risk, especially with the availability of the newer continence-preserving procedures (e.g., ileoanal anastomosis with pelvic pouch). On the other hand, more widespread expertise with colonoscopy has allowed closer surveillance for the flatter, more difficult to detect colon carcinomas of ulcerative colitis.

147. (A) (T), (B) (T), (C) (F), (D) (T), (E) (T)
Palliative resection of the primary tumor is indicated even in the presence of metastases. It reduces the possibility of obstruction, bleeding, fistula formation, infection, and continuous discharge from the primary tumor.

148. (A) (F), (B) (T), (C) (T), (D) (T), (E) (T)
The symptoms of heartburn and regurgitation are aggravated by postural changes, such as stooping or lying flat.

149. (A) (T), (B) (T), (C) (F), (D) (T), (E) (F)
Pneumococci were the most common cause. This now is gram-negative organisms. A diagnosis can be made by peritoneal aspiration and gram stain, but a confirmatory laparotomy usually is required.

150. (A) (T), (B) (F), (C) (T), (D) (T), (E) (F)
It may be impossible to feel these soft tumors on rectal examination. If invasive cancer is present, the prognosis has been reported to be somewhat worse than for ordinary rectal or colon cancer.

151. (A) (T), (B) (T), (C) (F), (D) (T), (E) (T)
Retroperitoneal fibrosis is two to three times more common among men than women.

152. (A) (T), (B) (T), (C) (T), (D) (T), (E) (F)
The contribution of the intestinal phase to total stimulation of acid secretion may be far more important than was formerly suspected.

153. (A) (T), (B) (T), (C) (F), (D) (T), (E) (T)
A fever above 38°C is unusual.

154. (A) (T), (B) (T), (C) (T), (D) (F), (E) (F)
Ultrasound cannot differentiate between a thyroid adenoma and thyroid carcinoma. Needle biopsy is a very valuable study, but it cannot differentiate between benign and malignant neoplasms.

155. (A) (T), (B) (T), (C) (T), (D) (F), (E) (T)
Marginal ulcers are notoriously difficult to treat.

156. (A) (T), (B) (T), (C) (F), (D) (F), (E) (T)
The surgical treatment of medullary carcinoma of the thyroid is total thyroidectomy. Metastases from medullary carcinoma of the thyroid are radioresistant.

157. (A) (T), (B) (T), (C) (T), (D) (F), (E) (T)
Retroperitoneal hematomas adjacent to the duodenum must be opened and explored.

158. (A) (F), (B) (T), (C) (T), (D) (F), (E) (F)
These are false diverticula consisting of mucosa and submucosa. A one-stage operation is preferred and carries minimal risk even in debilitated patients. These diverticula are usually located on the left side of the neck.

159. (D) Maneuvers, such as striking the choking adult on the back or turning a choking child upside down, may make it more difficult for the choking person to handle the problem successfully and may convert the situation into one that is less easily managed. A child may be struck on the back.

160. (A) Carcinoma of the colon is not a complication of diverticulitis, although the two problems may be present together.

161. (D) There is no evidence that a rigid dressing accelerates maturity of the stump. That is the time before a definitive prosthesis can be fitted. Such a dressing benefits the stump in other ways.

162. **(E)** Pass the stripper from the ankle to the groin. It is important to introduce the stripper at the distal incision because mistakes have occurred when it is introduced at the groin.

163. **(B)** The complement system (11 serum proteins in the classic pathway, 3 in the alternate pathway) is activated by the binding of the initially small amount of specific serum antibody to bacterial antigen (or in some cases by the antigen itself). The proteins link to become a complex, which damages or lyses the bacterial cell wall, releases chemoattractants for phagocytes, produces immune adherence, and identifies and prepares the bacteria for phagocytosis, a process called opsonization. The complement complex does not inject lysozymes into the bacterium. Those enzymes act within the phagocyte.

164. **(D)** The hormone gastrin causes gallbladder contraction, not relaxation.

165. **(C)** This injury is caused by sudden deceleration when the heart and aortic arch are projected forward and upward.

166. **(A)** Hypovolemia is associated with a lowered blood pressure, central venous pressure, and pulmonary capillary wedge pressure.

167. **(E)** The hypoglossal nerve (XII) should be identified whenever the internal carotid artery is mobilized.

168. **(A)** The majority of surgical wound infections are caused by staphylococci.

169. **(C)** Nearly all patients with the Mallory-Weiss syndrome stop bleeding spontaneously. Sixty percent show an association with alcohol and 90% with vomiting. There is no indication for vagotomy. Admission to a hospital because of upper gastrointestinal bleeding usually is required.

170. **(C)** Most patients receiving radiation at these sites develop transient and self-limiting diarrhea. Simple supportive therapy often is effective, a defunctioning colostomy is rarely required, rectovaginal fistulas are rarely self-healing, and steroids are beneficial.

171. **(C)** The arterial blood flow is not increased by the action of the calf muscle pump.

172. **(D)** Release of the highly antigenic cyst fluid poses a great risk of anaphylaxis. Seeding of daughter cysts is a significant threat but is not an immediate, life-threatening problem.

173. **(C)** Induced vomiting and gastric lavage are contraindicated because of the danger of compounding the original injury.

174. **(C)** During ejaculation, the internal sphincter of the urinary bladder contracts. After injury to the preortic and preiliac autonomic nerves, this sphincter does not contract during ejaculation.

175. **(B)** Hematomas after thyroid or carotid surgery must be evaluated under sterile conditions before ventilation is compromised. Small hematomas may resorb, but they increase the incidence of wound infection.

176. **(B)** Local anesthesia is excellent for augmentation mammaplasty. If a hematoma develops, it should be promptly evacuated with good antibiotic coverage, infection is rare, and all breast tissue should be removed when a subcutaneous mastectomy is performed.

177. **(D)** As pounds are shed serum cholesterol drops an average of 40% and triglycrides 35%.

178. **(B)** The syndrome is characterized by diarrhea.

179. **(A)** Anal fissures are local in the midline posteriorly on the posterior commissure of the anal canal. In women, they may occur in the midline anteriorly.

180. **(C)** Massive postsplenectomy sepsis occurs with an incidence 60 times greater than sepsis in the general population, with a risk as high as 1% per year. This risk is greatest in children under 4, and 80% of cases occur within 2 years of splenectomy. The patient typically has a history of febrile upper respiratory infection, nausea, vomiting, headache, and confusion, leading rapidly to shock and coma. Death commonly occurs within 24 hours. The absence of the two splenic opsonins tuftsin and properdin increases susceptibility to encapsulated bacteria. Fifty percent of cases involve the pneumococcus, with *Neisseria, Escherichia coli,* and *Haemophilus influenzae* following in incidence. Polyvalent pneumococcal vaccine should be administered well before splenectomy, and penicillin should be given prophylactically or at the onset of a febrile upper respiratory infection.

Second Examination
Questions

DIRECTIONS (Questions 1 through 39): Each question consists of an introduction followed by five statements. Mark T (true) or F (false) after each statement.

1. Sometimes secondary lung cancer is curable. This is most likely to be achieved if a coin lesion is present in the lung. Resection of such a solitary metastasis is indicated under certain criteria.

   (A) the primary tumor must be controlled
   (B) a waiting period of at least 3 months is advisable before thoracotomy if the primary lesion was treated within 2 years
   (C) lung metastases from melanoma and breast carcinoma in general do the best
   (D) a CT scan of the lung must be obtained to rule out more than one metastasis
   (E) the outlook improves as the interval between control of the primary lesion and appearance of the metastasis increases
   (1:314–315)

2. The following statements concern abdominal wall defects in newborn infants.

   (A) gastroschisis occurs with exposed bowel
   (B) an omphalocele is a congenital failure of development of the abdominal wall
   (C) the contents of an omphalocele are exposed
   (D) umbilical hernias occur because the linea alba fails to close after the cord atrophies
   (E) an umbilical hernia should be repaired as soon as possible *(2:1279–1281, 1295)*

3. Necrotizing enterocolitis (NEC) is the most common cause of nonobstructive acute abdominal disease in the newborn. The following statements concern this problem.

   (A) most victims have a birth weight below 1500 g
   (B) the abdomen is not distended
   (C) gas in the bowel wall or portal vein may be seen on an abdominal x-ray
   (D) treatment at first consists of stopping feeding, nasogastric tube aspiration, intravenous antibiotics, and intravenous fluid replacement
   (E) evidence of perforation is a clear indication for surgery *(3:1288)*

4. The following statements are in regard to respiratory distress due to a Bochdalek hernia.

   (A) there is a posterolateral diaphragmatic defect
   (B) the defect occurs with equal frequency on the right and left side
   (C) the lung on the affected side is compressed but of normal size
   (D) gastrointestinal distention increases the respiratory problem
   (E) improved survival appears to correlate with the preoperative correction of acidosis, hypercarbia, and hypoxia *(2:1641–1642)*

5. The following are some of the advantages of the abdominal approach in the repair of a Bochdalek hernia in the newborn.

   (A) a more secure closure of the diaphragmatic defect is obtained
   (B) duodenal bands can be identified and corrected
   (C) a gastrostomy is easily performed
   (D) it is easier to compensate for the small size of the abdominal cavity
   (E) a chest tube is not needed *(2:1642)*

6. Biliary atresia is usually due to complete obliteration of the extrahepatic bile ducts. In these patients, there are no visible bile ducts, and only tiny fibrous cords are found. The following statements concern this difficult problem.

   (A) the Kasai procedure consists of dividing the remnants of the hepatic ducts and anastomosing a loop of jejunum to this region
   (B) the intestinal conduit is brought to the skin alone or with a Roux loop as a Mikulicz double-barrel enterostomy
   (C) closure of this stoma is performed at the age of 18 to 24 months
   (D) earlier closure of the stoma results in ascending cholangitis
   (E) prophylactic antibiotics are given continuously for the first 2 to 3 years of life   (3:1284)

7. Hirschsprung's disease is caused by absence of ganglion cells of the myenteric plexus of Auerbach in the involved segment of colon. The following statements concern this problem.

   (A) absence of these ganglion cells causes a functional intestinal obstruction, which may occur as acute intestinal obstruction in a neonate or as delay in moving the bowels
   (B) enterocolitis is a dangerous complication of Hirschsprung's disease
   (C) in infants with enterocolitis, the best treatment is to bring bowel with ganglion cells down to the anus. A preliminary colostomy is rarely required in this age group
   (D) the best diagnostic test is punch biopsy; absence of ganglion cells is diagnostic
   (E) in older children, Hirschsprung's disease must be distinguished from other more frequent causes of constipation (3:1273-1276)

8. These statements are in regard to pneumothorax in the infant.

   (A) it is a rare occurrence
   (B) it must always be treated by chest tube to ensure survival
   (C) it is a common complication of hyaline membrane disease
   (D) tension pneumothorax is treated by catheter aspiration of air
   (E) the air leak seals promptly after catheter aspiration of tension pneumothorax (3:1262)

9. After a massive resection of the intestine, a patient develops the short bowel syndrome. The following statements concern this problem.

   (A) if the terminal ileum and ileocecal valve are preserved, a greater length of intestine can be resected than if they are not preserved
   (B) if all of the ileum is missing, bile salts are excreted instead of being recirculated
   (C) the key to treatment is the control of diarrhea and steatorrhea
   (D) a high pH in the bowel interferes with digestion and shortens the transit time
   (E) Lomotil and codeine, which reduce intestinal motility, are helpful   (2:1163)

10. The following complications of staphylococcal pneumonia in the infant commonly require tube drainage or surgical intervention

   (A) pneumatoceles that cause respiratory distress
   (B) pneumatoceles that persist after successful treatment of the pneumonia
   (C) pneumothorax
   (D) pleural effusion
   (E) marked pleural thickening that restricts ventilation   (3:1262)

11. The following statements are in regard to the operative treatment of tracheoesophageal fistula (TEF).

   (A) the infant should always be operated on as soon as possible after the diagnosis is made
   (B) a gastrostomy does not help prevent reflux of gastric contents into the esophagus in most instances
   (C) if there is an unavoidable delay in operating following diagnosis, it is imperative that repair be accomplished no longer than 24 hours after diagnosis
   (D) sump catheter decompression of the proximal esophageal pouch is useful
   (E) at the first operation, the TEF is closed, but it is usually unwise to attempt esophageal anastomosis   (3:1264-1266)

12. The following statements are in regard to duodenal obstruction in the neonate.

   (A) bile vomiting is characteristic
   (B) contrast studies are not needed if there is air in the intestine distal to the duodenum

(C) it is usually wise to spend several days preparing the infant before undertaking operation

(D) most infants with duodenal stenosis have Down's syndrome

(E) the upright film of the abdomen shows the double-bubble sign   *(3:1269–1272)*

13. The following statements are in regard to intestinal atresia distal to the duodenum.

(A) the most common site of atresia is the ileum

(B) squamous cells are not found in the intestinal lumen distal to the site of atresia

(C) atresia is probably due to an in utero vascular accident

(D) the gut in these infants is usually shorter than normal

(E) one does not expect to find adhesions at the time of laparotomy to correct the atresia   *(3:1272)*

14. Insulinoma in most cases occurs with the classic diagnostic (Whipple's) triad of hypoglycemic symptoms produced by fasting, blood glucose below 50 mg when symptomatic, and relief of symptoms by intravenous glucose. The following statements concern insulinoma.

(A) weight gain is common

(B) fasting hypoglycemia occurs in the presence of inappropriately high levels of insulin

(C) transhepatic venous catheterization assists in localizing the tumor

(D) surgery should take place after a trial of diazoxide to suppress insulin release

(E) tumors in the head of the pancreas usually can be enucleated   *(1:537–538)*

15. The following statements concern the diagnosis of the acute abdomen.

(A) the writhing patient in obvious pain often has ureteral or intestinal colic

(B) the patient with general peritonitis lies motionless

(C) the abdomen becomes distended early in patients with infarcted bowel

(D) corticosteroids do not affect the diagnosis of acute abdominal disease

(E) patients with paralytic ileus often have an area of localized abdominal tenderness   *(1:395–397)*

16. Nearly three quarters of the patients with pheochromocytomas experience symptomatic attacks. Common symptoms and signs of these attacks include:

(A) headache

(B) palpitation

(C) excessive perspiration

(D) fever

(E) flushing   *(3:679–686)*

17. The healing of a surgical wound may be delayed by which of the following.

(A) cancer chemotherapy with cytotoxic drugs

(B) heavy irradiation

(C) large doses of corticosteroids

(D) protein depletion

(E) ascorbic acid deficiency   *(1:8–9)*

18. The following are characteristic of pancreatic gastrinomas that cause the Zollinger-Ellison syndrome.

(A) the tumors are usually benign

(B) in the pancreatic tissue not involved in the tumor, the islet cells are hyperplastic

(C) if metastases are present, they may disappear following total gastrectomy

(D) relatives of patients with this type of endocrine tumor do not have endocrinopathies on a genetic basis

(E) the gastric hypersecretion caused by these tumors can be controlled by cimetidine   *(2:1367–1368)*

19. The following statements concern Cushing's syndrome.

(A) hypertension occurs in most patients

(B) the limbs are thin; the trunk and face are obese

(C) muscle weakness and backache are common

(D) total bilateral adrenalectomy is the indicated surgical treatment

(E) osteoporosis and pathologic fractures are frequent in advanced cases   *(3:670)*

20. Carcinoid tumors occur in the

(A) lung

(B) stomach

(C) pancreas

(D) ileum

(E) rectum   *(3:949–952)*

21. Fear and anxiety are normal before and after surgery. The following statements concern more severe psychiatric problems after a surgical operation.

(A) postoperative psychoses are most common after abdominal surgery
(B) drugs such as meperidine hyrochloride, cimetidine, and corticosteriods play a role in development of postoperative psychoses
(C) postoperative psychosis usually develops during the first 2 postoperative days
(D) first symptoms often include confusion, fear, and disorientation as to time and place
(E) postoperative emotional disturbances may be avoided by appropriate counseling of the patient by the surgeon before the operation   *(1:35)*

22. The following statements concern the concept of debulking a malignant tumor arising from the ovaries.

(A) with widespread pelvic involvement, surgical removal of the rectum and bladder in addition to the uterus and ovaries has not been found helpful
(B) maximum tumor reduction by surgery is beneficial if it does not expose the patient to life-threatening complications
(C) reduction of tumor mass appears to be helpful in improving the response to chemotherapy and irradiation
(D) an attempt should be made to remove all sites of tumor, including local peritoneal metastases
(E) the primary treatment is hysterectomy and bilateral salpingo-oophorectomy *(2:1770)*

23. The treatment of a patient with intraperitoneal abscesses consists of prompt drainage.

(A) percutaneous drainage is the preferred method
(B) percutaneous drainage is possible in about 75% of patients
(C) percutaneous drainage works best in well-localized lesions that do not contain solid debris
(D) open drainage is used when percutaneous drainage has failed or is inappropriate
(E) an untreated residual abscess is fatal in most patients   *(1:411)*

24. Atelectasis is the most common pulmonary complication of abdominal surgery. The following statements concern this problem.

(A) fever, tachypnea, and tachycardia in the first 48 hours after surgery indicate atelectasis
(B) obstructive causes include secretions and, occasionally, a malpositioned endotracheal tube
(C) an uncommon cause is closure of the bronchioles
(D) postoperative atelectasis can be largely prevented by early mobilization, coughing, frequent changes of position, and the use of a blow-bottle apparatus
(E) treatment consists of clearing the airway by coughing, percussion, and endotracheal suction   *(1:25-26)*

25. The following findings may be noted in a patient with early respiratory failure after an injury or major surgical operation.

(A) tachypnea, 25 to 30 breaths per minute
(B) tidal volume of less than 4 ml/Kg
(C) arterial hypertension
(D) PcO_2 above 45 mm Hg
(E) Po_2 below 60 mm Hg   *(1:17)*

26. The following statements concern the differentiation of diverticulitis from colon cancer as seen on a barium enema.

(A) diverticulitis usually involves a long segment of colon and carcinoma involves a short segment
(B) in carcinoma, the transition from normal bowel both above and below is abrupt; in diverticulitis, it is gradual
(C) in diverticulitis, the bowel is not spastic
(D) the mucosal pattern is destroyed in carcinoma
(E) diverticulae in other areas favors diverticulitis but does not rule out carcinoma   *(2:1187)*

27. The first signs of the malignant hyperthermia syndrome during anesthesia include

(A) respiratory acidosis
(B) metabolic acidosis
(C) bradycardia
(D) sustained muscle contracture after induction of anesthesia
(E) it is an inherited disease   *(1:172)*

28. A patient in the early postoperative period after coronary artery bypass is stable but develops severe abdominal pain. He has developed an acute abdomen.

(A) the patient is a relatively good risk for operative intervention
(B) an attempt should be made to avoid operation until 1 week after the bypass
(C) the risk of laparotomy is greater than the risk of sepsis
(D) operation is indicated for a perforated duodenal ulcer but not for acute acalculous cholecystitis
(E) in the patient described, the decision to operate is no different from the same patient prebypass   *(16:1824-1831)*

29. The following statements are in regard to pyogenic liver abscesses in the USA.

(A) a solitary abscess is more likely to be in the right lobe rather than in the left lobe
(B) abscesses due to biliary tract obstruction usually are solitary abscesses
(C) abscesses due to portal infections usually are solitary abscesses
(D) the diabetic is at higher risk for developing a hepatic abscess than is the nondiabetic
(E) trauma and shock put patients at high risk for developing hepatic abscesses   *(17:369-380)*

30. The following presenting symptoms occur in more than one half of the patients with pyogenic liver abscesses.

(A) right shoulder pain
(B) right upper quadrant pain
(C) anorexia
(D) diarrhea
(E) fever   *(17:369-380)*

31. The following laboratory and radiologic findings are reported in more than half of the patients with pyogenic liver abscesses.

(A) leukocytosis
(B) serum bilirubin greater than 2 mg/dl
(C) hypoalbuminemia
(D) abnormal liver–spleen scan
(E) elevated serum alkaline phosphatase   *(17:369-380)*

32. In patients at high risk of developing acute disseminated candidiasis, the following local measures to treat high density colonization of *Candida* are useful.

(A) nystatin suspension 400,000 units, "swish and swallow" qid
(B) miconazole vaginal suppositories
(C) remove catheter from vein
(D) irrigation of abscess cavity with amphotericin B 50 mg in 1000 ml 5% dextrose in water
(E) remove catheter from bladder and irrigate with solution mentioned in **D** via 3-way catheter   *(2:194)*

33. The following statements are about antibiotics.

(A) allergic reactions are frequent when penicillin is injected
(B) vestibular nerve damage and deafness may follow the administration of streptomycin
(C) chloramphenicol may produce aplastic anemia, thrombocytopenia, or neutropenia
(D) amphotericin B is neurotoxic
(E) erythromycin is associated with the development of gastrointestinal and hepatic disturbances   *(3:270-271)*

34. The following statements are in regard to the use of vasopressin for upper gastrointestinal bleeding.

(A) vasopressin therapy improves survival rate
(B) continuous intravenous infusion is as effective as intraarterial infusion
(C) when added to standard therapy to control upper gastrointestinal bleeding, vasopresin therapy more often results in cessation of bleeding than does standard therapy alone
(D) vasopressin therapy should not be continued for more than 48 hours
(E) "buying time" is the chief value of vasopressin therapy   *(19:743)*

35. The following statements concern intraoperative and postoperative myocardial infarction.

    (A) the incidence is higher if the operation is for some other manifestation of atherosclerosis
    (B) patients who have had a myocardial infarction within 3 months of a surgical operation are likely to suffer reinfarction and even death
    (C) in selected patients, a coronary artery bypass graft should precede an elective operation on another organ
    (D) most postoperative myocardial infarctions are symptomatic
    (E) the treatment of myocardial infarction in such patients includes the use of anticoagulants   *(1:29)*

36. Stage IV carcinoma of the breast may be treated by hormone manipulation. The following statements concern this form of therapy.

    (A) hormone manipulation is usually more successful in premenopausal women than in those who are postmenopausal
    (B) the response is better in those whose tumor contains estrogen receptors than it is in those with both estrogen and progesterone receptors
    (C) a favorable response to hormone manipulation can be expected in patients with rapidly growing tumors
    (D) younger patients respond better than do the very old
    (E) it is usually best to try chemotherapy before hormone manipulation   *(1:269)*

37. The following statements concern gallstone ileus.

    (A) episodes of partial intestinal obstruction precede complete obstruction
    (B) an x-ray may show air in the biliary tree
    (C) the gallstone usually passes from the gallbladder to the jejunum
    (D) treatment is to remove the gallstone and correct the fistula if possible
    (E) the most common site of obstruction is the proximal ilium   *(3:1164–1165)*

38. The following statements concern operations for cancer of the colon and rectum.

    (A) bilateral oophorectomy should be a part of operations for colorectal cancer unless contraindicated
    (B) for cancers of the descending colon, the segment supplied by the left colic vessels is removed
    (C) for cancers of the sigmoid colon, the left colic vessels are preserved when possible
    (D) lesions of the midtransverse colon are segmentally removed with the midcolic vessels
    (E) after resection of the right colon, an iliotransverse colostomy restores continuity of the gastrointestinal tract   *(2:1198–1202)*

39. Liver trauma is a problem in North America today.

    (A) the blunt trauma of an automobile accident tends to produce an explosive injury of the liver
    (B) a high-velocity missile injury shatters the liver parenchyma over a wide area from the wound track
    (C) in the case of a knife wound, bleeding is usually continuing at the time of operation
    (D) stress ulcers are common after hepatic trauma
    (E) a severe pulverizing injury may require formal hepatic lobectomy   *(1:462)*

DIRECTIONS (Questions 40 through 160): Each of the numbered items or incomplete statements in this section is followed by answers or by completions of the statement. Select the ONE lettered answer or completion that is BEST in each case.

40. Many drugs are toxic to the kidney. Of the following drugs or combination of drugs, which is LEAST likely to damage the kidney?

    (A) gentamicin
    (B) aspirin and ibuprofen
    (C) methicillin
    (D) amphotericin B
    (E) aspirin   *(1:88)*

41. In rehabilitation following an above-the-knee amputation (AK), special emphasis must be placed on exercise of the

    (A) hip flexors
    (B) hip extensors
    (C) hip abductors
    (D) back extensors
    (E) external rotators of the thigh   *(2:2052)*

42. A 1-year-old male child has an abdominal mass and an osteolytic lesion of the skull. The most likely diagnosis is

(A) Wilms' tumor
(B) hypernephroma
(C) Hodgkin's disease
(D) hepatoma
(E) neuroblastoma   *(2:1533)*

43. Malignant melanoma is a skin lesion that has the potential for early diagnosis. One of the following is INCORRECT.

(A) 1 to 5 years or longer may elapse before a superficial spreading melanoma becomes malignant
(B) melanomas are common among blacks
(C) nodular malignant melanomas occur on all body surfaces
(D) subungual melanomas occur most commonly under the nails of the thumb and great toe
(E) of the three types of melanoma (nodular, superficial spreading, and lentigo maligna), the nodular type is the most virulent

44. A patient has a carcinoma of the cecum and proximal ascending colon. Which of the following symptoms is UNUSUAL in such a patient?

(A) right lower quadrant pain
(B) indigestion
(C) anorexia and weight loss
(D) symptoms due to intestinal obstruction
(E) symptoms due to anemia   *(2:1199)*

45. The following statements concern malignant pleural effusion in patients with carcinoma of the breast. Which statement is INCORRECT?

(A) malignant pleural effusion develops at some time in almost 15% of patients with carcinoma of the breast
(B) when severe, the best treatment is closed chest tube drainage and instillation of a sclerosing agent
(C) a chest tube is inserted in a low interspace, and suction drainage is started
(D) 500 mg of tetracycline in 30 ml of saline is the best sclerosing agent
(E) fluid reaccumulation, if it occurs, may be treated by repeating the procedure after a few weeks   *(1:270)*

46. Following correction of a double aortic arch, a 6-month-old infant developed chylothorax.

Through a small polyethylene tube, about 150 ml of chylous fluid was drained daily until the thoracic duct was ligated on the tenth day. The most important consideration in advising operation is

(A) continuing loss of lymphocytes
(B) lung dysfunction from pachypleuritis
(C) depletion of plasma proteins
(D) threat of empyema
(E) loss of neutral fats and cholesterol
                                         (2:657-658)

47. Rupture of the spleen may occur from a number of causes, including each of the following. Which is out of order in frequency of occurrence?

(A) penetrating trauma
(B) blunt trauma
(C) delayed rupture
(D) iatrogenic rupture
(E) spontaneous rupture   *(1:552)*

48. The indications to surgically explore the bile ducts during the operation of cholecystectomy can be absolute or relative. Which of the following is an absolute indication?

(A) preoperative demonstration of small stones in the gallbladder
(B) the presence of a palpable common bile duct stone or stones
(C) jaundice, with a bilirubin over 7.0
(D) dilated common bile duct
(E) cholangitis   *(1:506)*

49. Platelet function is in part controlled by the prostaglandins. One of the following statements concerning the role of prostaglandins in blood coagulation is NOT CORRECT.

(A) the specific prostaglandin responsible for blood clotting is thromboxane A2
(B) thromboxane A2 is synthesized by platelets and causes platelet aggregation and vasoconstriction
(C) prostacyclin PGI2 is synthesized by endothelial cells and is a potent vasodilator
(D) prostacyclin PGI2 does not alter the ability of platelets to aggregate
(E) arachidonic acid is the major precursor of both thromboxane A2 and prostcyclin PGI2   *(3:501)*

50. Vascular ring anomalies of the aorta can best be diagnosed by

(A) barium swallow
(B) esophagoscopy
(C) bronchoscopy
(D) bronchogram
(E) cardiac catheterization   *(2:755-757)*

51. Suppurative thrombophlebitis is a serious and sometimes fatal condition. All of the following statements concerning this condition are correct EXCEPT

(A) a high fever is common
(B) blood cultures often are positive
(C) local signs of inflammation are present
(D) treatment with antibiotics usually is successful
(E) treatment consists of excising the affected vein proximal to the first open collateral and leaving the wound open   *(1:37)*

52. A patient is comatose, and it is suspected that an abdominal injury is present as well as a head injury. The objective of a peritoneal lavage is to

(A) exclude an extraperitoneal hematoma
(B) exclude the presence of peritonitis
(C) confirm that blood is present or is not present in the peritoneal cavity
(D) make the diagnosis of a ruptured spleen
(E) diagnose the presence of a ruptured hollow viscus   *(3:307)*

53. Which of the following statements best describes the situation with trench foot or immersion foot?

(A) trench foot and immersion foot occur after prolonged exposure to a wet and cold environment with temperatures above freezing
(B) trench foot and immersion foot occur after prolonged exposure to a wet and cold environment with temperatures below freezing
(C) both deep and superficial tissue destruction commonly occurs
(D) after rewarming, hyperemia may develop, but this is unusual
(E) after rewarming, the part is anesthetic, and edema rarely develops   *(3:240)*

54. Indirect inguinal hernias should always be repaired unless there are specific contraindications because the complications of incarceration, obstruction, and strangulation pose a greater risk than an operation. Of the following statements about the operation, which is NOT accurate?

(A) correct any obvious causes, such as chronic cough, before the operation
(B) it is essential to excise the sac of an indirect inguinal hernia
(C) in infants and young adults, the only repair usually necessary is reduction of the size of the internal ring
(D) bilateral repair is preferred whenever possible
(E) the Bassini repair leaves the spermatic cord in its normal anatomic position *(1:652)*

55. Multiple endocrine adenomatosis type I (MEA I) consists of involvement of the chromophobe cells of the pituitary, the islet cells of the pancreas, the parathyroid glands, and less frequently the adrenal cortex and the thyroid. Which of the following statements is FALSE?

(A) the most frequent presentation is peptic ulcer disease or its complications
(B) manifestations of hypoglycemia are the second most common presenting feature
(C) parathyroid chief cell hyperplasia is the characteristic pathologic lesion of the parathyroid glands
(D) adrenal cortical hyperfunction often occurs in patients with MEA
(E) the standard accepted surgical procedure for patients with the Zollinger-Ellison syndrome associated with non-beta cell pancreatic tumors is total gastrectomy   *(3:611)*

56. An infant with hypertrophic pyloric stenosis vomits repeatedly and has an inadequate intake of formula. The serum CO_2 is high, and the serum chloride is low. The serum potassium concentration is most likely to be

(A) 6.5 to 7.5 mEq/L
(B) 5.0 to 6.5 mEq/L
(C) 3.5 to 5.0 mEq/L
(D) 1.5 to 3.0 mEq/L
(E) of no importance in this patient   *(1:1110)*

57. A 12-year-old boy has sudden onset of pain in the thigh and starts limping. On examination, the limb is externally rotated, and there is limitation of passive internal rotation. Of the following, he is most likely to have

(A) displacement of the capital femoral epiphysis

(B) rheumatoid arthritis

(C) osteochondritis of the femoral head

(D) tuberculosis

(E) osteochondromatosis　　　　　*(1:991)*

58. Hyperparathyroidism is associated with all of the following EXCEPT

(A) nephrolithiasis

(B) diarrhea

(C) muscle weakness

(D) psychiatric disorders

(E) polyuria　　　　　*(3:623)*

59. Partial occlusion of one renal artery would likely manifest itself by causing

(A) hypertension

(B) gross hematuria

(C) pyrexia

(D) elevation of the blood urea nitrogen

(E) diminished urinary output　　　　　*(1:700)*

60. Over 90% of portasystemic shunts remain patent. Which is the best shunt for a patient who requires an elective portal decompression procedure?

(A) side-to-side portacaval

(B) end-to-side portacaval

(C) distal splenorenal

(D) central splenorenal

(E) mesocaval　　　　　*(1:480)*

61. An 18-year-old girl has tired easily and has had dyspnea on exertion since early childhood. She recently has become cyanotic. She has a grade III systolic murmur along the left sternal border. The electrocardiogram shows right axis deviation. A roentgenogram shows enlargement of both ventricles, enlargement of the pulmonary artery and its tributaries, and pulmonary congestion. The likely diagnosis is

(A) tetralogy of Fallot

(B) pulmonic stenosis

(C) aortic insufficiency

(D) ventricular septal defect

(E) aortic stenosis　　　　　*(2:767–769)*

62. Testicular tumors metastasize primarily to which lymph nodes?

(A) superficial inguinal nodes

(B) deep inguinal nodes

(C) periaortic nodes

(D) popliteal nodes

(E) celiac nodes　　　　　*(1:872)*

63. A 35-year-old woman complains of headache, muscle weakness, polydipsia, and nocturia. She has moderate hypertension but no retinopathy, and the rest of the physical examination is unremarkable except for severe muscle weakness. The most likely diagnosis is

(A) coarctation of the aorta

(B) fibromuscular hyperplasia of the renal arteries

(C) Cushing's syndrome

(D) malignant hypertension

(E) primary aldosteronism　　　　　*(1:662–664)*

64. Mediastinoscopy with biopsy of the paratracheal and carinal lymph nodes is almost invariably accurate in the diagnosis of

(A) pulmonary carcinoma

(B) sarcoidosis

(C) interstitial pneumonitis

(D) silicosis

(E) primary mediastinal tumor　　　　　*(1:308)*

65. Stress ulcer denotes a gastric or duodenal ulcer that develops in a patient as a result of stress. Which of the following is NOT a cause of stress ulcer?

(A) shock

(B) sepsis

(C) burns

(D) CNS trauma or tumors (Cushing's ulcer)

(E) aspirin　　　　　*(1:449)*

66. A 50-year-old man with a history of bouts of heavy drinking is thought to have acute pancreatitis. His serum analysis is 600 IU, and an abdominal x-ray shows an isolated loop of dilated small bowel. Which of the following treatment programs is NOT indicated?

(A) a full course of antibiotics in all such patients

(B) oral intake withheld

(C) large volumes of fluid given intravenously

(D) supplemental oxygen therapy

(E) total parenteral nutrition in all but mild attacks　　　　　*(1:524)*

67. Following splenectomy for congenital spherocytosis in childhood, all of the following would be expected EXCEPT

    (A) a transient leukocytosis
    (B) a transient rise in platelet count
    (C) persistence of spherocytes in the peripheral blood
    (D) persistence of increased red blood cell fragility
    (E) decreased life span of the erythrocytes

    (2:1379-1380)

68. A 55-year-old man is recovering from an acute myocardial infarction when he suddenly develops severe diffuse abdominal pain that does not respond to narcotics. His abdomen on examination is not unduly rigid or tender. You diagnose mesenteric infarction. At operation 6 hours later, you find ischemic intestine. Which of the following is NOT appropriate?

    (A) use the laser Doppler system to estimate bowel viability
    (B) use the qualitative fluorescein test to estimate bowel viability
    (C) use the oxygen electrode system to estimate bowel viability
    (D) resect nonviable bowel
    (E) plan a second-look operation if there is doubt about the viability of the remaining bowel

    (1:581)

69. In North America, obstruction of the small intestine is due to many causes. The most common in descending order of frequency of occurrence are listed. Which one is out of order?

    (A) external hernia
    (B) intrinsic or extrinsic neoplasms
    (C) adhesions
    (D) intussusception
    (E) volvulus

    (1:568)

70. A 60-year-old woman is found to have a perforated carcinoma of the sigmoid colon. She has general peritonitis. Her management will include all of the following EXCEPT

    (A) resection of the primary tumor and end-to-end anastomosis
    (B) a Hartmann procedure after resection of the tumor
    (C) drainage of the peritoneal cavity
    (D) appropriate antibiotics
    (E) nasogastric aspiration and intravenous fluid replacement

    (1:601)

71. A man aged 55 has a carcinoma of the rectum. The distal margin is 3 cm from the anal epithelium. The tumor is clinically considered to be Dukes B. The best treatment is

    (A) abdominoperineal resection
    (B) low anterior resection
    (C) local excision
    (D) laser photocoagulation
    (E) radiation therapy

    (1:595-605)

72. A patient has an aortoenteric fistula 2 years after the insertion of a Dacron aortofemoral bypass graft. The safest method of treating this patient is

    (A) closure of the aortic defect. Closure of the enteric opening and the interposition of the great omentum
    (B) closure of the enteric defect. Thorough irrigation with an antibiotic solution and administration of systemic antibiotics and insertion of a new aortofemoral bypass graft
    (C) closure of the enteric fistula. Ligature of the aorta and removal of the Dacron aortofemoral bypass graft, followed by insertion of an extraanatomic axillary-bifemoral bypass graft
    (D) giving a prolonged course of antibiotics after culture to confirm the identity and sensitivity of the infecting organism
    (E) excision of the graft, ligature of the arteries proximal and distal to the anastomosis. Good care to encourage the collateral circulation and the insertion of an extraanatomic bypass after the patient has stabilized

    (5:755)

73. Disseminated intravascular coagulation (DIC) is often a consumption coagulopathy. The consumption coagulopathy of DIC is characterized by all of the following EXCEPT

    (A) decrease in fibroginogen
    (B) fall in number of platelets
    (C) decrease in fibroginogen degradation products
    (D) prolongation of the prothrombin time (PT) and partial thromboplastin time (PTT)
    (E) activation of fibrinolysis

    (3:103)

74. The testicular tumor most sensitive to radiotherapy is

    (A) choriocarcinoma

(B) seminoma
(C) embryonal carcinoma
(D) malignant teratoma
(E) melanoma   *(1:83)*

75. The indications for splenectomy include all of the following EXCEPT

(A) ruptured spleen
(B) hereditary spherocytosis
(C) many patients with thrombocytopenic purpura
(D) splenic vein thrombosis with esophageal varies
(E) primary splenic tumor   *(1:544, 553)*

76. A patient develops sudden, severe, excruciating abdominal pain. The LEAST likely diagnosis is

(A) myocardial infarction
(B) acute appendicitis
(C) perforated peptic ulcer
(D) ruptured abdominal aneurysm
(E) renal colic   *(1:396)*

77. A 75-year-old man tests positive for blood in the stools. A colonoscopy removes three polyps (two adenomatous, one villous adenoma) from the sigmoid colon. At a follow-up examination, another polyp is removed that contains carcinoma. Resection of the involved segment is indicated if

(A) the gross margin is clear at endoscopy
(B) the microscopic margin is clear
(C) the cancer is well differentiated
(D) there is no lymphatic or venous invasion
(E) there are malignant cells in the muscularis mucosa   *(1:604)*

78. The diagnosis of a gastrojejunocolic or gastrocolic fistula is suspected if the following symptoms or signs develop EXCEPT

(A) the patient has had an operation that included a gastroenterostomy
(B) severe diarrhea and weight loss have occurred
(C) feculent vomiting occasionally occurs
(D) an upper gastrointestinal series fails to demonstrate the fistula
(E) malnutrition may be severe   *(1:433)*

79. Technetium scan is capable of demonstrating what percentage of Meckel's diverticula?

(A) 10%
(B) 30%
(C) 50%

(D) 70%
(E) 90%   *(3:947)*

80. A 20-year-old man after an abdominal gunshot wound develops an intestinal cutaneous fistula. He is transferred to your care 2 weeks after the injury, and you are told that the output from the fistula is 600 ml/day. His management consists of the following EXCEPT

(A) restore blood volume and correct fluid and electrolyte imbalance
(B) control fistula usually with an ostomy appliance
(C) delineate fistula with x-ray contrast
(D) operate and close the fistula as soon as **A, B,** and **C** have been achieved
(E) drain any abscess that appears   *(1:579)*

81. Cancer of the breast complicates about 1 in 3000 pregnancies. One of the following statements concerning this problem is INCORRECT.

(A) breast changes occurring during gestation make detection more difficult
(B) breast cancer is more malignant during pregnancy
(C) self-examination performed regularly and frequently aids earlier detection
(D) mammography in pregnant patients is a valuable and effective study
(E) if the cancer is confined to the breast, the prognosis is good; if the lymph nodes are involved, the outlook is poor   *(1:58)*

82. At least 50% of patients with a hiatal hernia are asymptomatic and require no treatment. Which of the following statements concerning symptomatic patients is INCORRECT?

(A) the head of the bed should be raised on 4- to 6-inch blocks; raising the head on pillows is ineffective
(B) frequent, small, high-protein and low-fat meals are advised
(C) the value of cimetidine is as yet undetermined
(D) the most effective operation is the Nissen fundoplication
(E) the most effective operation for a symptomatic acquired short esophagus is the Nissen fundoplication   *(1:389)*

83. Which of the following injuries is most likely to have caused a traumatic arterial thrombosis?

(A) fracture-dislocation of the knee joint
(B) fracture of the shaft of the femur
(C) fracture of the neck of the femur
(D) dislocation of the hip joint
(E) fracture of the patella   (4:484)

Questions 84 through 87

An 8-year-old girl is hospitalized for severe jaundice and upper abdominal pain. During the past 3 years, she has had four previous episodes of pain, jaundice, and fever, with spontaneous remission. Her temperature is 38.3°C (101°F). A firm mass is present just inferior to the right lobe of the liver. The bilirubin is 7.0 mg%, and the alkaline phosphatase is elevated.

84. The most likely diagnosis is

(A) hepatoma
(B) hepatitis
(C) congenital atresia of the bile duct
(D) choledochal cyst
(E) echinococcus cyst   (2:1310)

85. If left untreated, the probable outcome would be

(A) death within a few weeks
(B) recovery with no further difficulty
(C) severe biliary cirrhosis within 3 years
(D) a stationary course with persistent jaundice but no pain or less severe pain
(E) slow recovery with likely recurrence in the future   (2:1310)

86. Appropriate therapy would be

(A) low protein diet, bedrest, and antibiotics
(B) emetine hydrochloride
(C) isolation, stool culture, low-protein diet, no antibiotics
(D) internal drainage of the lesion
(E) excision and Roux-en-Y choledochojejunostomy   (2:1310)

87. This lesion

(A) does not cause biliary cirrhosis
(B) does not rupture spontaneously
(C) is more common in females than in males
(D) is not associated with biliary stone formation
(E) is of infectious origin   (2:1310)

88. Which of the following well-identified complications of ulcerative colitis does not require an urgent operation?

(A) toxic megacolon
(B) massive unrelenting hemorrhage
(C) fulminating acute ulcerative colitis
(D) obstruction secondary to stricture
(E) evidence of colon carcinoma   (3:1018-1019)

89. Only one of the following statements concerning hemorrhoids is correct.

(A) bleeding when it occurs is dark in color and of the venous type
(B) hemorrhoids are a common cause of anemia. In such patients, treatment of the anemia includes hemorrhoidectomy as primary therapy
(C) injection therapy consists of injecting 5% phenol in arachic oil into the feeding vein through insensitive columnar epithelium above the hemorrhoid
(D) it is important to exclude a proximal bowel carcinoma as a cause of hemorrhoids
(E) prolapse of hemorrhoids with defecation rarely returns spontaneously   (3:1038-1043)

90. Hemobilia was first described by Sandblom in 1948. Which of the following statements concerning hemobilia is true?

(A) in hemobilia, the basic lesion is an arteriobiliary fistula
(B) the usual cause is blunt trauma that has produced a deep rupture in the liver
(C) occlusion of the feeding artery by a radiologist is appropriate primary treatment
(D) the classic triad of symptoms is sudden severe right upper quadrant colicky pain followed in a few minutes by hematemesis or melena and then by jaundice
(E) all of the above   (3:1092-1095)

91. Hyperlipidemia (Frederickson types 1, 4, and 5) has been linked with pancreatitis, and the mechanism is postulated to be

(A) obstruction of the pancreatic microcirculation with micelles of fat
(B) intrapancreatic conversion of triglycerides to toxic free fatty acids by pancreatic lipase
(C) atherosclerotic occlusion of the pancreaticoduodenal arcade

(D) increased blood viscosity causing pancreatic microcirculatory sludging

(E) Rouleau formation with blockage of pancreatic microvessels   *(3:1178)*

Questions 92 through 94

A 31-year-old woman is admitted for diagnosis of the cause of a cough productive of a small amount of mucoid sputum and intermittent hemoptysis. Since her symptoms first began 3 years earlier, she has had recurrent respiratory infections with purulent sputum, for which she has been treated successfully with short courses of antibiotics. Chest films show a 2.5-cm rounded lesion close to the right lower lobe bronchus on both PA and lateral views.

92. The most likely diagnosis of the primary disease is

    (A) tuberculosis
    (B) bronchiectasis
    (C) bronchial carcinoid tumor
    (D) histoplasmosis
    (E) bronchogenic carcinoma   *(2:707–709)*

93. The most useful initial diagnostic procedure would be

    (A) cytologic examination of the sputum
    (B) laminography
    (C) bronchogram
    (D) bronchoscopy
    (E) acid-fast stain of the sputum   *(2:707–709)*

94. The definitive treatment of choice would be

    (A) postural drainage
    (B) appropriate chemotherapy alone
    (C) pneumonectomy
    (D) radiation therapy
    (E) lobectomy   *(2:707–709)*

95. Pseudomembranous enterocolitis may occur from bacterial overgrowth following clindamycin administration. The organism increasingly implicated in this condition is

    (A) *Bacteroides*
    (B) *Clostridium difficile*
    (C) *Escherichia coli*
    (D) *Klebsiella*
    (E) *Salmonella*   *(3:276)*

96. A reflex (automatic) neurogenic bladder may be expected in

    (A) meningomyelocele
    (B) diabetic neuropathy
    (C) cerebrovascular accident with cortical destruction
    (D) transection of the spinal cord
    (E) tabes dorsalis   *(2:1692)*

Questions 97 through 99

Four days after an uneventful Billroth II gastric resection, the patient, a 55-year-old man, suddenly has severe upper abdominal pain. On examination, his abdomen is rigid and he has a fever.

97. The probable diagnosis is

    (A) duodenal stump leak
    (B) acute pancreatitis
    (C) postoperative acute cholecystitis
    (D) wound infection
    (E) delayed rupture of a contused spleen *(1:432)*

98. The most helpful diagnostic procedure would be

    (A) barium swallow
    (B) serum amylase and lipase
    (C) 2-hour urinary amylase
    (D) white blood cell count
    (E) paracentesis   *(1:432)*

99. The treatment would be

    (A) splenectomy
    (B) nasogastric suction and anticholinergic medication
    (C) cholecystectomy
    (D) immediate abdominal drainage
    (E) nasogastric suction for 2 days followed by suture of the duodenal stump   *(1:432)*

Questions 100 through 103

A 57-year-old man, known for 5 years to have cirrhosis of the liver, is seen in surgical consultation because of esophageal varices demonstrated by barium swallow and confirmed by esophagoscopy. He has never had gastrointestinal bleeding, been in a coma, or required paracentesis. Both the liver and the spleen are enlarged. The serum bilirubin is 1.8 mg%, the SGOT is slightly elevated, BSP retention is 15%, and the prothrombin time is 14.5 seconds (control: 11.8 seconds).

100. It may be assumed that all of the following statements regarding this patient are true EXCEPT

    (A) portal hypertension above 30 cm of saline exists
    (B) there is a high probability of gastrointestinal bleeding in the future
    (C) the varices usually will not disappear
    (D) a portacaval shunt might not be possible because of portal vein thrombosis
    (E) a prophylactic portacaval shunt should be performed   *(1:471-481)*

101. If the patient should bleed massively from his varices, the immediate treatment might include all of the following EXCEPT

    (A) laxatives
    (B) enemas
    (C) tamponade of the lower esophagus and cardia of the stomach
    (D) vasopressin
    (E) morphine   *(1:471-481)*

102. All of the following statements concerning angiographic procedures in the cirrhotic patient are true EXCEPT

    (A) selective celiac or splenic artery angiography does not usually demonstrate active bleeding from esophageal varices
    (B) the portal vein and its tributaries can be visualized by selective celiac artery angiography
    (C) splenic pulp manometry is the safest method of determining whether or not the patient has portal hypertension
    (D) the wedged hepatic vein pressure accurately reflects portal vein pressure except in the presence of a presinusoidal block
    (E) the procedure to determine the wedged hepatic vein pressure has almost no morbidity   *(1:471-481)*

103. The patient recovers after a massive hemorrhage from varices, and with good nutrition his liver function improves. Which of the following statements is true?

    (A) it is unlikely that he will bleed a second time if his prothrombin time has returned to normal
    (B) an elective shunt should be recommended
    (C) a shunting procedure should be performed at the time of a second massive hemorrhage
    (D) a portacaval shunt will decrease the probability of the patient's developing hepatic encephalopathy during a second massive hemorrhage from varices
    (E) if the patient gives up alcohol and maintains good nutrition, it is probable he will have a normal life span   *(1:471-482)*

104. The petechiae associated with fat embolism are typically found

    (A) evenly distributed over the whole body
    (B) on the palms and soles
    (C) subungually
    (D) over the upper half of the body
    (E) on dependent areas   *(3:1768-1770)*

105. In 1950, Elden J. Gardner described a syndrome that bears his name. It consists of connective tissue lesions, skin lesions, bony tumors, multiple polyps of the large intestine, and a high risk of developing colon carcinoma. It is inherited as a mendelian dominant. One of the following statements concerning this syndrome is NOT correct.

    (A) the implications of Gardner's syndrome present the surgeon with a problem in cancer prevention
    (B) carcinoma of the large intestine is the most common cause of death
    (C) epidermal inclusion cysts should be excised because of the high risk of future malignancy
    (D) after colotomy and ileorectal anastomosis, the remaining polyps in the rectal segment regress
    (E) the definite familial pattern requires study of all members of the family   *(3:1028-1033)*

106. The most common cause of nonunion of a fracture is

    (A) malnutrition
    (B) corticosteroid therapy

(C) extensive soft tissue destruction at the fracture site or infection

(D) interposition of soft tissue between the bone ends

(E) idiopathic osteoporosis *(2:1955)*

Questions 107 through 112

Carcinoma of the breast is discovered during the first trimester of the second pregnancy of a 32-year-old woman. The tumor is 1.5 cm in size, is located in the upper, outer quadrant of the left breast, and produces dimpling of the skin. There are no clinically suspicious axillary nodes and no evidence by physical and radiologic examination of metastases. Blood chemistries are normal.

107. What is the proper approach to the treatment of this patient?

(A) biopsy and treatment should be delayed until the baby is delivered at term

(B) the pregnancy should be interrupted and a mastectomy performed 2 months later

(C) biopsy and mastectomy should not be delayed

(D) 5-fluorouracil should be used as the primary mode of treatment

(E) before consideration of mastectomy or other treatment, the response to oophorectomy should be determined

(1:258–270)

108. The TMN staging of the patient would be

(A) T1, N0, M0
(B) T1, N1, M1
(C) T2, N1, M0
(D) T2, N0, M0
(E) T3, N0, M0 *(2:534)*

109. The clinical staging of this patient would be

(A) stage I
(B) stage II
(C) stage III
(D) stage IV
(E) stage V *(1:258–270)*

110. This patient had a mastectomy. Thirty-two axillary nodes were included with the specimen, and none contained tumor. You would recommend

(A) prophylactic radiation therapy
(B) observation but no further treatment
(C) abortion and oophorectomy if the

mastectomy were performed while the patient was pregnant

(D) oophorectomy following the delivery of the baby

(E) prophylactic chemotherapy *(1:258–270)*

111. Three years after mastectomy, the patient develops lytic lesions in the lumbar spine and in the right femur. You would advise as your initial treatment

(A) tamoxifen or oophorectomy
(B) radiation therapy
(C) androgen therapy
(D) estrogen therapy
(E) corticosteroids *(1:258–272)*

112. Concerning pregnancy and contraception, what advice would you give the patient before the development of metastases?

(A) subsequent pregnancy has no effect on prognosis

(B) avoid pregnancy for a minimum of 1 year

(C) use contraceptive pills

(D) subsequent pregnancy has a beneficial effect on prognosis

(E) following the next pregnancy, suppress lactation *(3:562)*

113. The condition characterized by decreased esophageal motility and failure of lower esophageal sphincter (LES) relaxation is

(A) diffuse esophageal spasm
(B) achalasia
(C) scleroderma
(D) hypertensive LES
(E) postvagotomy dysphagia *(3:709–724)*

Questions 114 through 117

A 35-year-old man is admitted with a fever of 101°F, right flank pain, proteinuria, and hematuria. The serum creatinine is 3.8, the blood sugar is 180, and the serum uric acid is 12.2. Uric acid crystals are present in the urine. The intravenous pyelogram shows a dilated left ureter with a filling defect at the level of the pelvic brim and delayed filling of the right ureter.

114. The primary problem in this patient is

(A) oxalate calculi
(B) uric acid calculi
(C) renal vein thrombosis
(D) acute glomerulonephritis
(E) diabetic nephritis *(1:849–853)*

115. The next procedure in this patient is

    (A) PAH clearance test
    (B) renal arteriograms
    (C) renal venograms
    (D) repeat intravenous pyelogram
    (E) cystoscopy and ureteral catheterization
                                        (2:1698-1699)

116. The treatment of this patient is

    (A) bedrest, observation, and antibiotics
    (B) drainage of right ureter with ureteral catheter
    (C) thrombectomy of the renal vein
    (D) bilateral ureterolithotomy
    (E) right nephrostomy   *(2:1699)*

117. The long-term management of the patient is

    (A) make the urine alkaline
    (B) raise the pH of the urine to 7.00 or more and administer allopurinol
    (C) anticoagulate with heparin and coumadin
    (D) control of the diabetes
    (E) refer to the nephrology unit for long-term management   *(2:1701)*

Questions 118 and 119

A 20-year-old boy is injured in an automobile accident and suffers a closed fracture of the tibia and fibula. This is reduced, and the leg is placed in a cast. Ten days later, the patient develops left upper quadrant abdominal pain and arterial hypotension.

118. The most likely diagnosis is

    (A) rupture of the spleen
    (B) osteomyelitis
    (C) septicemia
    (D) a pulmonary embolus
    (E) fat embolism   *(2:1378)*

119. What diagnostic study would you perform just after a clinical examination?

    (A) urinalysis
    (B) plain x-ray of the abdomen and chest
    (C) abdominal aortography with visualization of the branches of the abdominal aorta
    (D) radioisotope scans
    (E) peritoneal tap   *(2:1378)*

Questions 120 through 122

A 60-year-old man developed right lower quadrant pain and tenderness. An appendectomy was performed for acute appendicitis. On the tenth postoperative day, he had sudden pain in the left chest, and a left pleural friction rub could be heard.

120. All of the following would be indicated EXCEPT

    (A) electrocardiogram
    (B) chest x-ray
    (C) examination of the legs
    (D) thoracentesis
    (E) anticoagulants   *(2:983-984)*

121. The best treatment would be

    (A) anticoagulants plus bedrest
    (B) anticoagulants plus ambulation
    (C) antibiotics and bedrest
    (D) ligature of the inferior vena cava
    (E) ligature of both femoral veins *(3:1731-1746)*

122. What would be the expected eventual outcome?

    (A) recurrent episodes
    (B) complete recovery
    (C) empyema
    (D) pneumonia
    (E) severe prolonged dyspnea   *(3:1731-1746)*

123. At the conclusion of the operation of thromboendarterectomy, the residual arterial wall consists of

    (A) adventitia and media
    (B) adventitia and external elastic lamina
    (C) adventitia, external elastic lamina, and outer layers of the media
    (D) adventitia, external elastic lamina, media, and internal elastic lamina
    (E) adventitia, media, and intima   *(4:358)*

124. Barrett's esophagus occurs when the normal squamous lining of the distal esophagus has been displaced by a metaplastic epithelium in response to esophageal reflux. Which of the following statements concerning this problem is INCORRECT?

    (A) ulcers and strictures often are present
    (B) heartburn is similar to that seen in reflux esophagitis
    (C) persistent Barrett's esophagus is a premalignant condition
    (D) esophagoscopy shows a pink lining to the distal esophagus
    (E) the diagnosis should be confirmed with a biopsy   *(1:390)*

125. A black woman aged 20 has a round, firm, discrete, relatively mobile, painless mass 2 cm in diameter in her breast. The most likely diagnosis is

    (A) fibrocystic disease
    (B) fibroadenoma
    (C) carcinoma
    (D) duct papilloma
    (E) fat necrosis   *(1:268)*

126. The prognosis of lung cancer depends mainly on the cell type and the stage of the disease. It is less favorable in all of the following situations EXCEPT

    (A) tumor of the squamous cell type
    (B) the tumor is visible bronchoscopically
    (C) cytology biopsy shows the tumor to be of the oat cell type
    (D) the tumor involves the chest wall by direct extension
    (E) the presence of the superior vena cava syndrome   *(1:309–311)*

127. Lung cancer may involve the mediastinum, when a variety of symptoms may develop that include all of the following EXCEPT

    (A) pleural effusion
    (B) retrosternal pain
    (C) hoarseness of the voice
    (D) swelling of the head and neck
    (E) swelling of the arms   *(1:310)*

128. The following statements concern a 55-year-old patient who complains of symptoms considered to be mesenteric angina. Which of these statements is NOT correct?

    (A) the superior mesenteric artery is completely occluded, with normal celiac and inferior mesenteric arteries in most patients
    (B) weight loss will be obvious
    (C) a lateral view of the aorta usually is essential in establishing the diagnosis
    (D) the pain occurs soon after eating
    (E) the food–pain relationship soon leads to reluctance on the part of the patient to eat   *(1:702)*

129. The most frequent site for lodging of a clinically significant peripheral arterial embolus is

    (A) brachial artery
    (B) femoral artery
    (C) distal aorta

(D) popliteal artery
(E) axillary artery   *(4:449)*

130. In the United States, a pyogenic liver abscess is most likely to be secondary to

    (A) carcinoma metastatic to the liver
    (B) pylephlebitis
    (C) trauma
    (D) biliary tract obstruction
    (E) perforated appendicitis with generalized peritonitis   *(17:369–380)*

131. The organism most commonly found in the abscess described in the question above is

    (A) *Escherichia coli*
    (B) *Staphylococcus aureus*
    (C) *Proteus*
    (D) *Klebsiella-Enterobacter*
    (E) *Enterococcus*   *(17:369–380)*

132. Cardiac conditions can masquerade as abdominal surgical problems, in which case the correct diagnosis is important. Which of the following statements is NOT correct?

    (A) the subacute onset of right heart failure may mimic gallbladder disease
    (B) many patients with angina pectoris think that they are suffering from indigestion
    (C) hemorrhoids or esophageal varices frequently are secondary to undiagnosed right heart failure
    (D) nausea and vomiting can result from digitalis therapy
    (E) slowly developing right heart failure can cause symptoms that appear to justify a diagnosis of carcinoma of the stomach
                                       (1:43)

133 The use of prophylactic antibiotics is now wide-spread before and during surgical operations. Which of the following statements is INCORRECT?

(A) the antibiotic selected should be appropriate for the infecting organism
(B) for clean operations in which a prosthesis is inserted, the antibiotic should be selected to combat the likely hospital infecting organism
(C) multiple antibiotics are better than using a single drug
(D) antibiotic prophylaxis cannot eliminate bacteria
(E) in urologic surgery, the antibiotic should be chosen on the basis of preoperative urine culture   *(1:106)*

134. Which of the following statements about secondary and tertiary hyperparathyroidism is NOT correct?

(A) in secondary hyperparathyroidism, there is an increase in parathyroid hormone secretion in response to a low plasma concentration of ionized calcium
(B) secondary hyperparathyroidism with renal osteodystrophy is a frequent complication of hemodialysis
(C) secondary and tertiary hyperparathyroidism are treated by operation on the parathyroid glands
(D) successful renal transplantation usually makes surgery on the parathyroid glands unnecessary
(E) tertiary hyperparathyroidism occurs when a patient with secondary hyperparathyroidism develops relatively autonomous parathyroid glands   *(1:254-255)*

135. The development of a recurrent peptic ulcer after surgery for peptic ulcer may be due to

(A) an insufficient operation
(B) incomplete vagotomy
(C) retained antrum
(D) Zollinger-Ellison syndrome
(E) all of the above   *(1:432)*

136. The cause of death after a major pelvic fracture is most frequently

(A) fat embolism
(B) injury to rectum
(C) injury to urethra
(D) pulmonary embolism
(E) uncontrolled hemorrhage   *(1:926)*

137. With reference to partial interruption of the inferior vena cava (Greenfield filter), all of the following statements are correct EXCEPT

(A) measurable leg edema is an early complication
(B) significant protection is afforded against later major pulmonary embolization
(C) major enlargement of collateral channels is common
(D) the vein becomes occluded below the site of the clip in most cases
(E) minor pulmonary emboli may occur postoperatively   *(1:726)*

138. A patient with atrial fibrillation undergoes a successful popliteal embolectomy. Just before the embolectomy, the venous blood from that lower limb showed a pH of 7.31, Po_2 19.3, Pco_2 45.8, K 4.7, and creatinine phosphokinase (CPK) 200. Five minutes after the embolectomy, the findings from the blood in the same vein were pH 6.80, Po_2 34.8, Pco_2 77.3, K 7.2, and CPK 77. Which of these postoperative findings is INCORRECT?

(A) pH
(B) Po_2
(C) Pco_2
(D) K
(E) CPK   *(13:231-237)*

139. A little boy aspirated a peanut and is cyanotic. On expiration, his mediastinum shifts to the right. Where is the peanut located?

(A) right mainstem bronchus
(B) left mainstem bronchus
(C) esophagus
(D) trachea
(E) lung parenchyma   *(3:1322)*

140. In an infection from a human bite, which of the following organisms is least likely to be found?

(A) spirochete
(B) pneumococcus
(C) staphylococcus
(D) streptococcus
(E) bacteroides   *(3:289)*

141. In Cushing's syndrome, purple striae and muscle wasting of the lower limbs are due to

(A) nitrogen depletion (protein)
(B) hypertension

(C) psychoneurosis

(D) excessive sodium retention

(E) excessive potassium loss in the urine

(3:662-671)

142. A patient is being operated on under general anesthesia. The abdomen is open and the diaphragm starts to jerk because of

(A) hypoxia

(B) anesthetic plane being too deep

(C) anesthetic plane being too shallow

(D) acidosis

(E) recent administration of muscle relaxant

(3:160-164)

143. A 50-year-old female with a 30% third degree burn and a 25% second degree burn develops anuria. Which of the following changes would occur in the blood chemistry?

(A) increased calcium

(B) increased potassium

(C) decreased potassium

(D) decreased sodium

(E) decreased chloride

(3:218-220)

144. A child with a hernia and cryptorchidism is operated on through the usual inguinal incision. No testicle is found in the inguinal canal. The surgeon should

(A) repair the hernia and do no more at that time

(B) repair the hernia and use hormones

(C) explore the retropubic space and repair the hernia

(D) explore the retropubic space up to the renal pedicle, and if the testicle is found and cannot be replaced in the scrotum, leave the testicle in position and repair the hernia

(E) do the same as in **D** but excise the testicle if it cannot be replaced in the scrotum

(3:1675)

145. The indications for colonoscopy may be diagnostic or therapeutic. Which of the following is NOT as yet a therapeutic indication or procedure?

(A) excision of polyp or polyps

(B) control of bleeding

(C) drainage of an inflamed diverticulum

(D) detorsion of volvulus

(E) removal of foreign body

(1:592)

146. The following statements concerning the anatomy of an intercostal space all are incorrect EXCEPT

(A) there are two intercostal arteries in each space

(B) each intercostal nerve has three cutaneous branches

(C) there are two intercostal muscles in each space

(D) the neurovascular bundle is located just above each rib

(E) the intercostal nerves consist of one main trunk

(1:277)

147. The following statements concerning the dumping syndrome all are correct EXCEPT

(A) shortly after eating, the patient experiences palpitations, sweating, dyspnea, and flushing

(B) gastrointestinal symptoms include nausea, abdominal cramps, belching, vomiting, and diarrhea

(C) this syndrome may occur after an operation that impairs the ability of the stomach to regulate the rate of emptying

(D) the cause is often postprandial reactive hypoglycemia

(E) if a second operation is required, the most effective is reconstruction of the pylorus when this is possible

(1:434)

148. The surgical treatment of choice for vascular compression of the duodenum is

(A) duodenal division and reanastomosis anterior to the superior mesenteric vessels

(B) division and retroduodenal anastomosis of superior mesenteric vessels

(C) mobilization of ligament of Treitz

(D) duodenojejunostomy

(E) total duodenal mobilization

(3:878)

149. Excision of the autonomic nerve plexus on the front and sides of the infrarenal abdominal aorta and common iliac arteries causes

(A) vasodilation of the perineal skin

(B) impotence in the male

(C) decreased sweating of the buttocks and perineum

(D) retrograde ejaculation in the male

(E) all of the above

(14:41)

Questions 150 through 154

A female patient, age 54, complained of pain and numbness in the right hand for 4 months. The pain was worse at night and caused the patient to wake and rub and move her hand and fingers for relief. On examination, there was some wasting of the right thenar muscles and reduced sensation to pin prick on the palmar surfaces of the index and middle fingers.

150. The lesion causing this problem most likely would be found in which of the following regions?

    (A) spinal cord
    (B) cervical spine
    (C) brachial plexus
    (D) shoulder
    (E) wrist   *(3:1549)*

151. The most useful diagnostic procedure would be

    (A) nerve conduction tests
    (B) lumbar puncture
    (C) phlebogram
    (D) arteriogram
    (E) myelogram   *(3:1549)*

152. The most likely diagnosis would be

    (A) cervical disc
    (B) cervical degenerative arthritis
    (C) Raynaud's phenomenon
    (D) degenerative myopathy
    (E) carpal tunnel syndrome   *(3:1549)*

153. The best treatment for the patient would be

    (A) a cervical collar
    (B) surgery
    (C) physiotherapy
    (D) cortisone injections
    (E) wrist splint   *(3:1549)*

154. The best operation would be

    (A) excision of cervical disc
    (B) spinal fusion
    (C) division of the transverse carpal ligament
    (D) upper dorsal sympathetic ganglionectomy
    (E) transposition of the ulnar nerve   *(3:1549)*

Questions 155 through 158

A 65-year-old white man is admitted to the hospital with moderate bleeding into the alimentary tract. During the past 4 days, he has had two similar episodes of hematemesis and melena. On admission, he has a fever of 101.5°F, his pulse rate is 106, and his blood

pressure 120/80. His hematocrit is 30, and his white blood cell count 19,500. He has a long midline abdominal scar that is well healed. There is tenderness and an indefinite mass in the abdomen centrally and above the umbilicus. He states that 1½ years before, an aneurysm of the abdominal aorta was resected and he was well until about 2 weeks before this admission.

155. Which of the following studies would be the most useful?

    (A) upper gastrointestinal series 1
    (B) barium enema
    (C) gastroscopy
    (D) sigmoidoscopy
    (E) abdominal arteriography   *(4:828-834)*

156. An arteriogram of the abdominal aorta is performed in the patient. This demonstrates an aortoenteric fistula arising from the proximal aortic anastomosis and communicating with the duodenum or proximal jejunum. The best treatment is

    (A) under maximum local and systemic antibiotic cover, remove the aortic prosthesis and insert another combined with meticulous closure of the enteric perforation
    (B) give the maximum possible doses of antibiotics; transfusion and supportive care until the fever subsides and the fistula closes
    (C) operate with full antibiotic cover, close the aortic fistula, close the enteric fistula, separate them with the greater omentum
    (D) remove the aortic prosthesis, ligature the aorta proximally and the iliac arteries distally, close the enteric fistula, and insert axillary femoral bypass grafts
    (E) operate, close the aortic fistula, close the enteric fistula, and perform a gastroenterostomy   *(4:828-834)*

157. The patient does well. His fever subsides, his wounds heal, he has good ankle pulses, and he leaves the hospital eating well and gaining weight. One and one-half years later, he returns with sudden onset of coldness of the right leg and foot. The foot is viable, but he develops intermittent claudication in the right calf after walking 50 feet. There are good pulses in the left lower limb; the right is pulseless. A diagnosis of thrombosis of the right axillary femoral bypass graft is made. The best treatment is

(A) conservative care, anticoagulants, and vasodilator drugs
(B) restore a flow through the occluded right axillary femoral bypass graft and, if necessary, replace it with a new graft
(C) insert a bypass from the side of the distal thoracic aorta to each common iliac artery
(D) perform a right lumber sympathectomy
(E) replace the original aortic prosthesis with a similar but slightly longer graft

(4:828-834)

158. Which is LEAST likely following infection of an iliofemoral prosthetic arterial bypass graft?

(A) thrombosis
(B) false aneurysm
(C) distal gangrene
(D) hemorrhage
(E) arteriovenous fistula *(4:828-834)*

159. In a patient with a mycotic aneurysm of the common femoral artery, the following statements would apply EXCEPT

(A) it occurs predominantly in young people
(B) the rest of the arterial tree is normal
(C) treatment of choice is resection and replacement by a prosthetic vascular graft
(D) bacterial endocarditis is a possible cause
(E) it will prove fatal to the patient if untreated *(4:841-846)*

160. One of the following statements concerning neurospinous claudication is NOT correct.

(A) about 5% of patients referred because of intermittent claudication have neurospinous disease
(B) the pain develops after walking but is not relieved by standing still
(C) pain in the back is common
(D) the pain is not relieved by sitting or lying down
(E) the peripheral pulses will be normal unless there is associated arterial disease *(3:1301)*

DIRECTIONS (Questions 161 through 180): Each question consists of an introduction followed by five statements. Mark T (true) or F (false) after each statement.

161. Internal hemorrhoids are classified as follows: 1st degree, bleeding; 2nd degree, prolapse that reduces itself; 3rd degree, prolapse that has to be reduced by the patient; 4th degree, prolapse

that cannot be reduced by the patient. The following statements concern the treatment of hemorrhoids.

(A) most 1st and 2nd degree hemorrhoids can be treated medically
(B) injection treatment consists of injecting sclerosant into the lumen of the veins
(C) rubber band ligation is a good method for 3rd degree hemorrhoids
(D) cryosurgery is a popular technique
(E) hemorrhoidectomy is used for 3rd and 4th degree cases *(1:634)*

162. The following statements refer to thymoma.

(A) thymoma is the most common mediastinal lesion
(B) 10 to 50% of patients with thymomas have myasthenia gravis
(C) 10 to 40% of patients with myasthenia gravis have thymomas
(D) younger patients with thymomas are more likely to have myasthenia gravis
(E) men with myasthenia gravis are twice as likely to have a thymoma as are women with myasthenia gravis *(23:1029)*

163. By definition, acute pancreatitis refers to acute inflammation occurring in a normal gland. When several such episodes occur, it becomes acute relapsing pancreatitis. The following statements relate to these conditions.

(A) complete or partial obstruction of the pancreatic ducts is the cause of this disease
(B) this is frequently a relatively benign, self-limiting disease
(C) if acute pancreatitis is resolving in a patient with gallstones, a chocystectomy should be performed immediately
(D) a raised serum amylase is a reliable diagnostic test
(E) in severe acute hemorrhagic pancreatitis, the abdomen may be rigid, and tachycardia and hypotension occur *(3:1376-1377)*

164. Signs of tentorial herniation of the brain include

(A) unilateral unreactive pupil
(B) absent corneal reflex
(C) depressed level of consciousness
(D) absent oculocephalic (Doll's eye) reflex
(E) contralateral spastic weakness   *(9:239)*

165. Cancer in the recipient of a renal allograft is an unexpectedly frequent complication.

(A) the incidence of cancer is not high enough to contraindicate transplantation
(B) some cancers have been transplanted with the kidney from the donor, their existence being unsuspected
(C) most of these cancers are primary tumors that appear in the immunosuppressed patient
(D) it has been estimated that the risk is greatest for the development of epithelial and lymphoid cancers
(E) about 75% of the cancers arising in immunosuppressed recipients arise in the lungs or alimentary tract   *(3:424)*

166. The prevention of septic complications is far more practical than treating them.

(A) as many as 50% of the members of a surgical team puncture their gloves during an operation
(B) organisms reaching the wound from the patient's skin can be kept to a minimum by preparation of the skin for 10 minutes
(C) active and passive immunization procedures for the prevention of surgical infections have merit in special situations, such as tetanus
(D) a patient with a heavily contaminated wound should receive antibiotics as soon as possible
(E) prophylactic antibiotics are usually ineffective in patients with indwelling central venous lines   *(3:263)*

167. Meckel's diverticulum is found in 0.3% of autopsy examinations. This condition is addressed in the following statements.

(A) the most common clinical problem associated with Meckel's diverticulum is intestinal obstruction
(B) the second most common symptom associated with Meckel's diverticulum is bleeding

(C) Meckel's diverticulitis accounts for the problem in about 20% of patients with symptoms from a Meckel's diverticulum
(D) bleeding from a Meckel's diverticulum comes from a peptic ulcer in the adjacent ileal mucosa
(E) when found incidentally, a Meckel's diverticulum should be removed when feasible   *(3:946-948)*

168. The following statements are related to carcinoma of the stomach in the USA.

(A) in 1950, the death rates for cancer of the stomach, lung, and large intestine were approximately equal, at 18 to 20 per 100,000 of the male population
(B) there are no symptoms of early carcinoma of the stomach
(C) in 1980, the death rates for cancer of the stomach, lung, and large intestine for males were, respectively, 5, 55, and 20 per 100,000
(D) fiberoptic gastroscopy combined with biopsies and cytology can make the diagnosis with an accuracy greater than 95%
(E) the only method offering hope of cure is excision of the involved portion of the stomach   *(3:881-889)*

169. Carcinoid tumors may be associated with the carcinoid syndrome. The following statements concern carcinoid tumors of the alimentary tract.

(A) the most frequent locations are the appendix and the jejunoileum
(B) less than 3% of carcinoid tumors of the appendix metastasize
(C) less than 10% of jejunoileal carcinoid tumors cause the carcinoid syndrome
(D) the carcinoid syndrome includes cutaneous flushing, abdominal cramps and diarrhea, and attacks similar to asthma
(E) the chemical cause of this syndrome includes the production by the tumor of histamine, kallikrein, prostaglandins, and serotonin   *(3:949-952)*

170. The following statements concern pheochromocytoma.

(A) hypertension is frequent; it may be persistent or paroxysmal
(B) diaphoresis is a frequent symptom

(C) CT is an excellent method of locating adrenal tumors larger than 1 cm in diameter
(D) hypertensive episodes may occur during the mobilization of the tumor. Sodium nitroprusside is an effective drug to treat this problem
(E) pheochromocytomas occur more frequently in males than females   *(3:679–686)*

171. The following statements relate to Crohn's disease.

(A) most patients will require surgery at some stage of the disease
(B) the reoperation rate is 50% per year
(C) recurrence after surgery is random and unrelated to duration of disease
(D) recurrence is typical at or proximal to a prior anastomosis
(E) resection should be carried back to histologically normal bowel   *(3:925)*

172. Besides alcohol and gallstone passage, the following have been associated with acute pancreatitis.

(A) hypercalcemia
(B) a sex-linked gene
(C) steroids
(D) hypovolemic shock
(E) ERCP   *(3:1179)*

173. Cystadenoma of the pancreas

(A) is always benign
(B) is not considered premalignant
(C) is rapid growing
(D) is difficult to differentiate from cystadenocarcinoma
(E) is best treated by internal drainage   *(3:1188)*

174. The following statements concern the blood supply of the large intestine.

(A) the inferior mesenteric vein is a tributary of the portal vein
(B) the middle colic artery supplies the hepatic flexure and proximal transverse colon
(C) the left colic artery is a branch of the superior mesenteric artery
(D) the middle and inferior hemorrhoidal arteries are branches of the hypogastric artery
(E) the colic arteries form arcades about 2.5 cm from the bowel, which communicate and form the marginal artery of Drummond   *(1:587)*

175. Implants of metal and plastic are being used with increasing frequency by surgeons. The following statements concern such implants in general.

(A) metallic mesh implants for herniorrhaphy eventually fragment; Dacron or polypropylene mesh does not fragment
(B) the metallurgy of solid metal implants is now a refined science
(C) Silastic is the material of choice for many solid implants, but contraction of the capsular scar is still a problem
(D) infection of all kinds of plastic prosthesis remains a major problem
(E) vascular access using implants was in the past doomed to fail in 1 or 2 weeks because of infection. The development of well-tolerated plastics with fabric rings has increased the period of usefulness to months or even years   *(1:93–94)*

176. The following statements concern surgical suture materials.

(A) silk sutures are slowly absorbed over a period of years
(B) stainless steel wire sutures retain their strength longer than synthetic, nonabsorbable sutures
(C) catgut made from the submucosa of the intestine of sheep is absorbed in a predictable time
(D) synthetic absorbable sutures have predictable rates of loss of tensile strength
(E) skin closure with adhesive tapes minimizes the probability of infection by avoiding the presence of foreign bodies in the form of skin sutures   *(1:93)*

177. The following statements concern the intestinal blind loop syndrome.

(A) bacterial overgrowth occurs in the blind loop
(B) steatorrhea and diarrhea are common
(C) microcytic anemia develops
(D) malnutrition occurs
(E) most patients can be helped by surgical correction   *(1:565)*

178. The following statements concern volvulus of the colon.

    (A) the most common segment involved is the sigmoid colon
    (B) abdominal colic occurs, with persistent pain between spasms
    (C) abdominal distention may be marked
    (D) if the sigmoid colon is viable at operation, it may be returned to the abdomen
    (E) the mortality is 50% if perforation has occurred   (1:616)

179. Many clinicians recommend a staging laparotomy in patients with early Hodgkin's disease. The following statements concern this.

    (A) radiation injury to left kidney and left lung is avoided
    (B) oophoropexy can prevent radiation injury to the ovaries
    (C) hypersplenism is a contraindication to staging laparotomy

    (D) staging laparotomy is not indicated in patients with stage IV disease
    (E) staging laparotomy is indicated in patients with non-Hodgkin's lymphomas   (1:551)

180. The following statements concern decubitus ulcers, a disastrous complication of immobilization.

    (A) hospital-acquired decubitus ulcers are nearly always the result of inadequate nursing care
    (B) decubitus ulcers result from prolonged pressure that robs tissue of its blood supply
    (C) decubitus ulcers are common in drug addicts
    (D) most decubitus ulcers are preventable
    (E) the first step in treatment is the incision and drainage of any infected spaces   (1:95)

Answers and Explanations

1. **(A) (T), (B) (T), (C) (F), (D) (T), (E) (T)**
Lung metastases from melanoma and the breast in general do badly. Very few 5-year survivals have been achieved by resection of lung metastasis from these primaries.

2. **(A) (T), (B) (T), (C) (F), (D) (T), (E) (F)**
The bowel is exposed in gastoschisis, and it is covered by the layers of umbilical cord in an omphalocele. Rupture may occur, however, which will expose the viscera. An umbilical hernia usually closes spontaneously, so repair should be deferred.

3. **(A) (T), (B) (F), (C) (T), (D) (T), (E) (T)**
The abdomen is distended in infants with NEC.

4. **(A) (T), (B) (F), (C) (F), (D) (T), (E) (T)**
The Bochdalek hernia is a posterolateral defect in the diaphragm, a persistent pleuroperitoneal canal. Ninety percent occur on the left side. Air swallowing, which begins at birth, increases the volume of the gut in the chest and leads to lung compression, mediastinal shift, and increased pulmonary vascular resistance. The affected lung is smaller then normal. Preoperative perforation decreases survival.

5. **(A) (T), (B) (T), (C) (T), (D) (T), (E) (F)**
In the transthoracic approach, the diaphragmatic closure is difficult because one is faced with pushing the abdominal viscera into a too small abdominal cavity. Other defects of intestinal rotation can be identified and corrected, if necessary, with the abdominal approach. If the abdominal cavity is too small, it is necessary to create a ventral hernia by closing only the skin. Sometimes a prosthesis must be used for temporary closure.

6. **(A) (T), (B) (T), (C) (T), (D) (T), (E) (T)**
All these statements are true.

7. **(A) (T), (B) (T), (C) (F), (D) (T), (E) (T)**
Resection of the aganglionic segment of bowel and anastomosis of normal bowel to the anus is not well tolerated in infants with enterocolitis. A preliminary proximal colostomy is required.

8. **(A) (F), (B) (F), (C) (T), (D) (F), (E) (F)**
Pneumothorax in the newborn is not rare. Most air collections are small and need not be treated. Ventilatory support of the infant with hyaline membrane disease commonly causes pneumothorax. Tension pneumothorax is best treated with an intercostal catheter connected to an underwater seal because the air leak does not seal for 3 to 5 days. Needle aspiration may be lifesaving for a patient in extremis.

9. **(A) (T), (B) (T), (C) (T), (D) (F), (E) (T)**
A low intestinal pH shortens the transit time. Hypersecretion of hydrochloric acid by the stomach follows massive intestinal resection. This reduces the pH of the intestinal contents and shortens the transit time through the remaining intestine.

10. **(A) (T), (B) (F), (C) (T), (D) (T), (E) (F)**
Pneumatoceles occurring during the course of staphylococcal pneumonia do not require drainage unless they cause respiratory distress. Those that persist after resolution of pneumonia gradually regress without treatment. Pneumothorax and pleural effusion are best treated by catheter drainage. Even the marked pleural thickening that restricts ventilation usually gradually resolves and seldom necessitates decortication.

11. **(A) (F), (B) (F), (C) (F), (D) (T), (E) (F)**
Many infants with TEF have pneumonia at the time of diagnosis. Such a patient may require several days of treatment before the operation can be performed safely. Treatment consists of antibiotics, fluids, decompressive gastrostomy to minimize gastroesophageal reflux, and drainage of the esophageal pouch to prevent further aspiration. Esophageal anastomosis usually can be accomplished at operation, but staged repair should be considered for premature infants and infants with associated anomalies.

12. **(A) (T), (B) (F), (C) (F), (D) (F), (E) (T)**
Bile vomiting in the neonate is characteristic of duodenal obstruction, and the double-bubble sign on x-ray confirms the suspicion. Contrast studies are usually not indicated unless there is air distal to the duodenum. About one third of patients with duodenal obstruction have Down's syndrome. Diagnosis is often prompt so that the patient does not require extended preoperative preparation.

13. **(A) (T), (B) (F), (C) (T), (D) (T), (E) (F)**
Atresia of the ileum is more common than jejunal atresia and much more common than colonic atresia. Squamous cells in the intestinal lumen distal to the site of atresial indicate that the gut was patent at one time. Experimentally, interruption of the blood supply to a segment of intestine in the embryo results in intestinal atresia. Adhesions and even intraabdominal calcifications found at operation are thought to be further evidence of an intraabdominal in utero catastrophe. The gut often is shorter than normal.

14. **(A) (T), (B) (T), (C) (T), (D) (F), (E) (T)**
Surgery should be performed promptly for three reasons: with repeated attacks cerebral damage occurs, obesity increases, and the tumor is malignant in 10% of cases.

15. **(A) (T), (B) (T), (C) (F), (D) (F), (E) (F)**
Distention occurs late in patients with infarcted bowel. Corticosteroids may mask the clinical signs of even advanced peritonitis. In patients with paralytic ileus, localized abdominal tenderness is not seen.

16. **(A) (T), (B) (T), (C) (T), (D) (F), (E) (T)**
The most common symptoms of the attack are headache, palpitation, and excessive perspiration. Patients may experience either flushing of the skin or pallor. They may have abdominal pain and vomit.

17. **(A) (T), (B) (T), (C) (T), (D) (T), (E) (T)**
All of these are correct. In addition wound healing is delayed by severe anemia, marked dehydration, anemia, or local ischemia.

18. **(A) (F), (B) (T), (C) (T), (D) (F), (E) (T)**
The majority of tumors are malignant. The islet cells away from the tumor usually are hyperplastic, so resection of an apparently solitary tumor may well not cure the disease. Some metastases disappear following total gastrectomy. Relatives of patients with the Zollinger-Ellison's syndrome should be screened for genetic endocrinopathies. Cimetidine has been of great assistance in the care of these patients.

19. **(A) (T), (B) (T), (C) (T), (D) (F), (E) (T)**
At present total bilateral adrenalectomy is infrequently indicated as the primary treatment of patients with Cushing's syndrome. Removal of the pituitary tumor is better.

20. **(A) (T), (B) (T), (C) (T), (D) (T), (E) (T)**
Carcinoids occur in all of these locations. The first three sites given in the question involve foregut carcinoids, the fourth involves a carcinoid of the midgut, and the fifth, the hindgut.

21. **(A) (F), (B) (T), (C) (F), (D) (T), (E) (T)**
Postoperative psychosis is more common after thoracic surgery than after abdominal surgery. Most overt psychiatric derangements are observed after the third postoperative day. Clinical manifestations of psychosis are rare on the first postoperative day.

22. **(A) (T), (B) (T), (C) (T), (D) (T), (E) (T)**
All of these statements are correct.

23. **(A) (T), (B) (T), (C) (T), (D) (T), (E) (T)**
All of these statements are correct.

24. **(A) (T), (B) (T), (C) (F), (D) (T), (E) (T)**
Closure of the bronchioles is the most common cause of atelectasis. Bronchioles of 1 mm or less are prone to close when the lung volume reaches a critical point. Dependent portions of the lung are the first to experience bronchiolar closure.

25. **(A) (T), (B) (T), (C) (F), (D) (T), (E) (T)**
Early respiratory failure within 48 hours of an operation or injury may develop in a short period

without an obvious cause. The blood pressure is not raised.

26. **(A) (T), (B) (T), (C) (F), (D) (T), (E) (T)**
The bowel often is spastic in diverticulitis.

27. **(A) (T), (B) (T), (C) (F), (D) (T), (E) (T)**
There is a sustained contracture of the muscles following induction of anesthesia. Excess oxygen consumption and excess carbon dioxide production result in metabolic and respiratory acidosis. It is an inherited disease that often is fatal.

28. **(A) (T), (B) (F), (C) (F), (D) (F), (E) (F)**
A stable postoperative coronary bypass patient is a better surgical risk than is the same patient in the immediate prebypass period. If operation is delayed and the patient becomes or remains septic, the mortality rate is high.

29. **(A) (T), (B) (F), (C) (T), (D) (T), (E) (T)**
Hepatic abscesses due to biliary tract obstruction and infection are frequently multiple and respond poorly to abscess drainage. Relief of biliary obstruction must be accomplished, but even then the mortality rate is high. Many hepatic abscesses in the diabetic have no specific cause that can be determined. Immunologic incompetence, whatever the cause, puts the patient at risk of developing a hepatic abscess.

30. **(A) (F), (B) (T), (C) (F), (D) (F), (E) (T)**
All the symptoms listed are at times presenting symptoms of liver abscesses, but only fever and abdominal pain are presenting symptoms in more than half of the patients. The classic symptom of right shoulder pain is now reported only rarely.

31. **(A) (T), (B) (F), (C) (T), (D) (T), (E) (F)**
Surprisingly, just under half of 445 patients with pyogenic hepatic abscesses had elevated serum bilirubins, and an elevated alkaline phosphatase was present in just under half the patients. Leukocytosis was present in 70%, and an abnormal liver–spleen scan was present in 80%. An abnormal chest film was helpful to the diagnosis in just over half of the patients. Hepatic scintiscans have increased diagnostic accuracy from 19% to 78%. Ultrasound and CT scans may prove even more helpful.

32. **(A) (T), (B) (T), (C) (T), (D) (T), (E) (T)**
All of the measures listed can be helpful in treating areas of high density colonization of *Candida* in an attempt to prevent acute disseminated candidiasis.

33. **(A) (T), (B) (T), (C) (T), (D) (F), (E) (T)**
Amphotericin B is highly nephrotoxic. It is not neurotoxic.

34. **(A) (F), (B) (T), (C) (T), (D) (F), (E) (T)**
Vasopressin added to standard therapy can buy time. It does not obviate the need for the use of standard measures to control bleeding. If the dosage can be reduced and bleeding does not recur, vasopressin can be used for more than a week, but high doses are not tolerated for long periods of time. At the present time, it appears that intravenous infusion is as effective as arterial infusion.

35. **(A) (T), (B) (T), (C) (T), (D) (F), (E) (F)**
More than 50% of postoperative myocardial infarctions are asymptomatic. This may be due to the residual effects of anesthesia and to postoperative analgesics. Anticoagulation prevents the formation of mural thrombus and arterial embolism after myocardial infarction, but anticoagulation is dangerous during the first 4 days after surgery.

36. **(A) (F), (B) (F), (C) (F), (D) (F), (E) (F)**
Hormone manipulation is more successful in postmenopausal women. The response is better for those with estrogen and progesterone receptor-positive tumors than it is with estrogen receptor-positive tumors. A slowly growing tumor responds better than a rapidly growing tumor. Very old patients usually respond well to hormone manipulation. Since the quality of life after an endocrine-induced remission is superior to that following chemotherapy, it is usually best to try hormone manipulation first in patients when the estrogen receptors are positive or unknown.

37. **(A) (T), (B) (T), (C) (F), (D) (T), (E) (F)**
The gallstone usually enters the duodenum, and the most common site of intestinal obstruction is the distal ilium.

38. **(A) (T), (B) (T), (C) (T), (D) (T), (E) (T)**
In 1950, there was enthusiasm for radical operations. The expected improvement did not occur. Today the operation should be appropriate to the individual situation. Because gravitational

metastasis occurs in the ovaries, oophrectomy is indicated in most female patients with colorectal cancer.

39. **(A) (T), (B) (T), (C) (F), (D) (T), (E) (F)** The bleeding from a knife wound of the liver usually stops spontaneously. In the absence of active bleeding, these wounds should not be sutured. A pulverizing injury rarely requires formal lobectomy after debridement. If bleeding cannot be controlled, the area can be packed and the patient reexplored 2 or 3 days later under general anesthesia.

40. **(E)** Aspirin usually is not nephrotoxic when taken alone, but the combination of salicylates and ibuprofen may cause renal failure.

41. **(B)** One must guard against flexion contracture of the hip, and the patient is not allowed to sit until able to hyperextend the thigh.

42. **(E)** Thirty percent of neuroblastomas metastasize to bone, 11% to skull or brain. Wilms' tumors metastasize to the lungs. The other tumors are rare at this age.

43. **(B)** Melanomas are uncommon among blacks.

44. **(D)** Intestinal obstruction is unusual because the caliber of the ascending colon is twice that of the left colon.

45. **(A)** Malignant pleural effusion develops at some time in almost 50% of patients with breast carcinoma.

46. **(C)** A large chyle loss can lead to nutritional depletion. When closed drainage fails to stop the chylothorax due to thoracic duct injury, ligation is indicated.

47. **(D)** Iatrogenic rupture accounts for 20% of splenectomies for splenic rupture. It usually occurs during upper abdominal surgery.

48. **(B)** The only absolute indication to explore the common duct found at operation is a palpable common bile duct stone or common duct stones demonstrated by cystic duct cholangiogram. The presence of a dilated common bile duct is an indication for operative cholangiography.

49. **(D)** Prostacyclin PGI2 inhibits platelet aggregation.

50. **(A)** Barium swallow usually establishes the diagnosis by demonstrating a typical area of compression of the esophagus, usually at the level of T3 or T4. A lateral tracheogram may demonstrate anterior compression of the trachea a short distance above the carina.

51. **(D)** Antibiotics alone are rarely effective, and there is a real risk that infected pulmonary emboli and lung abscesses will follow conservative care.

52. **(C)** Peritoneal lavage has an accuracy rate of 90% for blood in the peritoneal cavity. This test is only valuable if positive. A negative result does not totally exclude a surgical problem in the abdomen.

53. **(A)** Trench foot and immersion foot occur after prolonged exposure to a wet and cold environment with temperatures above freezing. When the lower limbs are immobile and dependent in a wet, cold, but nonfreezing situation, trench or immersion foot develops. Tissue destruction is usually superficial. After rewarming, hyperemia and massive edema develop.

54. **(D)** Bilateral repair for bilateral small hernias may be recommended but not for bilateral large hernias because there may be greater tension, with an increased recurrence rate.

55. **(D)** Adrenal cortical hyperfunction rarely occurs clinically. Therefore, surgery for the adrenal adenomas is rarely required.

56. **(D)** The baby is likely to have developed hypochloremic, hypokalemic alkalosis.

57. **(A)** The idiopathic form of slipped epiphysis occurs between the ages of 10 and 16 and is possibly due to endocrine or metabolic dysfunction.

58. **(B)** Thirty-three percent of patients with hyperparathyroidism are constipated. Diarrhea is not a recognized symptom.

59. **(A)** Hypertension may result from any process that causes prolonged ischemia of one or both kidneys.

60. **(C)** The distal splenorenal (Warren) shunt is the first choice for elective portal decompression. It is not satisfactory if ascites is present and may be too difficult for emergency decompression.

61. **(D)** This protocol describes the history and the findings in a patient who has developed pulmonary hypertension with a consequent right-to-left shunt through a ventricular septal defect. With pulmonic stenosis, which could result in a similar history, there would be normal or decreased vascularity of the peripheral lung fields.

62. **(C)** The common lymphatic metastases are to the periaortic retroperitoneal nodes.

63. **(E)** Hypertension, headache, and muscular weakness should lead you to suspect primary hyperaldosteronism. Coarctation, Cushing's syndrome, and malignant hypertension would have other physical findings. Fibromuscular hyperplasia should remain in the differential diagnosis.

64. **(B)** In sarcoidosis, the diagnosis is almost always accurate. Metastatic tumor is found in about 40% of cases of lung cancer. This procedure should not be done when the diagnosis is primary mediastinal tumor.

65. **(E)** Aspirin ingestion can produce a deleterious effect on the gastric mucosa. However, the lesions produced by salicylates should not be termed stress ulcers.

66. **(A)** Antibiotics are not useful in the average patient with acute pancreatitis and should be reserved for suppurative complications.

67. **(E)** Leukocytosis and thrombocytosis persist for varying periods of time following splenectomy. The spherocytes and the increased osmotic fragility of the cells are not altered by splenectomy, but hemolysis ceases after operation and the erythrocytes have a normal life span.

68. **(B)** Both the qualitative fluorescein test and the Doppler ultrasound flowmeter have proved to be of little help in estimating bowel viability. On the other hand, the quantitative fluorescein test and the laser Doppler used from within the bowel lumen have been found to be useful.

69. **(C)** Adhesions are the most frequent and ac-

count for 60% of cases of small intestinal obstruction in adults in North America.

70. **(A)** An aggressive approach should be employed. The tumor should be resected if possible, but a primary anastomosis should not be performed. For a tumor of the sigmoid colon that has perforated, a Hartmann procedure is required.

71. **(A)** The best chance of cure is with an abdominoperineal resection.

72. **(C)** The surgical management of this problem generally requires complete excision of the prosthesis and restoration of the circulation to the extremities by an extraanatomic bypass.

73. **(A)** DIC is often a defibrination syndrome. In some cases, a moderate dose of heparin may slow or stop the resulting bleeding.

74. **(B)** Seminomas are highly radiosensitive.

75. **(A)** About 33% of patients with a ruptured spleen require splenectomy. In the majority, splenorrhaphy or the application of a hemostatic agent can be used to preserve the spleen.

76. **(B)** The pain of acute appendicitis is at first a visceral pain because of distention of the appendix. At this time, it is less severe than pain that develops a few hours later in the right lower quadrant.

77. **(E)** There are no lymphatics in the lamina propria of the large bowel, but they are present in the muscularis mucosae, so that the potential for metastasis exists.

78. **(D)** A barium enema unfailingly demonstrates the fistulous tract. An upper gastrointestinal series shows the marginal ulcer in 50% of patients but the gastrocolic fistulas in only 15%.

79. **(C)** Technetium is picked up by gastric mucosa that is found in approximately 50% of Meckel's diverticula.

80. **(D)** About 30% of fistulas close spontaneously. This is a high output fistula. Total parenteral nutrition and no oral intake should continue for at least 1 month, at which time most fistulas that are going to close will have begun to do so. This is the time for operation if the fistula is not closing.

81. **(D)** Mammography is not very helpful during pregnancy because of the increased radiodensity of the breast.

82. **(E)** The Nissen fundoplication when used with a short esophagus has been associated with frequent complications, particularly ulceration of the intrathoracic stomach. Fundoplication is the most effective for a hiatal hernia without a short esophagus.

83. **(A)** About one third of all patients with a dislocation of the knee joint have a thrombosis of the popliteal artery.

84. **(D)**

85. **(E)**

86. **(E)**

87. **(C)**

Answers 84 through 87

The choledochal cyst is a congenital anomaly more common in females. It may be symptomatic in childhood or asymptomatic until adulthood. Once symptomatic fever occurs, pain and jaundice tend to recur and become progressive. If untreated, biliary cirrhosis, biliary obstruction, cholecystitis, or rupture may occur. Excision and choledochojejunostomy is the treatment of choice.

88. **(C)** Fulminating acute ulcerative colitis should be treated with steroids, fluid, electrolyte replacement, etc. Only if this fails to control the acute problem should urgent surgery be performed.

89. **(D)** The bleeding is red in color and of an arterial type. Anemia is not often due to hemorrhoids, therefore, other causes should be sought. Injection therapy consists of an injection around and not into the feeding vein. Prolapse of hemorrhoids after defecation usually responds spontaneously or with manual assistance by the patient.

90. **(E)** All of the above.

91. **(B)** Although microcirculatory compromise may be an operative mechanism in shock-related pancreatitis, familial hyperlipidema is thought to injure the pancreas through cleavage of triglyceride to toxic free fatty acids by lipase.

92. **(C)**

93. **(D)**

94. **(E)**

95. **(B)** Pseudomembranous enterocolitis following administration of clindamycin or after a bowel preparation is increasingly caused by *C. difficile*. Treatment is with vancomycin. *Staphylococcus* sp. is the other commonly implicated organism.

Answers 92 through 95

Bronchial carcinoid tumors previously known as "bronchial adenomas" should be suspected as a cause of recurrent bouts of pulmonary infection, particularly between the ages of 20 and 40, and particularly in women. Bronchiectasis would cause more sputum production. The lesion may or may not show on chest films, and bronchoscopy is necessary to make the diagnosis of the lesion and its location. The carcinoid appears as a rounded, reddish or purple mass that is very vascular. Bronchotomy and plastic repair of the bronchus may be possible if it is not invasive, but lobectomy is the treatment of choice if secondary infection has produced a diseased lobe.

96. **(D)** When the area between T7 and C7 is involved, a well-functioning reflex bladder usually results. The uninhibited neurogenic bladder, dysfunction similar to that of the bladder of an infant, may be produced by cerebrovascular accidents and multiple sclerosis. This condition presents as urgent voiding almost without voluntary control. Meningomyelocele results in the centrally denervated neurogenic bladder with overflow incontinence, as do traumatic, neoplastic, or other congenital lesions of the sacral segments or cauda equina. Tabes dorsalis or combined cord degeneration may result in the sensory paralytic bladder; the patient is unaware of bladder filling.

97. **(A)**

98. **(E)**

99. **(D)**

Answers 97 through 99

Blowout of the duodenal stump, which should be a very rare complication if the surgeon is careful in his choice of operation, usually occurs 3 to 6 days after a Billroth II gastrectomy. Wound infection would not cause abdominal rigidity. The other diagnoses given are possibilities. A barium swallow would not aid in making any of the likely diagnoses, and there would be leukocytosis with all of the diagnoses. The level of the serum amylase and lipase and of the urinary amylase might or might not aid in differentiating pancreatitis from duodenal stump leakage. With stump leakage, one ought to be able to recover bile-stained fluid from the abdomen by paracentesis or by peritoneal lavage. Immediate reoperation to establish drainage is mandatory when the diagnosis is made or strongly suspected.

100. **(E)**

101. **(E)**

102. **(C)**

103. **(B)**

Answers 100 through 103
Prophylactic portacaval shunt in unselected patients does not improve longevity. The protection against hemorrhage is offset by a higher mortality from liver failure. Splenectomy has no permanent effect on portal pressure except in some cases of myeloid metaplasia and tropical splenomegaly. The patient has developed hepatic encephalopathy. Intestinal antibiotics are given to decrease intestinal bacteria that act on intestinal protein including blood. Blood volume must be maintained to avoid prerenal azotemia. Both umbilical vein catheterization and wedged hepatic vein pressure measurement have a lower morbidity than does splenic pulp manometry. At least two thirds of those who survive the initial hemorrhage will bleed again and the risk of dying from the second hemorrhage is 50 to 80%. It is principally for patients who survive the first hemorrhage that portacaval shunts are recommended. Hepatic encephalopathy is especially likely to occur after a portacaval shunt. About 30% of patients are dead within a year after the diagnosis of cirrhosis is established. Cirrhotics with varices have an even greater mortality rate.

104. **(D)** Petechiae from fat embolism have a distribution that favors the upper half of the body: over the chest and axillae and on the conjunctiva and uvula.

105. **(C)** These cysts require removal for cosmetic and other reasons. Removal of all cysts is not required.

106. **(C)** Fracture callus arises primarily from soft tissue surrounding the fracture site, and vascularization of the callus occurs from the same soft

tissue. Extensive local soft tissue destruction from the injury or subsequent infection is the most common cause of nonunion. Malnutrition and osteoporosis can result in delayed union or nonunion, and they contribute to the occurrence of pathologic fractures.

107. **(C)** At the present time, it is thought that the best treatment for this patient is mastectomy without delay. If the lesion is apparently confined to the breast, there is a 60% 5-year survival. If there are axillary node metastases, the 5-year survival is only 5 to 20%.

108. **(D)** The lesion shows skin attachment but not infiltration, ulceration, peau d'orange, etc. (T2). The nodes are clinically negative (N0), and there are no evident distant metastases (M0).

109. **(A)** Stage I, by both the International and American systems. The tumor is less than 5 cm in diameter, the axillary nodes are not suspected to contain metastases, and the skin shows only dimpling (incomplete fixation). No distant metastases are demonstrable. There is no Stage V in either system.

110. **(B)** Interruption of pregnancy and castration seem to have little beneficial effect. If radiation therapy is advised at all before evidence of recurrence or metastases, it would be reserved for patients with positive axillary lymph nodes. Prophylactic chemotherapy is not yet advised but may hold promise in the future.

111. **(A)** Tamoxifen is preferred as the initial treatment for multiple lesions in premenopausal women. It might be combined with oophorectomy or followed by radiation therapy to a symptomatic lesion. Estrogen therapy is contraindicated.

112. **(B)** Although the evidence is controversial, it is probably well to advise the patient to avoid pregnancy for a minimum of 1 year and to avoid hormone-containing medicines.

113. **(B)** Achalasia is characterized by a progressive decrease in coordinated contractions in the body of the esophagus associated with failure of the LES to relax at the appropriate time. The etiology is unclear, and the treatment is palliative: hydrostatic dilatation or esophagomyotomy to relieve LES spasm. Diffuse spasm, as the name

implies, is characterized by increased, discoordinated contractions throughout the esophagus. Fibrous replacement of smooth muscle in scleroderma results in both decreased peristalsis and decreased lower esophageal pressure, with resultant reflux. Patients with hypertensive LES as an isolated condition usually do not have decreased peristalsis. A small percentage (1 to 3.6%) of patients have a transient LES motility disturbance (spasm or atonicity as a result of injury to lower esophageal innervation during truncal vagotomy).

114. **(B)** Uric acid calculi are not radiopaque. They, therefore, show as filling defects and do not show on a plain x-ray film.

115. **(E)** Cystoscopy and retrograde ureteral catheterization, first, confirm the diagnosis of nonopaque ureteral calculi. Second, they may expedite the passage of these calculi.

116. **(A)** About 80% of ureteral calculi will pass spontaneously.

117. **(B)** Uric acid calculi are best treated on a long-term basis by changing the pH of the urine to 7.00 or more, limitation of purines in the diet, and a dose of allopurinol (Zyloprim) 300 mg every 12 hours.

118. **(A)** Evidence of rupture of the spleen usually occurs within a week of injury but can occur 3 or more weeks after an injury.

119. **(E)**

120. **(D)** Thoracentesis would not be of diagnostic value in this patient at this time.

121. **(A)** Anticoagulants and bedrest are the recommended treatment for a patient who has had one pulmonary embolus that was not catastrophic.

122. **(B)** Although recurrent episodes may occur, the most likely outcome is complete recovery.

123. **(C)** The operation of thromboendarterectomy is performed in a plane of cleavage in the media.

124. **(B)** In Barrett's esophagus, the most common symptom is heartburn, but the symptoms are milder than in patients without a changed epithelium. Presumably, the metaplastic epithelium is less sensitive than squamous epithelium.

125. **(B)** Fibroadenoma is a common benign tumor that is slightly more frequent and tends to occur at an earlier age in black women. Both breasts may be involved in more than 10% of patients.

126. **(A)** Tumors of the squamous cell type can be treated by a combination of radiotherapy and surgery with some success.

127. **(A)** Oat cell carcinoma frequently invades the lymphatics, producing a pleural effusion. Mediastinal involvement is not necessary for this development.

128. **(A)** Most patients with chronic isolated complete occlusion of the superior mesentric artery are asymptomatic. This is because of the excellent collateral circulation among the celiac, superior mesenteric, and inferior mesenteric arteries in most patients.

129. **(B)** The common femoral artery is the most frequent site of a significant peripheral arterial embolus.

130. **(D)** Appendicitis is no longer the leading cause of pyogenic liver abscesses. Biliary tract infections now cause one third of the abscesses, and portal infections account for 20%.

131. **(A)** *Escherichia coli* can be cultured from the pus of one third of cases of pyogenic liver abscess. The other organisms listed in the question follow as causes in the order listed, from **B** to **E**. However, anaerobic cultures were likely of poor quality during part of the 25-year period during which these data were gathered, and it is likely that anaerobes are present in more than the 6% of cases cited in this reference.

132. **(C)** Although both hemorrhoids and esophageal varices may, on rare occasions, follow the liver congestion secondary to right heart failure, the cardiac problem is obvious at this stage.

133. **(C)** The use of multiple antibiotics increases the risk of drug reactions and diminishes the effectiveness in the long run by promoting the emergence of resistant stains.

134. (C) Most patients with secondary and tertiary hyperparathyroidism can be treated medically. If a relatively normal serum calcium and phosphorus are maintained during dialysis and vitamin D is given, operation on the parathyroid glands usually is unnecessary. In tertiary hyperparathyroidism, operation on the parathyroid glands should be withheld if possible.

135. (E) Most recurrent ulcers probably develop because an inadequate operation was selected, such as a vagotomy and pyloroplasty, when an antectomy and vagotomy would have been better.

136. (E) Bleeding, particularly from the pelvic veins, may be uncontrollable in some patients with fractures of the pelvis. Therapeutic arteriographic intervention with embolization can be very helpful.

137. (D) In most patients, the vein remains patent both proximal and distal to the clip.

138. (E) CPK has a normal level of about 77. After a popliteal embolectomy, the level in the venous blood from that limb rises to a level of 650 or higher, indicating significant muscle damage.

139. (B) A peanut in the main bronchus will lead rapidly to obstructive emphysema. On expiration, the mediastinum shifts to the opposite side.

140. (B) Infection is the most severe complication of a human bite. The pneumococcus is an unlikely infecting organism.

141. (A) Excessive production of corticoids in Cushing's syndrome results in a catabolic effect that leads to protein depletion.

142. (C) Modern general anesthesia consists of the administration of a number of drugs. In the case described, the dosage required to control the diaphragmatic movement had not been maintained.

143. (B) An increasing serum potassium level is a frequent and hazardous complication of anuria.

144. (E) When it is impossible to bring a testicle to a palpable location in the scrotum or low in the inguinal canal, it is best to excise the testicle because of the very high incidence of carcinoma in abdominal testes.

145. (C) Diverticular disease may limit colonoscopy or lead to complications, such as perforation. Drainage of an inflamed diverticulum is not as yet a therapeutic procedure.

146. (B) There is one intercostal artery in each space that receives blood from both the aorta and the internal mammary artery. There are three intercostal muscles; two lie superficial and one deep to the neurovascular bundle, which is located just below each rib. The intercostal nerves divide into an anterior and a posterior ramus.

147. (D) Postprandial reactive hypoglycemia is not related to dumping. This condition is due to hypoglycemia developing 3 to 4 hours after eating. Dumping occurs soon after eating.

148. (D) Duodenojejunostomy is the most widely preferred surgical treatment for vascular compression of the duodenum. Division and reanastomosis of either duodenum or vessels would be complex and risky. Mobilization of the ligament of Treitz alone may not be sufficient. Mobilization of the duodenum and transposition to the right of the vessels may risk compromising the vascular supply to the duodenal wall.

149. (D) This nerve plexus may be excised or divided in operations on the abdominal aorta and during a radical lymph node dissection for a tumor of the testicle. During ejaculation, the internal sphincter of the urinary bladder closes; removal of these nerves abolishes this. The result is that the semen is ejaculated into the urinary bladder and not externally—so-called retrograde ejaculation. The sympathetic chains remain intact so that there are no vasomotor changes in the skin.

150. (E) These are the history and physical findings of a compression of the median nerve in the carpal tunnel at the wrist.

151. (A) Although no tests are absolutely reliable, nerve conduction tests are the best.

152. (E) The carpal tunnel syndrome consists of compression of the median nerve in the fibroosseous compartment behind the transverse carpal ligament.

153. (B) Decompression by surgery may produce dramatic relief if performed before nerve damage has occurred.

154. **(C)** The procedure for the carpal tunnel syndrome is division of that part of the tunnel formed by the transverse carpal ligament.

155. **(E)** It is likely that this patient has an aortoenteric fistula. The most useful test would be an arteriogram.

156. **(D)** The graft is infected when an aortoenteric fistula has developed. Healing may occur with surgery and antibiotics, but not always. Removal of the prosthesis is required to eradicate the infection with certainty.

157. **(C)** The advantage of an aortoiliac graft is that it restores good blood flow to both lower limbs.

158. **(E)** Infection of a prosthetic graft frequently leads to hemorrhage, thrombosis, false aneurysm, or distal gangrene. It rarely leads to the formation of an arteriovenous fistula.

159. **(C)** A mycotic aneurysm is caused by a bacterial infection that is likely to involve a prosthetic graft and cause secondary hemorrhages.

160. **(D)** The pain is relieved by sitting or lying down; it is not relieved by standing still.

161. **(A) (T), (B) (F), (C) (T), (D) (F), (E) (T)** Injection treatment consists of injecting the sclerosant into the loose areolar tissue above the internal hemorrhoids, not into the lumen of the vein. Cryosurgery has not gained wide acceptance because uncontrolled sloughs of the mucosa occur.

162. **(A) (F), (B) (T), (C) (T), (D) (F), (E) (T)** Thymoma is the second most common mediastinal lesion after neurogenic tumors and is usually seen in patients over 20 years of age. Up to half of patients with thymomas have myasthenia gravis; this increases to 80% for men over 50 and women over 60. Men with myasthenia gravis are twice as likely as women to have a thymoma. Ten to forty percent of patients with myasthenia have a thymoma. Myasthenia patients with and without thymoma benefit from thymectomy.

163. **(A) (F), (B) (T), (C) (F), (D) (T), (E) (T)** The incidence of ductal obstruction in postmortem examinations does not support the concept that ductal obstruction is the basic cause of this disease. If pancreatitis is resolving, it is better to wait until resolution is complete before operating for associated gallstones.

164. **(A) (T), (B) (F), (C) (T), (D) (F), (E) (T)** Tentorial herniation can compress the third cranial nerve (oculomotor) causing pupillary dilatation. Compression of the pyramidal (motor) tract within the cerebral peduncle abutting on the tentorium can cause contralateral spastic weakness. Herniation is associated with a decreased level of consciousness. The fifth (trigeminal) and seventh (facial) nerves are involved with the corneal reflex, and the eighth (acoustic) is necessary for the oculocephalic (Doll's eye) reflex. These reflexes are indices of brain stem function and do not signify tentorial herniation.

165. **(A) (T), (B) (T), (C) (T), (D) (T), (E) (F)** About 75% of these cancers are either lymphoid or arise in the epithelial cells of the skin, cervix of the uterus, or lips.

166. **(A) (F), (B) (T), (C) (T), (D) (T), (E) (T)** As many as 90% of a surgical team puncture their gloves during an operation.

167. **(A) (F), (B) (F), (C) (T), (D) (T), (E) (T)** The most common symptom is bleeding, and intestinal obstruction is the second most common clinical presentation.

168. **(A) (T), (B) (T), (C) (T), (D) (T), (E) (T)** In 1930, carcinoma of the stomach was very common, and carcinoma of the lung was very rare. By 1950, the incidence of cancer of the stomach, colon, rectum, and lung was equal. Today, carcinoma of the lung is very common, and carcinoma of the stomach is rare in the USA. The fiberoptic gastroscope has greatly increased the accuracy of the diagnosis of gastric cancer. Today, as in Billroth's time, surgical excision is the only method offering hope of cure in cancer of the stomach.

169. **(A) (T), (B) (T), (C) (T), (D) (T), (E) (T)** Carcinoid tumors occur most frequently in the appendix and jejunoileum. Those in the appendix rarely metastasize. Carcinoid tumors rarely cause the carcinoid syndrome—only 136 of 3718 reported by Sabiston. The syndrome when present includes all of the indicated symptoms. At one time, the syndrome was thought to be due to overproduction of serotonin. It is likely that increased production of histamine, kallikrein, and

prostaglandins is more important than serotonin in the production of symptoms.

170. **(A) (T), (B) (T), (C) (T), (D) (T), (E) (F)**
There is no sex predilection for pheochromocytoma.

171. **(A) (T), (B) (F), (C) (F), (D) (T), (E) (F)**
If followed long enough, virtually all patients with Crohn's disease will require surgery at some time in the course of the disease. The reoperation rate is between 5% and 15% a year, and the rate of recurrent problems requiring surgery is proportional to the duration of disease (the longer the duration, the higher the recurrence rate and the shorter the interval). Recurrence typically appears at and proximal to the prior anastomosis. Conservative resection to grossly normal bowel helps preserve bowel length (short bowel syndrome is a significant risk) and does not alter the outcome.

172. **(A) (T), (B) (F), (C) (T), (D) (T), (E) (T)**
The relationship of hypercalcemia to pancreatitis is well documented. The familial form of pancreatitis is associated with an autosomal dominant gene. Steroids as well as other drugs, such as furosemide, chlorothiazide, and sulfasalazine, have been linked with pancreatitis. Laboratory evidence that hypoperfusion due to small vessel occlusion can cause pancreatitis may explain the mechanism in shock. ERCP, as well as manipulation of the ampulla in common duct exploration, may precipitate pancreatitis.

173. **(A) (T), (B) (F), (C) (F), (D) (T), (E) (F)**
Cystadenoma is by definition a benign lesion but is difficult to distinguish from a cystadenocarcinoma. It is a slowly growing lesion that is considered premalignant and for that reason should be excised if possible rather than drained internally. If it proves to be a carcinoma, the cure rate with excision is reported as high as 68% for 5 years.

174. **(A) (F), (B) (T), (C) (F), (D) (T), (E) (T)**
The inferior mesenteric vein is a tributary of the splenic vein. The left colic artery is a branch of the inferior mesenteric artery.

175. **(A) (T), (B) (T), (C) (T), (D) (T), (E) (T)**
All of the statements are correct.

176. **(A) (T), (B) (F), (C) (F), (D) (T), (E) (T)**
Synthetic, nonabsorbable sutures generally are inert and retain their strength longer than wire. The reason is that repeated movement causes steel wire to undergo metal fatigue and eventually break. The resorption time of catgut is highly variable. There is little use for catgut in modern surgery.

177. **(A) (T), (B) (T), (C) (F), (D) (T), (E) (F)**
If macrocytic anemia develops, it is because of the binding of vitamin B_{12} by anaerobic bacteria, which prevents absorption of the vitamin. Most patients do not have a problem amenable to surgical correction, but when possible, surgical correction should be performed.

178. **(A) (F), (B) (T), (C) (T), (D) (F), (E) (T)**
The most common segment involved is the cecum. The cecum is involved in 50% of cases, whereas the sigmoid colon is involved in 45%. Most surgeons resect the sigmoid colon even if it is viable to prevent recurrence.

179. **(A) (T), (B) (T), (C) (F), (D) (T), (E) (F)**
Hypersplenism is an indication for splenectomy because removal of the spleen improves tolerance to chemotherapy. Staging laporotomy is rarely indicated in patients with non-Hodgkin's lymphoma because systemic treatment usually is required.

180. **(A) (T), (B) (T), (C) (T), (D) (T), (E) (T)**
All of the statements are correct.

Third Examination
Questions

DIRECTIONS (Questions 1 through 100): Each of the numbered items or incomplete statements in this section is followed by answers or by completions of the statement. Select the ONE lettered answer or completion that is BEST in each case.

Questions 1 and 2

A 65-year-old man enters the hospital with a 2-day history of pneumaturia. He is obese, and physical examination is completely negative. The white blood cell count is 13,000.

1. Which of the following tests would be LEAST likely to assist the diagnosis?

   (A) cystoscopy
   (B) proctoscopy
   (C) cystometrogram
   (D) plain abdominal x-ray film
   (E) intravenous pyelogram   (3:1660)

2. The most likely diagnosis in the patient described in the previous question is

   (A) carcinoma of the bladder
   (B) carcinoma of the colon
   (C) carcinoma of the prostate
   (D) diverticulum of the bladder
   (E) diverticulitis of the colon   (3:1660)

Questions 3 through 5

A 30-year-old male graduate student from India is admitted with dysuria. He has suffered from hematuria, dysuria, and frequency. The urine contains pus cells, but the culture is sterile.

3. The most likely diagnosis is

   (A) renal tuberculosis
   (B) carcinoma of the bladder
   (C) schistosomiasis (bilharzia)
   (D) ureteral calculus
   (E) urethral stricture   (2:1697)

4. The diagnosis is most directly made by

   (A) culture of the urine for acid-fast bacillus
   (B) cystoscopy
   (C) repeated urinalysis
   (D) intravenous pyelogram
   (E) biopsy of the kidney   (2:1697)

5. The best treatment of the patient is

   (A) antituberculosis chemotherapy for 2 years
   (B) sulfa drugs and diuretics
   (C) ureterolithotomy
   (D) full rest in a tuberculosis hospital
   (E) regular bladder irrigations   (2:1697)

6. A young man is stabbed at the base of his neck on the left side. There is subcutaneous and mediastinal emphysema, a small hemopneumothorax, and moderate dysphagia. Of the following procedures, which is likely to be the most important initially?

   (A) an arteriogram of the branches of the aortic arch
   (B) an exploratory operation
   (C) a contrast esophagogram
   (D) diagnostic aspiration of the left pleural cavity
   (E) observation with repeat chest film in 3 hours   (2:1099)

Questions 7 through 9

A 45-year-old white female is admitted to the hospital with recurrent right upper quadrant pain. Ten years previously, she had undergone a cholecystectomy and common bile duct exploration. One stone was removed from the common bile duct. About 5 years later, she began to develop intermittent attacks of crampy right upper quadrant pain that became progressively worse and more frequent in nature. There was no history of jaundice.

7. The most likely diagnosis is

   (A) biliary dyskinesia
   (B) chronic pancreatitis
   (C) cystic duct stump syndrome
   (D) biliary cirrhosis
   (E) recurrent common duct stone   *(2:1322)*

8. An intravenous cholangiogram is performed and shows no gallstones but does show a dilated common bile duct. The most likely diagnosis would be

   (A) recurrent common bile duct stone
   (B) carcinoma of the ampulla of Vater
   (C) carcinoma of the head of the pancreas
   (D) benign fibrosing stenosis of the common bile duct
   (E) chronic pancreatitis   *(2:1322)*

9. Which of the following statements is most likely to be true about this patient?

   (A) the stone probably formed in the common bile duct
   (B) the stone was probably residual and missed at the first operation
   (C) common duct stones are most usually found impacted at the ampulla of Vater
   (D) the stone was most likely formed in the intrahepatic bile ducts
   (E) the stone formed in the cystic duct at the point of ligature and division   *(2:1322)*

10. Hemoptysis is characteristic of which cardiac valvular pathologic condition?

    (A) pulmonic stenosis
    (B) aortic insufficiency
    (C) tricuspid stenosis
    (D) mitral stenosis
    (E) mitral regurgitation   *(3:2348)*

11. Echinococcosis (hydatid disease) is caused by the tapeworm *Echinococcus granulosus*. The

worm's adult phase is in the intestine of the dog and occasionally the fox. Ova are passed by the dog and are eaten by intermediate hosts, the sheep and humans. Larval cysts form in the intermediate host. The dog is reinfected by eating uncooked infected sheep. Which of the following statements concerning hydatid disease in humans is INCORRECT?

    (A) most human infections occur in adult life
    (B) cysts in the lung can be delivered by the anesthesiologist's inflating the lung after the surgeon had made an incision over the cyst
    (C) pulmonary cysts are more easily removed than are hepatic cysts
    (D) mebendazole or albendazole are of value in preventing recurrence and in patients with disseminated disease
    (E) hydatid cyst of the liver may be seen first after the cyst ruptures into the bile ducts, causing bilary colic and jaundice   *(1:116)*

12. Which of the following conditions does NOT predispose to the formation of renal calculi?

    (A) milk alkali syndrome
    (B) Paget's disease (osteitis deformans)
    (C) renal tubular acidosis
    (D) hyperparathyroidism
    (E) transverse myelitis   *(2:1609,1697,1925)*

13. Which of the following statements concerning multiple endocrine adenomatosis (MEA) is NOT correct?

    (A) MEA type 1 (Werner syndrome) is characterized by hyperparathyroidism, Zollinger-Ellison syndrome, pituitary tumor, adrenocortical tumor, and insulinoma
    (B) MEA type II (Sipple's syndrome) consists of hyperparathyroidism, medullary carcinoma of the thyroid, and pheochromocytoma
    (C) medullary carcinomas of the thyroid arise from cells of the ultimobranchial bodies, which also secrete calcitonin
    (D) treatment of medullary carcinoma of the thyroid is subtotal thyroidectomy
    (E) both MEA syndromes are familial
          (1:246-249)

14. Which of the following statements concerning the treatment of hyperparathyroidism is NOT correct?

(A) operation is the only successful treatment for hyperparathyroidism

(B) arteriography is the best method of localizing the problem

(C) the presence of a normal parathyroid indicates that the problem is an adenoma because in hyperplasia all the parathyroid glands are involved

(D) adenomas may be multiple

(E) in patients with multiple endocrine adenomatosis type I or II syndromes, total parathyroidectomy and autotransplantation to the forearm may be recommended   *(1:252)*

15. Inflammatory carcinoma is the most malignant form of breast cancer. Which of the following statements about this problem is WRONG?

(A) the overlying skin becomes erythematous, edematous, and warm

(B) a rapidly growing tumor forms, which enlarges the breast

(C) the inflammatory changes may be mistaken for an infectious process

(D) a biopsy shows invasion of the lymphatics

(E) treatment is mastectomy followed by radiotherapy and chemotherapy   *(1:261)*

Questions 16 through 18

16. The most common posterior-superior sulcus chest tumor in a 6-month-old child is

(A) ganglioneuroma

(B) cystic hygroma

(C) teratoma

(D) enteric cyst

(E) neuroblastoma   *(2:725)*

17. If left untreated, the most likely outcome in the patient described in the preceding question would be

(A) no change

(B) slow resolution of the lesion

(C) death from metastatic spread

(D) death from invasion of the trachea

(E) paraplegia from invasion of the spinal column   *(2:725)*

18. The treatment of choice for the tumor in the child is

(A) excision plus postoperative x-ray therapy

(B) x-ray therapy alone

(C) surgery alone

(D) x-ray therapy, chemotherapy, and surgery

(E) x-ray therapy plus dactinomycin   *(2:725)*

19. The following statements concern Paget's carcinoma of the breast; one is NOT correct.

(A) the basic lesion is a ductal carcinoma

(B) Paget's carcinoma is usually obvious and easily diagnosed

(C) the first symptom often is itching or burning of the nipple, with superficial erosions or ulcerations

(D) when a palpable breast tumor is present, the prognosis is worse than when nipple changes only are present

(E) the diagnosis is established by biopsy of the nipple lesion   *(1:261)*

20. A patient has a histologically confirmed bronchogenic carcinoma. A bronchoscopy is performed. Which one of the following findings does NOT indicate inoperability?

(A) vocal cord paralysis

(B) extension of the lesion above the carina

(C) fixation of the carina

(D) fixation of the bronchial tree

(E) abscess distal to the tumor   *(1:301–302)*

Questions 21 and 22

A 40-year-old man is injured in an automobile accident. On admission to the hospital, he is in severe respiratory distress and has coughed up blood. The breath sounds are decreased on the left side of the chest. The trachea is shifted to the left, and there is emphysema in the neck. The blood pressure is 100/70 and the pulse rate is 120.

21. The most likely diagnosis is

(A) tension pneumothorax

(B) hemopneumothorax

(C) pericardial tamponade

(D) bronchial laceration

(E) rupture of the aorta   *(2:201)*

22. The initial treatment of the patient should be

(A) continued observation

(B) immediate thoracotomy

(C) closed chest tube drainage

(D) repeated pleural aspiration

(E) antibiotics, blood transfusion, and supportive care   *(2:201)*

23. Postmenopausal patients with metastatic breast cancer may be managed in all of the following ways EXCEPT

    (A) tamoxifen 10 mg twice a day is now the treatment of choice
    (B) tamoxifen has fewer side effects than diethylstilbestrol and is just as effective
    (C) androgens are a useful alternative to tamoxifen
    (D) aminogluthethimide should be reserved for patients who have relapsed after an initial response to tamoxifen and then diethylstilbestrol
    (E) hypophysectomy and adrenalectomy are rarely used   *(1:270)*

24. Which of the following conditions is NOT associated with an increased incidence of carcinoma of the esophagus?

    (A) achalasia
    (B) Patterson-Kelly or Plummer-Vinson syndrome
    (C) corrosive esophagitis
    (D) gastric ulcer
    (E) tylosis palmari's and plantaris   *(2:1092)*

25. Tuberculosis remains the most common infectious cause of death worldwide. Since chemotherapy became available, the role of surgery in the management of pulmonary tuberculosis has diminished greatly. Which of the following statements concerning the role of surgery is NOT correct?

    (A) the performance of diagnostic procedures
    (B) resection for a destroyed lobe
    (C) persistent bronchopleural fistula
    (D) large tuberculous cavities
    (E) intractable hemorrhage   *(1:304)*

26. A 50-year-old man has superior vena cava obstruction. This is most likely due to

    (A) bronchogenic carcinoma
    (B) constrictive pericarditis
    (C) superior mediastinal fibrosis
    (D) thymoma
    (E) retrosternal thyroid   *(2:892)*

27. The following statements concern the prognosis of patients with lung cancer. Which is NOT correct?

    (A) without surgery, 95% of patients with lung cancer die within 2 years

    (B) the average reported delay between the first visit to a physician and operation is 4 to 6 months
    (C) the prognosis is best in young adults and women
    (D) the survival rates at 5 years are 35% following lobectomy and 20% after pneumonectomy
    (E) the overall operative mortality is now less than 5%   *(1:313)*

Questions 28 and 29

A 45-year-old woman develops sudden excruciating interscapular pain radiating into the right lower limb. On physical examination, the right femoral pulse is not felt and the left femoral pulse is weak. There is an aortic diastolic murmur.

28. The blood pressure is 120/90, and the pulse rate is 100. The most likely diagnosis is

    (A) myocardial infarction
    (B) embolus of the abdominal aorta
    (C) dissecting aortic aneurysm
    (D) pulmonary embolus
    (E) spontaneous pneumothorax   *(2:884-887)*

29. The most useful diagnostic test would be

    (A) electrocardiogram
    (B) chest x-ray
    (C) serum transaminase determination
    (D) hematocrit determination
    (E) aortography   *(2:884-887)*

30. The best treatment of a patient 3 weeks after chest trauma who has a clotted hemothorax and compressed lung is

    (A) apical lysis
    (B) decortication with tube drainage
    (C) pneumonectomy
    (D) injection of a lytic enzyme and repeated aspirations
    (E) thoracostomy with tube drainage   *(1:291)*

31. A clean, simple, penetrating wound of the cervical esophagus is treated by

    (A) antibiotics and nasogastric suction
    (B) simple repair of the esophagus and closure of the wound
    (C) repair of the esophagus and drainage of the wound

(D) cutaneous pharyngostomy for salivary drainage

(E) cutaneous esophagostomy   *(2:227)*

32. A 16-year-old boy has sustained a knife slash injury of the right parotid gland, and the right facial nerve is injured. Which of the following describes the best treatment?

(A) exploration and repair should be delayed 3 weeks to permit more adequate exploration of the nerve

(B) if the major salivary duct is injured it should be repaired over a stent, which is left in place for 2 weeks

(C) if a salivary fistula develops, it can be treated by irradiation

(D) primary repair of the facial nerve is indicated

(E) primary repair of the facial nerve is indicated only if the major salivary duct has not been injured   *(2:227)*

Questions 33 and 34

Following blunt trauma to the abdomen, the only intraabdominal injuries are three small lacerations of the edge of the right lobe of the liver. There is no active bleeding at the time of the operation.

33. The best operative procedure is

(A) suture of the lacerations without drainage of the area

(B) suture of the lacerations with drainage of the area

(C) packing of the lacerations with Gelfoam and drainage of the area

(D) packing of the lacerations with Gelfoam, suturing the lacerations over the Gelfoam, and drainage of the area

(E) drainage of the area alone without the use of liver sutures   *(2:243)*

34. A retroperitoneal hematoma is discovered during exploration for blunt trauma to the abdomen. What is the best course for the surgeon?

(A) explore the hematoma only when it is associated with a pelvic fracture

(B) explore only expanding hematomas

(C) explore no retroperitoneal hematoma

(D) explore the hematoma only if the source of bleeding has been determined preoperatively by angiography

(E) explore all retroperitoneal hematomas not associated with pelvic fractures   *(2:256)*

35. Which of the following tumors is LEAST radiosensitive?

(A) malignant melanoma

(B) Hodgkin's disease

(C) Ewing's sarcoma of bone

(D) epidermoid carcinoma

(E) basal cell carcinoma   *(2:343)*

36. The most common cause of respiratory and cardiac arrest during spinal anesthesia is

(A) anesthetic block of the phrenic nerve

(B) allergic hypersensitivity to the anesthetic agent

(C) increased relaxation of the peripheral arterioles

(D) operations performed in the head-up position

(E) preanesthetic medication overdosage   *(2:449)*

Questions 37 through 39

An 8-year-old boy has a swollen, painful knee, fever, and leukocytosis. He resists attempts to move the knee joint, which contains fluid. The skin on the medial side of the knee is erythematous, hot, and tender in an area 2 × 4 cm in size. There is a history of mild injury to the knee 1 week ago, and the child has had a cough and sore throat for several days.

37. The best treatment would be to

(A) clean the involved skin, dress the area, immobilize the knee with a compression bandage, start antibiotic treatment, and reexamine the child in 2 days, or sooner if symptoms become worse

(B) aspirate a few drops of fluid for culture and start antibiotic therapy

(C) aspirate the joint at the site of involved skin, attempt to aspirate all of the fluid, and await the results of culture

(D) aspirate the knee joint completely at a site away from the involved skin, attempt to remove all of the fluid, and start antibiotic therapy before the results of culture are known

(E) obtain a culture from the involved skin with a Pasteur pipette or a large-bore needle and syringe and start an antibiotic before the culture results are obtained   *(2:2011–2012)*

38. If treatment is begun before the results of culture are known, which antibiotic would you select?

    (A) ampicillin
    (B) gentamicin
    (C) penicillin G
    (D) tetracycline
    (E) methicillin   *(2:2011-2012)*

39. At some time in the patient's course, the diagnosis of septic arthritis is made. Which statement describes the most likely treatment of choice, in addition to appropriate antibiotic therapy?

    (A) aspiration of the knee joint again about a week later to make certain that the fluid is sterile or that a superimposed infection has not occured
    (B) surgical drainage of the knee joint
    (C) aspiration of the joint until dry and immediate immobilization in a plaster cast
    (D) surgical drainage with early active motion of the joint to prevent ankylosis
    (E) aspiration of the joint every other day, four times, then surgical drainage
                                        (2:2011-2012)

40. A patient is suspected of having an intraperitoneal abscess. Of the following studies used to locate such an abscess, which is the most useful?

    (A) x-rays with or without contrast
    (B) ultrasonography
    (C) CT scan
    (D) indium-labeled autologous leukocyte scan
    (E) gallium-67 citrate scan   *(1:411)*

41. A serious complication of resection of an aneurysm of the descending thoracic aorta, even with adequate bypass perfusion, is

    (A) stress peptic ulcer
    (B) paraplegia
    (C) cerebral embolism
    (D) congestive cardiac failure
    (E) hepatic failure   *(2:881)*

42. Paradoxical motion, or flail chest, causes all of the following EXCEPT

    (A) disturbed cardiac output
    (B) increased respiratory work
    (C) irregular distribution of air to the lungs
    (D) decreased alveolar-capillary gradient
    (E) increased alveolar oxygen level   *(2:633-634)*

43. The only communication between the bronchial arteries and the pulmonary circulation is

    (A) patent ductus arteriosus
    (B) interlobar and segmental pulmonary veins
    (C) pre- and postarteriolar capillary plexus
    (D) small muscular pulmonic arteries
    (E) a tributary of an arteriovenous fistula
                                        (15:1398)

44. The etiology of Bell's palsy is

    (A) local vasospasm leading to an intratympanic entrapment syndrome
    (B) a viral disease
    (C) ischemic neuritis
    (D) trauma
    (E) unknown   *(1:796)*

45. Vitamin B_{12} deficiency would be most likely to follow which of the following operations?

    (A) partial gastrectomy
    (B) partial gastrectomy with resection of the duodenum and head of the pancreas
    (C) resection of the jejunum
    (D) resection of the ileum
    (E) total colectomy   *(3:920)*

46. After splenectomy for spherocytic anemia, one may expect all of the following EXCEPT

    (A) transient leukocytosis
    (B) the erythrocytes achieve a normal life span
    (C) persistence of the anemia
    (D) persistence of the osmotic fragility
    (E) persistence of the spherocytosis
                                        (2:1379-1380)

47. Which of the following statements concerning surgery in patients with hematologic malignant disorders is NOT correct?

    (A) the common anticancer chemotherapeutic agents interfere with wound healing (e.g., melphalan, cyclophosphamide, methotrexate)
    (B) patients with polycythemia vera have an increased risk of both hemorrhage and thrombosis
    (C) very high platelet counts may be encountered. If possible, platelet pheresis to a platelet count of below 1,000,000 should precede surgery

(D) the risks of surgery are not increased if the patient is in hematologic remission

(E) if excessive bleeding occurs during surgery, transfusions and platelet packs are used

(1:51)

48. In achalasia, the findings on esophageal manometry include all of the following EXCEPT

(A) the pharyngoesophageal sphincter has a normal action

(B) the esophagus is devoid of primary peristaltic waves

(C) the pressure in the gastroesophageal sphincter is about 80 mm Hg

(D) the subcutaneous injection of bethanechol produces forceful sustained contraction of the lower two thirds of the esophagus

(E) the response to bethanecol is absent in normal individuals

(1:372)

49. The lesion responsible for subclavian steal syndrome is

(A) common carotid artery occlusion

(B) subclavian artery occlusion proximal to the origin of the vertebral artery

(C) vertebral origin stenosis

(D) internal carotid stenosis

(E) thrombosis of the second part of the subclavian artery

(2:948)

50. Which of the following is the more frequent cause of hypothyroidism?

(A) nodular goiter

(B) carcinoma of the thyroid

(C) lymphadenoid goiter (Hashimoto's thyroiditis)

(D) Riedel's thyroiditis

(E) subtotal thyroidectomy

(2:1560)

51. The extracolonic manifestations seen in association with ulcerative colitis include each of the following EXCEPT

(A) skin lesions, such as erythema

(B) uveitis

(C) thyroiditis

(D) arthritis

(E) pericarditis

(1:618)

52. At this time resection is the best method of cure for carcinoma of the lung but is not possible in two thirds of the cases. Which of the following statements concerning the management of lung cancer by radiotherapy is NOT accurate?

(A) radiotherapy is most effective for patients with Pancoast tumors

(B) radiotherapy is used for the palliation of patients with lung cancer

(C) radiotherapy cures 7 to 10% of lung cancer

(D) preoperative radiation exceeding 3000 rads has been implicated in bronchial stump problems where the operative area has been treated directly

(E) postoperative radiotherapy may benefit patients with mediastinal involvement or Pancoast tumor

(1:312)

53. A man aged 50 complains of weight loss and pain in the abdomen. He also has pain in the back. The pain is made worse by lying down and improved when he sits up and leans forward. The pain is not improved by morphine but is partially relieved by aspirin. The most likely diagnosis is

(A) carcinoma of the stomach

(B) abdominal aortic aneurysm

(C) carcinoma of the body of the pancreas

(D) degenerative arthritis of the lumbar spine

(E) lymphoma of the abdominal nodes

(1:534)

54. A patient with symptomatic esophageal achalasia is usually treated first with

(A) medication

(B) controlled forceful dilatation

(C) surgery

(D) combined therapy

(E) an antireflux operation

(2:1069)

55. Oliguria in a burn patient, during the first 24 hours, is probably explained by

(A) inadequate hydration

(B) corticosteroid secretion elevation

(C) infection

(D) vasoconstriction

(E) apprehension

(2:271–272)

56. Hyperkalemia causes

(A) an elevated ST segment

(B) a depressed ST segment

(C) renal failure

(D) hypoproteinemia

(E) constipation

(2:56)

Questions 57 and 58

A 40-year-old man has vomiting and fever of short duration, gross hematuria, and pain in the right flank. An intravenous pyelogram is done, which shows delayed visualization of the right kidney and a filling defect in the normally visualized left renal pelvis

57. The correct diagnosis is

    (A) carcinoma of the renal pelvis
    (B) glomerulonephritis
    (C) uric acid stones
    (D) calcium oxalate stones
    (E) calcium phosphate stones   *(2:1697–1670)*

58. The correct step in the management of the patient would be

    (A) right nephrostomy
    (B) cystoscopy and retrograde catheterization
    (C) nephrectomy
    (D) bilateral nephrostomy
    (E) lithotripsy   *(2:1697–1670)*

59. Which of the following Nobel Prize winners won the prize for introducing a surgical operation?

    (A) Sir Frederick Grant Banting
    (B) Emil Theodore Kocher
    (C) Charles Huggins
    (D) Antonio Eges Moniz
    (E) George Hoyt Whipple   *(11:8,743)*

60. Splenectomy may be expected to be most beneficial in

    (A) erythroblastosis fetalis
    (B) Christmas disease
    (C) splenosis
    (D) absence of factor VII
    (E) chronic idiopathic thrombocytopenic purpura   *(2:1382)*

61. In the carpal tunnel syndrome, the patient would have compression of the

    (A) radial artery
    (B) median nerve
    (C) basilic vein
    (D) radial nerve
    (E) ulnar nerve   *(2:2087–2088)*

62. In congenital wryneck (torticollis)

    (A) the first manifestations of the disease are usually not present until the child is 2 years old

    (B) 20% of patients have hip dysplasia
    (C) x-ray examination is not necessary
    (D) early operation is not indicated even in severe cases
    (E) in the early stages of development, the lesion is not tender, and manipulation of the neck is not painful   *(2:1892–1893)*

63. Which of the following statements about amebic hepatitis abscess is true?

    (A) they are usually multiple
    (B) metronidazole 750 mg orally three times a day for 10 days usually cures this abscess
    (C) incision and drainage often are necessary
    (D) the left lobe of the liver is the usual site
    (E) in most patients the pus from the abscess contains the trophozoites of *Entamoeba histolytica*   *(2:1265)*

64. An injured patient suspected of having a cervical spine injury should be transported to the emergency room with the

    (A) neck immobilized in 45° of flexion
    (B) neck immobilized in 45° of extension
    (C) head turned toward the side of the painful injury
    (D) head turned away from the side of the painful injury
    (E) head immobilized with a semirigid cervical collar and a backboard   *(9:259)*

65. A 65-year-old female patient was admitted to the hospital with a blue-black lesion under the great toenail, which was 4 mm in diameter and not painful. The lesion was noticed 4 months before and had not changed in size during this period. Which of the following would be the best initial treatment?

    (A) amputation of the toe and a radical groin dissection
    (B) amputate the toe
    (C) remove the toenail and do a wide local excision
    (D) perform a hindquartet amputation
    (E) perform an above-knee amputation   *(2:518)*

66. A 21-year-old patient has a chest x-ray during a routine physical examination. He is found to have a tumor located in the right paravertebral gutter posteriorly. He is completely asymptomatic. Which of the following is the most likely diagnosis?

(A) neurogenic tumor
(B) lymphosarcoma
(C) teratoma
(D) bronchogenic carcinoma
(E) intrathoracic goiter   *(2:724)*

Questions 67 and 68

A patient develops a septic tenosynovitis of the thumb, which is untreated. He then develops pain in the palm over the first metacarpal.

67. The most likely diagnosis is infection of the

   (A) midpalmar space
   (B) thenar space
   (C) radial bursa
   (D) ulnar bursa
   (E) retroflexor space of the wrist   *(2:2081)*

68. The treatment of choice would be incision

   (A) through the distal palmar crease on the ulnar side of the hand
   (B) over the area of maximum tenderness
   (C) at the radial side of the wrist
   (D) at the ulnar side of the wrist
   (E) on the dorsum of the hand distally, in the space between the thumb and index finger
                                             (2:2067)

69. Surgeons customarily divide wound healing into certain types. Which of the following statements concerning these types of wound healing is NOT correct?

   (A) healing by first intention (primary) occurs when a clean wound is reapproximated and heals without complication
   (B) healing by second intention (secondary) occurs when an open wound granulates and is eventually covered by migration of epithelial cells
   (C) secondary closure is the same as healing by second intention
   (D) granulation tissue contains new collagen blood vessels, fibroblasts, and inflammatory cells, especially macrophages
   (E) delayed primary closure is the closure of a wound 4 to 7 days after operation or injury   *(1:86)*

70. One of the following statements concerning the prevention and treatment of clostridial myositis is NOT correct.

   (A) clostridial infections are preventable by early debridement, leaving the wound open, and support of the circulation
   (B) modern treatment (e.g., antibiotics, surgery) obviates amputation in most patients
   (C) most surgeons have abandoned the use of polyvalent gas gangrene antitoxin
   (D) early use of hyperbaric oxygenation can reduce tissue loss
   (E) suspicion should be directed at a wound inflicted out of doors that is contaminated with a foreign body, soil, or animal or human feces in which muscle is injured
                                             (1:111)

71. In a patient with stenosis of the origin of the internal carotid artery, the most frequent cause of a transient ischemic attack of cerebral insufficiency is

   (A) reduction of the cerebral blood flow due to the arterial stenosis
   (B) thrombosis of the stenosed carotid artery, followed by the formation of an adequate collateral circulation
   (C) microembolization from the atheromatous plaque
   (D) transient obstruction of the carotid artery
   (E) transient reduction in cardiac output *(2:942)*

72. In which of the following conditions would you NOT expect a significant shift of the extracellular fluid?

   (A) acute pancreatitis
   (B) severe third degree burn
   (C) inflammatory carcinoma of the breast
   (D) peritonitis
   (E) acute intestinal obstruction   *(2:48-49)*

Questions 73 through 77

A young Mississippi Valley farmer, while working in his barn, dropped a power saw on his right foot. Two toes were bruised, and the fifth toe was lacerated. He applied a small dressing and, by changing to a loose old shoe, was able to continue working. The bruises subsided, and the laceration was healing well. Eight days later, he noted the recurrence of pain in the lacerated toe and had severe generalized headaches. He was restless and unable to work and went to bed.

73. The next day, this patient might be expected to manifest

    (A) irritability and repeated clonic spasms of all the skeletal muscles
    (B) severe spreading cellulitis of the right leg
    (C) chills, fever, rapid pulse, and spreading cellulitis with raised edges
    (D) malaise, fever, prostration, right inguinal adenopathy, and several small vesicles on the right fifth toe
    (E) mania, paralysis of the muscles of deglutition, and severe spasms on coughing and taking fluids by mouth
    (2:186–188)

74. The potent toxin produced in the infection characteristically

    (A) demyelinates the nerves of the brain and spinal cord
    (B) produces acute peripheral neuritis
    (C) acts at the neuromuscular junction and at the neurons centrally
    (D) passes along the nerve axis cylinders to the central nervous system
    (E) produces lesions in the gray matter of the spinal cord
    (2:186–188)

75. In the presence of the symptoms of severe toxicity, the lacerated right fifth toe should be

    (A) amputated
    (B) carefully debrided
    (C) treated conservatively
    (D) cauterized
    (E) widely excised and packed at the wound
    (2:186–188)

76. One of the important features of the management of the patient would be

    (A) control of the convulsions with sedation and relaxants, plus tracheostomy and control of respiration
    (B) maintenance of the patient on a respirator
    (C) very intensive antibiotic therapy
    (D) wide incision and drainage of the tissues of the leg
    (E) midthigh amputation
    (2:186–188)

77. If death occurs, it would be due to

    (A) generalized flaccid paralysis
    (B) progressive respiratory failure
    (C) overwhelming septicemia
    (D) cardiac arrest due to the convulsions
    (E) bacterial endocarditis
    (2:186–188)

Questions 78 through 80

A 40-year-old man has undergone a Billroth II partial gastrectomy. On the third postoperative day, this patient becomes shocky. On the sixth postoperative day, he has a purulent, foul-smelling drainage from the wound, which opens. At this time, he complains of pain in the left shoulder.

78. The most likely cause of this situation is

    (A) intraabdominal hemorrhage
    (B) wound infection
    (C) pancreatitis
    (D) dehiscence of the duodenal stump
    (E) coronary thrombosis
    (2:479)

79. In this patient, the most appropriate test to establish the diagnosis would be

    (A) an upper gastrointestinal series
    (B) upright chest and abdominal films
    (C) serum amylase determination
    (D) white blood cell count
    (E) electrocardiogram
    (2:479)

80. The best treatment of the patient would be

    (A) immediate operation and sump suction drainage
    (B) immediate operation and resuture of the duodenal stump
    (C) conservative care with gastric aspiration, antibiotics, intravenous fluid, and electrolyte replacement
    (D) observe to see if a local abscess will form
    (E) apply suction to the draining wound *(2:479)*

81. A 60-year-old woman is in shock with a major acute hemorrhage from the rectum. She has passed red blood in large quantities. Which of the following is the LEAST likely cause of bleeding of this type from the large bowel?

(A) diverticulosis of the left colon
(B) carcinoma of the colon
(C) angiodysplasia
(D) ulcerative colitis
(E) ischemic colitis   *(1:612)*

82. A man aged 50 has a curative resection of a Dukes B carcinoma of the sigmoid colon with an anastomosis at the rectosigmoid junction. Ideally, the follow-up should include all of the following EXCEPT

(A) carcinoembryonic antigen levels every 2 months
(B) fecal blood every 6 months
(C) barium enema every year
(D) colonoscopy every year
(E) clinical examination if possible every 6 months   *(1:602)*

Questions 83 and 84

A 30-year-old white female has suffered from three bouts of pneumonia during the past year. She suffers from coughing spells at night. She notices difficulty with swallowing, particularly when emotionally upset. There has been a 10-lb weight loss during the past year. Liquids are taken, but solids are difficult to swallow.

83. The most likely diagnosis is

(A) peptic esophagitis
(B) carcinoma of the esophagus
(C) achalasia of the esophagus
(D) peptic ulcer
(E) hiatal hernia   *(2:1068–1069)*

84. The initial treatment of the patient would be

(A) Heller's procedure
(B) esophageal dilatation
(C) partial gastrectomy
(D) esophagogastrostomy
(E) radiotherapy   *(2:1069–1069)*

85. In performing an esophagectomy for carcinoma of the lower third of the esophagus and in restoring continuity with an esophagogastrostomy, which pair of arteries should you preserve?

(A) left gastric and right gastric
(B) right gastric and right gastroepiploic
(C) right gastroepiploic and left gastroepiploic
(D) left gastric and right gastroepiploic
(E) left gastroepiploic and left gastric
                    (2:1094–1095)

86. A 65-year-old man complains of dysphagia that has been present for 9 months. He also regurgitates undigested food. The most likely diagnosis is

(A) pharyngoesophageal (Zenker's) diverticulum
(B) hiatal hernia
(C) carcinoma of the esophagus
(D) achalasia of the distal esophagus
(E) esophageal web   *(1:374–375)*

87. Treatment of a patient with peritonitis consists of fluid and electrolyte replacement, systemic antibiotics, and the operative control of sepsis. The following statements concern the operative management. Which is NOT correct?

(A) the incision is usually in the midline. The first step is to obtain aerobic and anaerobic cultures of the fluid
(B) the primary problem is then corrected
(C) the peritoneal cavity is lavaged with about 3 L of warm isotonic saline
(D) in severely infected patients, repeat operations may be required until all locations are drained
(E) prophylactic drainage should be employed in most patients   *(1:407)*

88. In an omphalocele, which of the following is/are correct?

(A) it is covered only by the peritoneum and the amniotic membrane
(B) it should be repaired immediately after birth
(C) the prognosis is poor if the amniotic membrane is ruptured
(D) it often contains part of the liver
(E) all of the above   *(2:1663)*

89. A 2-week-old infant is admitted with vomiting that commenced at birth but has become progressively worse and has contained bile. The stools have been scanty and there has been a progressive refusal of food. The examination reveals a moderately distended upper abdomen. Which of the following would be the LEAST likely diagnosis?

(A) hypertrophic pyloric stenosis
(B) duodenal atresia
(C) annular pancreas
(D) superior mesenteric artery syndrome
(E) malrotation of the colon   *(2:1648–1649)*

90. The dumping syndrome after a partial gastrectomy is due primarily to

   (A) hyperosmolarity in the jejunum
   (B) hypoosmolarity in the jejunum
   (C) gastric achlorhydria
   (D) hypoglycemia
   (E) bile reflux into the stomach   *(2:1123-1124)*

91. The most important factor responsible for the prevention of gastroesophageal reflux is

   (A) intraabdominal position of the cardioesophageal junction
   (B) pinchcock action by the diaphragmatic crura
   (C) intrinsic lower esophageal sphincter
   (D) oblique entrance of the esophagus into the stomach (angle of His)
   (E) integrity of the phrenoesophageal ligament   *(2:1074)*

92. A young man was shot in the abdomen 4 hours before admission. The entry wound is in the left lower quadrant; there is an extensive wound of the sigmoid colon about 2 cm above the peritoneal reflexion. There are no other major injuries. Which of the following procedures should be carried out?

   (A) exteriorization of the injured colon
   (B) debridement and closure of the colon wound with proximal diverting colostomy and drainage
   (C) Hartmann's operation and drainage
   (D) debridement and closure of the colon with drainage and careful observation
   (E) debridement and closure of the colon wound with drainage and tube cecostomy   *(2:240-241)*

93. Malrotation of the cecum often is associated with

   (A) volvulus of the midgut
   (B) duodenal atresia
   (C) Meckel's diverticulum
   (D) tracheoesophageal fistula
   (E) intussusception   *(2:1651)*

Questions 94 through 96

A 40-year-old obese woman has suffered for some years from easy fatigability and bouts of confusion. She has found that the attacks have been relieved by eating. She has noticed episodes of hunger, weakness, and tachycardia. Recently, she has also suffered from attacks of fainting and mental confusion. Just before she was admitted, she went into coma.

94. The most likely diagnosis is

   (A) hepatic failure
   (B) islet cell tumor of the pancreas
   (C) Cushing's syndrome
   (D) aldosteronism
   (E) chronic nephritis   *(2:1365-1367)*

95. The most useful diagnostic test would be

   (A) tolbutamide test
   (B) fasting blood sugar
   (C) blood ammonia
   (D) serum sodium and potassium
   (E) blood urea nitrogen   *(2:1365-1367)*

96. The best treatment for the patient would be

   (A) resection of the pancreatic adenoma
   (B) total pancreatectomy
   (C) resection of the distal two thirds of the pancreas if no lesion is found
   (D) bilateral adrenalectomy
   (E) hemodialysis   *(2:1365-1367)*

97. A 50-year-old man complains of severe pain when he passes stool. The pain persists for 30 to 40 minutes. The most likely cause is

   (A) an anorectal fistula
   (B) an anal fissure
   (C) coccygodynia
   (D) carcinoma of the rectum
   (E) hemorrhoids   *(2:1224-1225)*

98. A 50-year-old man, a reformed alcoholic, is found to have esophageal varices. He has not bled. His serum albumin is 3.7, he is not jaundiced, he has no ascites, and his nutrition is excellent. He can be classified as Child's group A. Which of the following is the best management?

   (A) expectant treatment is the best treatment unless the patient is part of a clinical trial
   (B) prophylactic sclerotherapy
   (C) a total portacaval shunt
   (D) a distal splenorenal (Warren) shunt
   (E) treat the patient with propranolol prophylactically   *(1:477-478)*

Questions 99 and 100

A 65-year-old man is known to have a duodenal ulcer. He bleeds massively, suffering with hematemesis and melena. He is in mild shock with a hemoglobin of 6.5 g. He is blood group B, Rh negative. There is a shortage of group B, Rh-negative blood.

99. The best intravenous fluid to treat this patient would be

   (A) blood group B, Rh positive
   (B) dextran
   (C) plasma
   (D) serum albumin
   (E) blood group A, Rh negative   *(2:104)*

100. The patient responds well to treatment. The next step in treatment is either medical or surgical but should NOT include

   (A) subtotal gastrectomy
   (B) feeding and, if necessary, transfusion
   (C) vagotomy and hemigastrectomy
   (D) truncal vagotomy alone
   (E) gastric aspiration and transfusion, unless necessary   *(2:1128)*

DIRECTIONS (Questions 101 through 168): Each question consists of an introduction followed by five statements. Mark T (true) or F (false) after each statement.

101. Which of the following statements is/are true in regard to ventricular septal defects?

   (A) there is an increased susceptibility to bacterial endocarditis
   (B) they produce a to-and-fro murmur along the right sternal border
   (C) pulmonary blood flow exceeds systemic blood flow
   (D) operation is recommended when pulmonary vascular resistance is three-fourths systemic resistance
   (E) small defects need not be closed *(2:766-770)*

102. During the resection of an infrarenal abdominal aortic aneurysm, the surgeon notes that the inferior mesenteric artery is about 1 cm in diameter. The following statements concern the steps that should be taken.

   (A) palpate the origins of the celiac, superior mesenteric, and hypogastric arteries
   (B) divide the inferior mesenteric artery close

to the aorta and observe any changes in the left colon
   (C) preserve a cuff of aortic wall around the origin of the inferior mesenteric artery
   (D) observe the backflow from the inferior mesenteric artery
   (E) divide the inferior mesenteric artery and exteriorize a loop of sigmoid colon as a precaution   *(4:977-978)*

103. The postpericardiotomy syndrome is characterized by fever, malaise, and pericardial and pleural effusions.

   (A) fever during the first 5 days after cardiopulmonary bypass usually is due to atelectasis
   (B) low-grade aseptic pericarditis responds to aspirin or indomethacin
   (C) the postpericardiotomy syndrome can occur as late as 3 months postoperatively
   (D) thoracentesis may be necessary
   (E) hospital admission usually is required   *(1:320)*

104. The following statements concern the problem of breast cancer and pregnancy.

   (A) the data are insufficient to determine whether interruption of pregnancy improves the prognosis of patients found to have breast cancer during pregnancy
   (B) theoretically the increased levels of estrogen produced by the placenta could be detrimental in a patient with an estrogen receptor-positive tumor
   (C) pregnancy is, in general, inadvisable in patients with axillary node involvement at the time of treatment for breast carcinoma
   (D) theoretical considerations and not firm clinical evidence from controlled trials are the basis for opinions concerning pregnancy and breast cancer
   (E) in patients with inoperable or stage IV breast cancer, the harmful effects of hormone therapy, radiotherapy, and chemotherapy on the fetus are an added reason to advise interruption of an early pregnancy   *(1:267)*

105. In primary hyperaldosteronism

    (A) in most patients, adenomas are present in both adrenal glands
    (B) the cortex of the adrenal glands is usually hypoplastic
    (C) the plasma renin level is elevated
    (D) hypokalemic alkalosis is common
    (E) nephropathy may occur   *(2:1509-1512)*

106. Which statements are true concerning large, peripheral, traumatic arteriovenous fistula?

    (A) the immediate effect is a decrease in both systolic and diastolic blood pressure
    (B) the late effect is an increase in both systolic and diastolic blood pressure
    (C) obliteration of the fistula causes a decrease in pulse rate
    (D) they usually result in arterial insufficiency of the extremity distal to the fistula
    (E) ligation of the proximal artery is adequate treatment   *(2:931-934)*

107. Following the treatment of a supracondylar fracture of the elbow in a young child, the patient complains of severe pain, and the radial pulse is not palpable. Which of the following statements concerning the diagnosis and management of brachial artery spasm or thrombosis in this type of injury is/are true?

    (A) irreversible damage to the muscles of the forearm does not usually occur during the first 18 to 24 hours
    (B) active extension of the fingers causes pain, but passive extension does not
    (C) in the less severe cases, the ulnar nerve is more often damaged than is the median nerve
    (D) the greatest damage is usually to the flexor digitorum profundus and the flexor pollicis longus
    (E) the cast should be removed and fasciotomy performed   *(2:2083-2085)*

108. Stress fractures

    (A) are most commonly found in the middle-aged and elderly
    (B) often involve the metatarsals, proximal tibia, and distal fibula
    (C) are painless
    (D) when first symptomatic, may show only osteoporosis of the stressed area on x-ray examination
    (E) treatment is immobilization   *(2:1956)*

109. Which of the following statements is/are true regarding fractures in children as compared with fractures in the adult?

    (A) open or compound fractures are more common in children
    (B) nonunion of fractures occurs more commonly in children
    (C) in children, shaft fractures of the long bones should be treated by open reduction more often than similar fractures in the adult
    (D) similar fractures heal more rapidly in children than in adults
    (E) disturbance of epiphyseal growth leads to deformity   *(2:1952)*

110. The following statements concern the solitary nodule in the thyroid gland.

    (A) a solitary thyroid nodule is more likely to be malignant than is a multinodular goiter
    (B) low-dose radiation in infancy or childhood is associated with an increased incidence of thyroid cancer later in life
    (C) a thyroid nodule is more likely to be cancer in women than it is in men
    (D) hot thyroid nodules rarely are malignant
    (E) thyroid cancer is present in 10% of children with solitary cold thyroid nodules   *(1:244)*

111. In patients with endometriosis

    (A) an implant on the colon can produce recurring symptoms of partial bowel obstruction
    (B) small peritoneal implants can cause incapacitating pain
    (C) symptoms occur only after the onset of regular menstruation
    (D) menstrual aberrations occur in less than half of the symptomatic patients
    (E) the pathology is not always intraabdominal   *(2:1757-1758)*

112. The following statements concern rejection of a renal transplant.

    (A) most rejections occur in the first 3 months
    (B) acute rejection can be treated with an increased dosage of corticosteroids. It can be reversible
    (C) chronic rejection is resistent to treatment, and kidney loss eventually occurs

(D) hyperacute rejection is due to preformed cytotoxic antibodies against donor lymphocytes or renal cells; it can be reversed
(E) during rejection, the kidney becomes smaller   *(1:1173–1174)*

113. In 1872, Moritz Kaposi described a sarcoma that developed on the legs and feet. In 1981, the Center for Disease Control reported an outbreak of an aggressive form of Kaposi's sarcoma in male homosexuals. The following statements concern this lesion.

(A) in the mildest form, bluish red raised nodules occur predominantly on the legs
(B) renal transplant patients are reported to have a much greater incidence of Kaposi's sarcoma than the general population
(C) Kaposi's sarcoma is endemic in central Africa
(D) the severe aggressive form is associated with lymphadenopathy and visceral involvement
(E) most patients with Kaposi's sarcoma have acquired immunodeficiency syndrome (AIDS)   *(3:1591–1593)*

114. Morphine is the most widely used narcotic for the relief of postoperative pain. The following statements concern morphine.

(A) morphine depresses respiration
(B) pain is a powerful respiratory stimulant
(C) morphine stimulates intestinal activity
(D) morphine usually is given intravenously
(E) morphine given intramuscularly produces a peak analgesic effect in 30 minutes   *(1:20–21)*

115. Which of the following statements concerning the oxyhemoglobin dissociation curve are true? (A shift to the left indicates that less oxygen is released at a given tissue oxygen tension; a shift to the right indicates that more oxygen is released at a given tissue oxygen tension.)

(A) cooling shifts the oxyhemoglobin dissociation curve to the left
(B) hydrogen ions shift the dissociation curve to the right
(C) carbon dioxide shifts the dissociation curve to the right
(D) red cell diphosphoglycerate (DPG) shifts the curve to the right

(E) warming shifts the curve to the right   *(2:160–165)*

116. Carcinoma of the prostate has been diagnosed in a man aged 70. The following statements concern his treatment.

(A) a stage A_1 cancer requires observation only
(B) if the tumor is stage A_2 or B_1 or B_2, the best treatment is total prostatectomy and pelvic lymphadenectomy
(C) radiation therapy is the best treatment for stage C lesions
(D) a symptomatic patient with metastasis should receive estrogens
(E) transurethral prostatectomy usually is required in patients receiving palliation only   *(1:869–871)*

117. In idiopathic retroperitoneal fibrosis

(A) the first symptom is dull, noncolicky pain
(B) on pyelography, the ureters are displaced medially
(C) symptoms of intermittent claudication are due to compression of the aorta or iliac arteries
(D) ureteral obstruction is due to fibrous tissue invasion of the ureter
(E) peristalsis of the ureter is normal   *(3:787–788)*

118. The following statements concern villous adenomas of the rectum and colon.

(A) the first symptom often is the discharge of blood and mucus from the rectum
(B) invasive malignancy is found at the time of first treatment in about one third of patients
(C) a majority of patients pass numerous watery mucoid stools rich in electrolytes. Hypokalemia and hypochloremia result
(D) if invasive cancer is present, a formal resection for malignancy is required
(E) when invasive cancer is not demonstrable on biopsy, the lesion is locally excised and fully examined histologically. If malignancy is found, a resection for malignancy is required. If malignancy is not found, nothing further need be done   *(3:1003)*

119. The following statements refer to mitral stenosis.

(A) cardiac cachexia is characteristic
(B) pulmonary vascular resistance may be increased dramatically
(C) atrial fibrillation is a rare complication
(D) atrial fibrillation decreases cardiac output by 20%
(E) atrial fibrillation often is complicated by systemic embolization   *(3:2348)*

120. Protein loss after injury

(A) is due to impaired protein synthesis
(B) occurs primarily from muscle
(C) is commensurate with the protein catabolism needed to supply energy
(D) is greater in healthy young men than in debilitated, elderly men
(E) is greater in the malnourished than in the well nourished   *(2:27)*

121. Cancers of the thyroid gland exhibit a wide range of growth and malignant behavior. The following statements are about thyroid cancer.

(A) papillary adenocarcinoma occurs in young adults, grows very slowly, and is compatible with a long life even when metastasis are present
(B) undifferentiated carcinomas occur late in life, and the prognosis is very poor
(C) follicullar adenocarcinoma may be difficult to distinguish microscopically from normal thyroid tissue. The metastases often pick up radioactive iodine after total thyroid ablation
(D) carcinomas of the colon, prostate, and stomach are the most likely to metastasize to the thyroid gland
(E) subtotal and partial thyroidectomy are acceptable operations for papillary carcinoma of the thyroid   *1:246-247)*

122. Bacterial cholangitis can be a serious and sometimes fatal condition. The following statements concern this problem.

(A) Charcot's triad—biliary colic, jaundice, chills and fever—occurs in 70% of patients
(B) obstruction of the bile duct, either partial or complete, is always present
(C) most cases of bacterial cholangitis require drainage of the common bile duct
(D) cholangiography is an important investigation that should be performed in onset cases
(E) suppurative cholangitis requires immediate drainage of the common bile duct
          (1:503-504)

123. Primary carcinoma of the liver is common in East Asia and parts of Africa. It is uncommon in the USA.

(A) chronic hepatitis B infection is the principal etiologic factor worldwide
(B) ultrasound scanning combined with alpha-fetoprotein (AFP) measurement is a widely used screening method in the USA
(C) resection of the tumor offers the only possibility of cure
(D) palliative resection can be of value in selected cases
(E) about 25% of primary liver cancers are resectable, and the 5-year survival rate after curative surgery is about 30%
          (1:463-465)

124. The classic treatment of a caustic burn of the esophagus formerly was administration of antibiotics and corticosteroids followed by observation for the formation of late strictures. The introduction of very strong alkali solutions into the marketplace has changed this.

(A) determination of the extent of injury by esophagoscopy is important
(B) a first degree injury (mucosal hyperemia, edema, and superficial desquamation) may be treated without operation
(C) urgent laparotomy with inspection of the distal esophagus and stomach together with a full-thickness gastric biopsy is the best treatment for second and third degree injuries
(D) second and minor third degree injuries are treated by the insertion of a Silastic tube stent and a feeding jejunostomy
(E) severe third degree injuries require emergency esophagectomy, a cervical esophagostomy, and a feeding jejunostomy
          (1:378-379)

125. Solitary pulmonary nodules or coin lesions are circumscribed pulmonary lesions seen on x-ray. They are due to granulomatous disease or cancer.

(A) lesions less than 1 cm in diameter probably are benign
(B) the larger the lesion the greater the likelihood of malignancy

(C) a history of living in an area where granuloma is endemic favors the diagnosis of granuloma

(D) the 5-year survival in patients with malignant coin lesions after resection is about 20% if the lesion is less than 2 cm

(E) it is probable that the most useful study is a previous chest x-ray for comparison *(1:313–314)*

126. Systemic symptoms associated with radiation therapy (malaise, nausea, vomiting, and weakness) are related to the

(A) rate of delivery of the radiation
(B) volume of tissue irradiated
(C) dose delivered per session
(D) type of tissue treated
(E) total dose *(2:344)*

127. The cure rate of which of these malignancies is higher with surgery than with radiation therapy?

(A) adenocarcinoma of the lung
(B) ovary
(C) pancreas
(D) neuroblastoma
(E) renal cell carcinoma *(2:363–366)*

128. You would advise radiation rather than operative removal for most patients with which of the following tumors?

(A) inflammatory breast carcinoma
(B) oat cell carcinoma of the lung
(C) Hodgkin's disease
(D) actinic skin cancer
(E) renal cell carcinoma *(2:345)*

129. Peritoneal adhesions are now the most common cause of acute and recurrent small bowel obstruction in North America. How can adhesions be prevented?

(A) tissue ischemia, mechanical trauma, infection, and foreign body reaction predispose to adhesion formation

(B) precise and gentle operative technique reduces adhesion formation

(C) abdominal packs are satisfactory when well moistened

(D) the peritoneal floor should always be covered with peritoneum even if it means doing so under tension

(E) intraperitoneal irrigation with 200 ml of high molecular weight (70) dextran has

proved to be effective in preventing primary adhesions *(1:417)*

130. Renal allograft transplantation for end-stage renal disease is CONTRAINDICATED in a

(A) 45-year-old diabetic woman
(B) 69-year-old cirrhotic man with severe emphysema
(C) patient with Goodpasture's disease (antibodies to glomerular basement membrane)
(D) patient with a large carcinoma of the bladder
(E) patient well controlled on dialysis *(2:410)*

131. Hyperacute rejection of a renal allograft

(A) is unrelated to the number of blood transfusions received before transplantation
(B) is unrelated to the rejection of a previous transplant
(C) becomes apparent 2 to 3 days after transplantation
(D) is an indication for immediate nephrectomy
(E) is likely mediated by humoral antibody *(2:420)*

132. Complications of immunosuppressive therapy following renal transplantation include

(A) a susceptibility to bacterial infection
(B) iatrogenic Cushing's disease
(C) an increased incidence of malignancy
(D) an increased incidence of cataracts
(E) fungal infections *(2:391)*

133. Which of the following is/are characteristic of halothane anesthesia?

(A) the toxic concentration is eight times the concentration necessary to produce surgical anesthesia
(B) very high levels of oxygen may be administered with halothane
(C) halothane is one of the safest general anesthetic agents when anesthesia must be given by inexperienced personnel
(D) it is frequently associated with arterial hypotension
(E) it is safe to administer epinephrine when halothane is being used *(3:160–161)*

134. Which of the following statements is/are true in regard to fractures of the proximal humerus?

    (A) shoulder motion is started after 4 weeks in older patients, after 2 weeks in younger patients
    (B) fractures of the greater tuberosity should be reduced anatomically
    (C) humeral shaft fractures are more common than humeral neck fractures
    (D) in older people, proximal humeral fractures occur in the surgical neck rather than in the anatomic neck of the humerus
    (E) they occur in the anatomic neck in children   (2:1967)

135. In tubal pregnancy

    (A) the first symptom is shock in 70 to 80% of patients because of exsanguinating hemorrhage that occurs at the time of rupture
    (B) the patient usually has the symptoms and signs of early pregnancy and always has a history of recent menstrual irregularity
    (C) the uterus will be enlarged and soft even if there is no history of menstrual irregularity
    (D) a tubal mass may not be palpable even if the patient is symptomatic from a tubal pregnancy
    (E) a test for pregnancy will be positive   (2:1753)

136. When large transfusions are administered in a short period of time (massive transfusion)

    (A) patients who survive do not have a high probability of developing isoantibodies subsequently and, therefore, a high risk of subsequent transfusion reaction
    (B) warming the blood decreases the incidence of cardiac arrest
    (C) a high blood citrate level does not produce a bleeding diathesis
    (D) the large amount of potassium infused is unlikely to cause cardiac arrest unless the patient has oliguria
    (E) fresh frozen plasma should be given   (2:107-108)

137. The following statements concern hepatic encephalopathy.

    (A) elderly patients are more susceptible after a portal systemic shunt than are young individuals
    (B) encephalopathy is less common after a distal splenorenal shunt than other portal systemic shunts
    (C) alcoholics do worse than those with postnecrotic cirrhosis
    (D) patients with preoperative thrombosis of the portal vein do badly
    (E) constipation can be beneficial   (1:485)

138. Pneumothorax may be traumatic, spontaneous, or iatrogenic.

    (A) both open chest wounds and tension pneumothorax are surgical emergencies
    (B) iatrogenic pneumothorax may follow the insertion of a central venous pressure catheter
    (C) in young adults, spontaneous pneumothorax develops from emphysematous blebs usually near the apex of the upper lobe of the lung
    (D) chest pain frequently occurs and is referred to the shoulder or arm of the involved side
    (E) the key to treatment is reexpansion of the lung   (1:292)

139. The following statements deal with the preservation of donor kidneys for transplantation.

    (A) the kidney may be preserved with simple hypothermia or continuous pulsatile perfusion
    (B) simple hypothermia provides good preservation for 48 hours
    (C) continuous pulsatile perfusion provides good preservation for 3 days
    (D) the kidney should be removed immediately after cardiac arrest
    (E) the cadaver donor must have good kidney function   (1:1169-1170)

140. In a 15-year-old child who has a large, symptomatic pulmonary arteriovenous fistula, the following would be expected.

    (A) polycythemia
    (B) pulmonary artery hypertension
    (C) cyanosis
    (D) opacification of the lesion on arch aortography
    (E) low pulmonary venous pressure (2:668-669)

141. Because of the innervation of the abdomen and its contents with both visceral and somatic or parietal nerves, abdominal pain has some unusual patterns.

(A) pain caused by irritation of the undersurface of the diaphragm is felt at the tip of the shoulder blade (inferior angle of the scapula)

(B) pain at the commencement of acute appendicitis is felt around the umbilicus

(C) pain due to cholecystitis can be felt at the tip of the shoulder, having been referred via the phrenic nerve

(D) the later pain of acute appendicitis is a somatic (parietal) pain felt over the location of the appendix, usually in the right lower quadrant

(E) with a perforated peptic ulcer the pain may move down the right flank to the right lower quadrant   *(1:394)*

142. The following statements are about fat embolism.

   (A) most patients are symptomatic within 24 hours of the trauma that produced fat embolism

   (B) it occurs with soft tissue trauma as well as with fractures of the long bones

   (C) fever commonly occurs

   (D) in a patient with extensive trauma, an elevated serum lipase level in the first 48 hours is probably due to pancreatitis rather than to fat embolism

   (E) intravenous alcohol is the treatment of choice   *(2:470–472)*

143. The clinical diagnosis of fat embolism is suggested by

   (A) delirium
   (B) tachycardia
   (C) petechiae
   (D) a sudden rise in the hematocrit
   (E) respiratory distress syndrome   *(2:470–472)*

144. Following appendectomy, the patient develops a wound infection, and *Clostridium perfringens* is cultured from the pus. The patient has no clinical signs of clostridial myonecrosis (gas gangrene). Treatment should consist of

   (A) specific antitoxin
   (B) antibiotics
   (C) hyperbaric oxygen
   (D) open drainage
   (E) observation only   *(2:184–185)*

145. The treatment of a patient with tetanus includes

   (A) excision and debridement of the wound
   (B) control of convulsions

(C) antibiotics

(D) large doses of tetanus toxoid

(E) human tetanus immune globulin *(2:187–188)*

146. The following mediastinal lesions are characteristically found in the anterior mediastinum.

   (A) teratomas
   (B) thymic tumors
   (C) intrathoracic parathyroid adenomas
   (D) bronchogenic cysts
   (E) small cell anaplastic carcinomas
                            (2:692; 716–724)

147. A young adult has sustained blunt trauma to the abdomen. At operation, the pancreas is found to be completely transected, but the spleen and duodenum are intact. The following procedures would be considered good surgical treatment.

   (A) distal pancreatectomy; oversewing the proximal severed end

   (B) oversewing the distal severed end of the pancreas and pancreaticojejunostomy to the proximal end

   (C) pancreaticojejunostomy to both proximal and distal severed ends

   (D) thorough drainage of the area only

   (E) total pancreatectomy   *(6:700)*

148. The following statements concern disseminated intravascular coagulation (DIC).

   (A) DIC consumes enough of some clotting factors that diffuse bleeding may occur

   (B) a common clinical manifestation is bleeding from needle puncture sites

   (C) heparin may be necessary to stop the pathologic clotting

   (D) DIC is uncommon in patients having urologic procedures

   (E) DIC may follow massive trauma   *(1:53)*

149. The following statements concern the autologous transfusion of blood.

   (A) blood drawn at the rate of a unit per week can be predeposited before an elective surgical procedure

   (B) intraoperative autotransfusion may be a valuable adjunct in the management of major trauma

   (C) intracavity blood contains fibrinogen

   (D) systemic anticoagulation is required when intraoperative autotransfusion is used

   (E) embolii are a problem during intraoperative autotransfusion   *(1:53–54)*

150. The following statements concern hepatic resection.

    (A) removal of 85% of the liver is compatible with survival
    (B) the cirrhotic liver regenerates well
    (C) the serum albumin should be greater than 3 g/L before operation
    (D) in many patients, there is fever after the operation and no cause can be found
    (E) most elective hepatectomies require a thoracoabdominal incision   *(1:460–461)*

151. The treatment of patients with acute cholecystitis is controversial. The following statements concern this problem.

    (A) the disease resolves spontaneously in 60% of patients
    (B) an emergency is present as in acute appendicitis
    (C) the decision to perform a cholecystostomy should be made at the time of the operation
    (D) if perforation or empyema is suspected, emergency operation is indicated
    (E) in patients with poor general condition, percutaneous catheter cholecystostomy may be used   *(1:498–500)*

152. Gastric carcinoma develops in 25,000 patients in the USA each year. This has dropped from 75,000 30 years ago. The reason for this is unknown. The following statements concern gastric carcinoma.

    (A) the mean age at diagnosis is 50
    (B) it is found equally among men and women
    (C) the first symptom is often postprandial heaviness and discomfort
    (D) an upper gastrointestinal series is diagnostic in 90% of patients
    (E) the proximal stomach is the site of the tumor in 45% of patients   *(1:450–452)*

153. These statements are in regard to pneumothorax in the infant.

    (A) it is a rare occurrence
    (B) it is often treated by chest tube to ensure survival
    (C) it is a common complication of hyaline membrane disease
    (D) tension pneumothorax is treated by catheter aspiration of air

    (E) the air leak seals promptly after catheter aspiration of tension pneumothorax *(3:1262)*

154. In infantile lobar emphysema, the following are found on the chest film.

    (A) wedge-shaped densities adjacent to the affected lobe
    (B) radiodensity of the affected lobe
    (C) elevation of the ipsilateral diaphragm
    (D) mediastinal shift to the opposite side
    (E) retrosternal radiolucency   *(3:1262)*

155. The following statements concern the thymoma.

    (A) myasthenia gravis occurs only with the lymphocytic type of thymoma
    (B) most thymomas are first diagnosed by a routine chest x-ray in an asymptomatic patient
    (C) the treatment of choice is total thymectomy
    (D) following thymectomy, about one third of patients with myasthenia gravis achieve complete remission
    (E) the presence of malignancy can be established by a histologic examination of the tumor   *(1:298)*

156. The following statements are in regard to the operative treatment of tracheoesophageal fistula (TEF).

    (A) the infant should always be operated on as soon as possible after the diagnosis is made
    (B) a gastrostomy does not help prevent reflux of gastric contents into the esophagus in most instances
    (C) if there is an unavoidable delay in operating following diagnosis, it is imperative that repair be accomplished no longer than 24 hours after diagnosis
    (D) sump catheter decompression of the proximal esophageal pouch is useful
    (E) at the first operation, the TEF is closed, but it is usually unwise to attempt esophageal anastomosis   *(3:1264–1266)*

157. Cyclosporine is a fungal cyclic peptide that represents an entire new class of clinically important immunosuppressive agents.

    (A) it is an antimitotic agent
    (B) cyclosporine inhibits the production of cytotoxic T cells

(C) it is prescribed in combination with moderate doses of prednisone

(D) it is an alkylating agent

(E) it does not induce lymphoma in the recipient *(2:386-387)*

158. The following statements concern postoperative hepatic dysfunction.

(A) increased hemolysis often results from incompatible blood transfusion

(B) posttransfusion hepatitis develops soon after surgery

(C) anesthesia may cause hepatocellular insufficiency

(D) liver function tests are useful in determining the cause of post hepaticobilary obstruction

(E) renal function must be monitored closely in patients with postoperative jaundice *(1:33)*

159. Pyogenic osteomyelitis of the vertebral column

(A) causes severe back pain that is not relieved by rest

(B) is most common during adolescence and in young adulthood

(C) does not usually cause marked collapse of the vertebral bodies

(D) is most common in the thoracic region

(E) is most often due to *Staphylococcus aureus* infection *(3:1891-1892)*

160. Peritoneal lavage is used as a diagnostic procedure in an adult who has sustained blunt abdominal trauma. A liter of Ringer's lactate is infused into the peritoneal cavity. In the returned fluid, a positive test is indicated by

(A) bile in the fluid

(B) greater than 25,000 RBC/mm³

(C) greater than 500 WBC/mm³

(D) bacteria in the fluid

(E) fluid amylase of 25 units *(6:160)*

161. Instances in which parenteral hyperalimentation is indicated include

(A) an adult who remains decerebrate 8 weeks after an accident

(B) a patient with excessive metabolic requirements following severe injury

(C) as preparation of the bowel for left colectomy for carcinoma

(D) prolonged paralytic ileus following multiple operations for a pancreatic abscess

(E) preoperative treatment of severe relapsing pancreatitis *(2:75)*

162. The following are indications for exploration of penetrating wounds of the neck and thoracic inlet.

(A) thoracic wounds whose trajectory traverses the superior mediastinum or thoracic inlet

(B) radiologic evidence of a widened mediastinum

(C) a large hematoma

(D) any wound above the clavicle or manubrium that penetrates the platysma muscle

(E) a stab wound of the esophagus *(2:221)*

163. Empyema is the term used for an infected effusion within the pleural space.

(A) common causative organisms are *Staphylococcus aureus* and *Streptococcus pyogenes*

(B) the patient may be severely toxic

(C) needle aspiration with antibiotics is the preferred treatment

(D) metastatic brain abscesses are a common complication

(E) closed tube drainage with negative pressure reduces the size of the residual air space *(1:288-290)*

164. The evaluation of the patient who begins to bleed during or after surgical procedures may be an emergency situation that is difficult to solve.

(A) if large quantities of banked blood have been used, the patient should be assumed to be thrombocytopenic until proved otherwise

(B) bleeding from the surgical wound and not from cutdowns usually does not indicate a general hemostatic problem

(C) bleeding after use of extracorporeal bypass may be due to inadequate neutralization of heparin

(D) severe hemorrhagic disorders due to thrombocytopenia may occur in gram-negative sepsis

(E) a common cause of this problem is inadequate or ineffective hemostasis *(2:89)*

165. These methods of sterilizing surgical instruments are considered quite reliable.

    (A) autoclaving (saturated steam at 75 mm Hg and 120°C
    (B) boiling in water for 30 minutes
    (C) dry heat at 170°C for 1 hour
    (D) soaking in 2% aqueous alkaline glutaraldehyde
    (E) gas sterilization in 12% ethylene oxide and 88% freon for 105 minutes at 410 mm Hg and 55°C   *(2:195)*

166. Carbuncles develop from the confluent infection of hair follicles (furuncles) that spreads through the dermis to the subcutaneous tissue. As the carbuncle enlarges, the blood supply to the skin is destroyed, and the center becomes necrotic.

    (A) carbuncles are common
    (B) carbuncles are seen more often in diabetics
    (C) carbuncles must be treated with antibiotics and incision
    (D) carbuncles often are more extensive than they appear to be
    (E) carbuncles on the neck may lead to epidural abscess and meningitis   *(1:108–109)*

167. At present, the following procedures are thought to decrease the incidence of tumor spread at the time of surgery.

    (A) the use of 0.5% formaldehyde to prevent local recurrence from carcinoma of the cervix
    (B) the use of plastic drapes to protect the edges of the incision
    (C) electric cauterization of the cut surface of a tumor entered during the course of the operation
    (D) irrigation of the wound with sodium hypochlorite
    (E) early ligature of the arterial supply   *(6:230)*

168. The following statements concern the surgical treatment of lung cancer.

    (A) this usually involves laryngoscopy, bronchoscopy, and mediastinoscopy
    (B) often the possibility for resection can be determined only during the operation
    (C) lobectomy is the treatment of choice in good-risk patients with localized disease
    (D) lasers can be used to restore a lumen to an obstructed bronchus, which may give effective palliation

    (E) bronchoplastic procedures can be used for bronchial adenomas   *(1:308–313)*

DIRECTIONS (Questions 169 through 180): Each of the numbered items or incomplete statements in this section is followed by answers or by completions of the statement. Select the ONE lettered answer or completion that is BEST in each case.

169. Cancer of the lung can cause manifestations that are extrathoracic and not due to metastases. Which of the following statements is INCORRECT?

    (A) connective tissue syndromes, such as dermatomyositis, scleroderma, or hypertrophic pulmonary osteoarthropathy, may develop
    (B) carcinoid syndrome with weight loss, anorexia, explosive diarrhea, cutaneous flushing, and tachycardia may develop
    (C) clubbing of the digits or hypertrophic pulmonary osteoarthropathy have an adverse prognostic significance
    (D) migratory thrombophlebitis may occur
    (E) oat cell carcinomas may cause hyperadrenocorticism and the inappropriate production of antidiuretic hormone   *(1:310)*

170. Which of the following comments on the anatomy of the blood supply of the stomach or duodenum is INCORRECT?

    (A) the inferior pancreaticoduodenal artery is a branch of the gastroduodenal artery
    (B) the left gastric artery is a branch of the celiac artery
    (C) the fundus of the stomach along the greater curvature is supplied by short gastric arteries (vasa brevia)
    (D) venous blood from the stomach drains into the portal vein via the coronary, gastroepiploic, and splenic veins
    (E) the right gastric artery is a branch of the hepatic artery   *(1:423)*

171. The stomach contributes to the digestion of food in many ways. Which of the following statements about the role of the stomach is INCORRECT?

    (A) the cephalic phase of gastric secretion is abolished by vagotomy
    (B) the presence of food in the small intestine releases entero-oxyntin, which stimulates gastric acid secretion

(C) a meal with a high fat content leaves the stomach in less than 3 hours in most individuals

(D) a pH below 2 to 5 in the antrum inhibits the release of gastrin

(E) the presence of food in the stomach stimulates the release of gastrin from the antrum *(1:425–426)*

172. An otherwise healthy woman aged 60 is found after an x-ray taken during a routine physical examination to have several medium-sized (5 cm) gallstones. You would NOT

(A) advise elective cholecystectomy

(B) do a cholecystogram

(C) advise cholecystectomy if the gallbladder was not functioning

(D) advise cholecystectomy if the gallbladder was calcified

(E) advise cholecystectomy if a large radiolucent stone was demonstrated in addition to the medium-sized stones *(1:496–498)*

173. Of the following statements concerning the portal venous circulation, which is true?

(A) the portal vein is formed by the junction of the superior and inferior mesenteric veins

(B) the pressure in the portal vein is usually 10 to 15 cm of water

(C) sudden occlusion of the portal vein results in a fall in the hepatic artery flow

(D) occlusion of the hepatic artery causes the portal venous pressure to rise

(E) the left gastric vein drains into the splenic vein *(1:471–472)*

174. A woman aged 30 has a massive infarction of the small intestine. After resection, she is left with 1.5 m (4 feet) of small intestine. The proximial jejunum has been anastomosed to the ileum 10 cm from the iliocecal valve. Her postoperative management will include all of the following EXCEPT

(A) massive fluid and electrolyte replacement

(B) total parenteral nutrition

(C) cimetidine 200 mg every 6 hours intravenously

(D) loperamide to control the diarrhea

(E) oral feeding as soon as possible *(1:565–567)*

175. The treatment of a documented acute compartment syndrome of the leg is

(A) elevation

(B) fasciotomy

(C) antibiotics

(D) support hose

(E) physical therapy *(2:1990)*

176. Malignant tumors of the anus are uncommon, and some types are rare. Which of the following tumors does NOT arise from the anus?

(A) epidermoid carcinoma

(B) adenocarcinoma

(C) malignant melanoma

(D) Bowen's disease

(E) basal cell carcinoma *(1:647)*

177. Which statement is true concerning total joint replacement?

(A) longevity of the replacement is best in younger patients

(B) infection is not a problem

(C) longevity of the replacement is best in older patients

(D) bilateral replacements cannot be performed because of the technical considerations

(E) component breakage is not a problem *(2:1995)*

178. Spondylolisthesis is

(A) an anterior subluxation of one vertebral body on another

(B) an idiopathic osteolysis of the posterior bony elements of the spine

(C) associated only with a herniated nucleus pulposis

(D) not seen before the fourth decade of life

(E) a terminal diagnosis before paraplegia develops *(2:1885)*

179. Of the following statements about hormone manipulation in the premenopausal patient, all are correct EXCEPT

(A) in the past, bilateral oophorectomy was the usual first choice for hormonal manipulation in premenopausal women
(B) the antiestrogen tamoxifen is used instead of oophorectomy
(C) those who respond to tamoxifen and then relapse may subsequently respond to aminoglutethimide (secondary hormonal therapy)
(D) aminoglutethimide inhibits adrenal hormone synthesis. When combined with a corticosteroid, aminoglutethimide provides an effective medical adrenalectomy
(E) megestrol acetate is no longer used in premenopausal patients   *(1:270)*

180. The frequency of pseudomembranous enterocolitis following use of clindamycin is

(A) 1%
(B) 5%
(C) 10%
(D) 15%
(E) 20%   *(18:794–795)*

Answers and Explanations

1. **(C)** A cystometrogram gives information on bladder capacity and innervation. It is not useful in a suspected colovesical fistula. A barium enema is the best study.

2. **(E)** Pneumaturia is usually due to colovesical fistula, and diverticulitis is the most common cause.

3. **(A)** The finding of sterile pyuria is highly suggestive of renal tuberculosis, a disease that is still quite common in India.

4. **(A)** The diagnosis is made most directly by a culture of the sediment of a 24-hour specimen of urine for acid-fast bacilli.

5. **(A)** Tuberculosis must be treated as a general disease. This is best done with chemotherapy for 2 years.

6. **(C)** Perforation of the esophagus should be ruled in or out.

7. **(E)** Once a patient has had a stone removed from the common bile duct, there is always the possibility of recurrence.

8. **(A)** Again, there is a history of a previous common bile duct stone coupled with a dilated common bile duct. Even if a stone is not visualized, it is still the most likely cause of the problem.

9. **(B)** Stones may form in the common bile duct, but common sense indicates that it is more likely that a small stone was not removed at the first procedure.

10. **(D)** Mitral stenosis causes pulmonary venous hypertension, and hemoptysis is often a sign of the resulting pulmonary congestion.

11. **(A)** Most human infections occur in childhood after the ingestion of material contaminated by dog feces.

12. **(B)** Although the urinary excretion of calcium occasionally is raised in Paget's disease of bone, the serum calcium and phosphorus usually are normal, and there is not an increased incidence of urinary calculi.

13. **(D)** Medullary thyroid carcinoma has such a high incidence of nodal involvement that, in addition to total thyroidectomy, a central lymph node dissection should be performed, followed by concomitant or interval prophylactic neck dissection, especially if the serum calcitonin remains elevated after thyroidectomy.

14. **(B)** Arteriography is now rarely used, but digital subtraction angiography can be useful for mapping the venous pattern.

15. **(E)** Mastectomy is seldom if ever indicated because metastases occur early and widely. Radiotherapy, chemotherapy, and hormone therapy are the most valuable measures. This lesion is rarely curable.

16. **(E)** Common tumors in this location are neurogenic tumors. In young children, the neuroblastoma is the most common.

17. **(C)** Metastases to the liver and subcutaneous tissues are frequent in young children with neuroblastomas.

18. **(D)** A localized neuroblastoma should be excised if possible and the area irradiated. However, most tumors are unresectable when first seen. The best treatment is then radiotherapy and chem-

otherapy, followed by surgery if the tumor becomes resectable.

19. **(B)** Paget's carcinoma frequently is diagnosed as dermatitis, causing an unfortunate delay of treatment.

20. **(E)** Carcinoma of the lung is a cause of lung abscess. The presence of such an abscess does not indicate inoperability.

21. **(D)** The presence of emphysema in the neck, combined with the history and physical signs, indicates a rupture of the bronchus.

22. **(B)** The treatment of rupture of the bronchus is initially closed chest drainage. If the lung does not remain expanded, thoracotomy and repair of the bronchus are indicated.

23. **(C)** Androgens have many side effects and should rarely be used.

24. **(D)** There is no association between gastric ulcer and carcinoma of the esophagus. All of the other conditions are considered to be precancerous.

25. **(D)** Most cavities, even large ones, resolve with efficient medical treatment, but occasionally surgery may be necessary to rule out other diseases, such as cancer.

26. **(A)** Bronchogenic carcinoma is the most common cause of superior vena cava obstruction.

27. **(C)** The prognosis is poor in young adults, women, and children, probably because adenocarcinomas and undifferentiated tumors predominate in these patients.

28. **(C)** The history given is indicative of a dissecting thoracic aortic aneurysm.

29. **(E)** Aortography will establish the diagnosis in most patients with dissecting aneurysms of the aorta.

30. **(B)** The results of decortication are best if the procedure is not unduly delayed.

31. **(C)** Simple repair and drainage (because of the high incidence of salivary leak) is the treatment for the wound described. Massive loss of tissue (e.g., gunshot wounds) may require cutaneous pharyngoscopy and cutaneous esophagostomy.

32. **(D)** Primary repair of the facial nerve is indicated unless there is gross contamination or massive loss of tissue. The major duct is repaired over a stent, which is then removed. If repair is impossible, the duct is ligated. Irradiation to cause gland atrophy would be contraindicated in a patient this young.

33. **(E)** These small lacerations of the liver are adequately and best treated by drainage alone. Packing with Gelfoam can prolong bile drainage, and unnecessary sutures can restart bleeding. Adequate drainage is a required part of the treatment of any traumatic liver injury.

34. **(E)** Modern surgical and radiographic techniques have improved our handling of the retroperitoneal hematoma due to blunt trauma. Massive retroperitoneal hematomas following pelvic fractures are best not explored. This can cause uncontrollable bleeding and prevent spontaneous tamponade. Embolization or thrombotic therapy through an angiographic catheter may prove to be the treatment of choice. With modern surgical techniques, all other hematomas are best explored to find and control the bleeding point and to identify injuries to adjacent hollow and solid viscera.

35. **(A)** Probably the only surprise in this list is the very radiosensitive Ewing's sarcoma of bone. The low cure rate by radiation alone is related to the frequency of distant metastases, not to its lack of sensitivity to ionizing radiation.

36. **(D)** Decreased cardiac output due to venous pooling of blood is accentuated by the head-up position and is overcome by the head-down position. Decreased venous return often due to the head-up position is the most common cause of respiratory and cardiac arrest during spinal anesthesia.

37. **(D)** You should suspect pyogenic arthritis rather than cellulitis with a secondary knee effusion. Aspiration is necessary for diagnosis. Aspiration until the joint is as dry as possible is good therapy. Because your diagnosis of pyogenic arthritis may be wrong, do not aspirate through the involved skin. It is a good idea to begin therapy with a well-selected antibiotic before the culture results are known.

38. **(A)** Because *Haemophilus* is suspect, ampicillin should be the antibiotic of choice among the

agents listed. Methicillin might well be selected for an adult in whom related findings suggested the possibility of penicillin-resistant staphylococci. The likelihood of coliform infection, possibly requiring gentamicin therapy, is remote. There are other reasons for avoiding tetracycline therapy in young children, even when the organism is sensitive.

39. **(B)** In a child and in most adults, surgical drainage is necessary. Removing and preventing the reaccumulation of pus in the joint is a necessary part of therapy. In streptococcal infections, daily aspiration may be successful. The joint must be put at rest. Skin traction would be used for this patient.

40. **(C)** A CT scan of the abdomen is the best study. It is highly sensitive and specific, being accurate in more than 95% of cases.

41. **(B)** Paraplegia is a serious complication of this operation, the risk of which is minimized by adequate bypass perfusion. Nevertheless, paraplegia may still occur from ligature of the intercostal arteries arising from the aneurysm.

42. **(E)** One of the major consequences of flail chest is oxygen desaturation caused by a functional right-to-left shunt created by the failure of the lung under the flail segment to ventilate.

43. **(C)** The bronchial arteries give branches that form a capillary plexus in the muscular coat of the bronchial tubes. Branches are given off from this plexus to a second plexus that communicates with the pulmonary circulation.

44. **(E)** Paralysis of the facial nerve may result from trauma, including surgical operations. It may be associated with viral infections, including herpes zoster, or it may be caused by tumors, particularly of the cerebellopontine angle. When the cause of this paralysis is not known, it is called Bell's palsy.

45. **(D)** Vitamin B_{12} (cyanocobalamin) binds with intrinsic factor in the stomach. This makes vitamin B_{12} unavailable to intestinal microorganisms. This vitamin B_{12}–intrinsic factor complex becomes dissociated in the ileum where the water-soluble vitamin B_{12} is absorbed.

46. **(C)** Splenectomy for spherocytosis does not change the osmotic fragility or shape of the red cells. A transient leukocytosis occurs, and the erythrocytes achieve a normal life span. As a result, the anemia does not persist and is relieved.

47. **(A)** The common anticancer drugs do not interfere with wound healing as long as the total granulocyte count is at least 1500.

48. **(C)** The pressure in the gastroesophageal sphincter is normally 20 mm Hg. In achalasia, it may rise to 40 mm Hg or twice normal, not to 4 times the normal level.

49. **(B)** The subclavian steal syndrome is due to thrombosis of the subclavian artery proximal to the origin of the vertebral artery.

50. **(E)** In about one quarter of the patients with hypothyroidism, the cause is subtotal thyroidectomy, usually for thyrotoxicosis, although the indication for the operation may have been a nodular goiter. An increasingly frequent cause of hypothyroidism is ^{131}I therapy for hyperthyroidism.

51. **(C)** All of the manifestations occur in patients with ulcerative colitis except thyroiditis.

52. **(C)** Radiotherapy alone cures 1 to 2% carcinoma of the lung.

53. **(C)** Carcinoma of the body of the pancreas may cause pain of this type.

54. **(B)** It is usual to try controlled forceful dilatation before a surgical operation.

55. **(A)** Renal failure in a recently burned patient is probably due to tubular obstruction by protein precipitate. This can be prevented by maintaining, with a sufficient water load, a urine output of 30 to 50 ml per hour.

56. **(B)** An elevated serum potassium causes the following changes in the electrocardiogram: high peaked T waves, a widened QRS complex, and depressed ST segments. At higher levels, heart block and diastolic cardiac arrest occur.

57. **(C)** Uric acid stones are nonopaque to x-rays and would explain the filling defect in the left renal pelvis and the probable obstruction to the right ureteropelvic junction.

58. (B) It is important to establish the diagnosis of nonradiopaque urinary calculi.

59. (D) Antonio Moniz was a neuropsychiatrist who won the Nobel Prize for introducing the operation of prefrontal obotomy. This operation has been abandoned.

60. (E) Idiopathic thrombocytopenic purpura in a child is best treated conservatively because remission may occur. Steroids also are of value. If the disease becomes chronic, splenectomy is indicated.

61. (B) The following structures lie within the carpal tunnel: the flexor sublimis and profundus tendons, the flexor pollicis longus, and the median nerve.

62. (B) One fifth of the patients with congenital wryneck also have hip dysplasia. The condition first becomes evident in the early months of life, and x-ray examination is useful to exclude vertebral anomalies as the cause. Excision of the tender swelling when the child will tolerate the procedure eliminates the cause of subsequent changes. The first sign is a tender swelling in the lower part of the sternocleidomastoid muscle. Stretching the muscle is painful and increases the tenderness.

63. (B) The abscess is usually large and single. Treatment consists of the administration of metronidazole together with aspiration or incision and drainage when necessary. The pus is positive for *Entamoeba* in less than one third of patients.

64. (E) At the scene of the accident, the exact nature of the injury, if any, cannot be determined. Half the injuries occur in hyperextension. The safest course is to immobilize the neck with a semirigid cervical collar and backboard.

65. (B) Wide local excision of the primary—in this case, by amputation of the toe—is recommended. Prophylactic groin dissection is not advised as a routine procedure.

66. (A) Neurogenic tumors are the most common asymptomatic tumors of the costovertebral region or paravertebral gutter.

67. (B) The thenar space is separated from the midpalmar space by a septum from the palmar fascia to the third metacarpal. The tendon sheath of the index finger does not connect with other tendon sheaths or bursae.

68. (E) The thenar space is best drained by an incision on the dorsum of the hand just behind the web between the thumb and index finger.

69. (C) Secondary closure is the approximation of a wound more than 7 days after it occurs. This requires skin grafting or excision of the wound margins, mobilization of the skin edges, and approximation with sutures. It is a bigger procedure than delayed primary suture. It is not the same as healing by second intention.

70. (B) With adequate treatment, deaths are unusual, but the outlook for limb salvage is not so favorable, and many affected limbs have to be amputated.

71. (C) To be hemodynamically significant, a stenosis of the internal carotid artery must occlude more than 75% of the lumen. Microemboli from a plaque occur even when the lumen is less compromised, and they are common.

72. (C) The extracellular fluid changes significantly in all of the conditions except inflammatory carcinoma of the breast.

73. (A) This patient is likely to have tetanus.

74. (C) The exotoxin of tetanus causes muscular contractions and spasms by acting at the neuromuscular junction and stimulating the neurons centrally.

75. (A) The wound would be excised. When the tetanus-infected wound is on the fifth toe, amputation is the most effective way of obtaining an adequate wound excision.

76. (A) Control of the contractions plus tracheostomy and control of respirations is important because the main cause of death in these patients is respiratory arrest.

77. (B) Respiratory arrest is the main cause of death in tetanus.

78. (D) Blowout of the duodenal stump is the most common cause of death after a Billroth II gastrectomy.

79. **(B)** The presence of free air in the upper abdomen is valuable evidence of duodenal stump blowout in such patients.

80. **(A)** Immediate reoperation is mandatory, as is a sump suction drain placed in the region of the leaking duodenal closure.

81. **(B)** Benign or malignant neoplasms rarely cause acute massive exsanguinating hemorrhage.

82. **(C)** Barium enema examinations are not used routinely in most follow-up programs.

83. **(C)** "Spillover pneumonitis" in a patient age 40 with the symptoms noted is usually due to achalasia of the esophagus or cardiospasm.

84. **(B)** Mechanical hydrostatic dilatation has been found a useful technique and is the preferred initial method of management.

85. **(B)** Reconstruction is performed by anastomosing the stomach to the esophagus high in the thorax, usually proximal to the divided azygos vein. This is done by forming a gastric pouch that is sufficiently mobile to be moved into the upper thorax and that has a blood supply sufficient for the esophagogastric anastomosis to heal. The mobility is achieved by dividing the left gastric and the left gastroepiploic arteries, and the blood supply is retained by preserving the right gastric and the right gastroepiploic arteries.

86. **(A)** The likely diagnosis is a pharyngoesophageal diverticulum. A barium x-ray usually is diagnostic. It is of interest that many patients have a hiatal hernia in addition to a diverticulum and that esophageal webs can produce almost the same symptoms but are uncommon.

87. **(E)** Drainage of the free peritoneal cavity is ineffective and often undesirable.

88. **(E)** Omphalocele is a rare defect of the periumbilical abdominal wall in which the coelomic cavity is covered only by the peritoneum and the amniotic membrane.

89. **(A)** The infant with hypertrophic pyloric stenosis does not vomit bile. With duodenal atresia, the bile duct sometimes enters distal to the obstruction when the vomitus does not contain bile.

90. **(A)** The dumping syndrome is largely due to distention of the jejunum by an outpouring of extracellular fluid into the bowel lumen, which is the result of the premature entry into the proximal bowel of hypertonic chyme.

91. **(C)** In spite of the demonstration of an intrinsic lower esophageal sphincter, there remains considerable controversy as to the exact method by which gastroesophageal reflux is prevented. Although other factors play a part, the intrinsic sphincter, which functions best when in the normal position, is the most important.

92. **(B)** The principles of management of patients with wounds of the colon are well established. It is recommended that severe wounds of the left colon be either exteriorized as a colostomy or repaired and returned to the peritoneal cavity, with a proximal diverting colostomy being performed at the time of the initial surgery. It is not possible to exteriorize the colon 2 cm from the peritoneal reflexion. Therefore, the treatment is repair and immediate diverting colostomy.

93. **(A)** From the sixth to eleventh week of intrauterine life, part of the midgut protrudes into the umbilical cord. The midgut is then withdrawn into the peritoneal cavity and rotates in a counterclockwise direction. Incomplete rotation leaves the cecum in the right upper quadrant. This is associated with a failure of fixation of the mesentery, and volvulus of the whole midgut may result.

94. **(B)** Patients with insulinomas have a wide variety of symptoms, and they often are obese from overeating in attempts to prevent the attacks. The symptoms vary from sweating and hunger to mental confusion and coma.

95. **(B)** In a patient with an insulinoma, prolonged fasting invariably will produce a blood sugar of below 50 mg per 100 ml. This is the most valuable test. The response of the blood sugar to oral or intravenous tolbutamide also is useful. Patients with an insulinoma have a greater and more prolonged depression of the blood sugar than normal.

96. **(A)** It is essential to mobilize the pancreas and explore it very carefully. The adenoma, if found, should be excised. Controversy arises if the adenoma is not found, and since authorities differ, it is not possible to state whether total or distal

pancreatectomy is the best treatment when this problem arises.

97. **(B)** An anal fissure causes severe burning or tearing pain when passing stool. The pain subsides a little when the stool has passed, but this is followed by spasm of the sphincter muscles, which causes the pain to return for half an hour or more.

98. **(A)** Patients with varices that have not bled have a 25% chance of bleeding, with a mortality of 50% for those who bleed. It is possible that prophylactic sclerotherapy may be of value, but clinical trials have not been completed.

99. **(A)** A few units of Rh-positive blood can be administered to Rh-negative recipients if compatible on a Coombs' crossmatch. This must never be done in girls or women of childbearing age.

100. **(D)** Although most would advise surgery in this patient, medical treatment would be given a trial by many. Truncal vagotomy without a limited gastrectomy or a drainage procedure would be a mistaken form of therapy.

101. **(A) (T), (B) (F), (C) (T), (D) (F), (E) (F)**
There is an increased risk of developing bacterial endocarditis (15 to 30%), and this is possibly an indication for considering the closure of small, asymptomatic defects. The characteristic murmur is a pansystolic murmur along the left sternal border. Pulmonary blood flow does exceed systemic blood flow. Early correction of the defect in symptomatic patients is recommended to prevent the great increase in pulmonary vascular resistance. When pulmonary vascular resistance is greater than one-half systemic resistance, the risk of operation is very great, and the chance of improvement is small.

102. **(A) (T), (B) (F), (C) (T), (D) (T), (E) (F)**
A large inferior mesenteric artery indicates probable disease of the celiac and superior mesenteric arteries. Such inferior mesenteric arteries should be reimplanted. In this situation, it is wise to preserve a cuff of the aneurysmal wall around the origin of the inferior mesenteric artery. This facilitates reimplantation. It is wise to observe the backflow from the inferior mesenteric artery. An indication for exteriorization of the left colon is ischemia. Reimplantation of the inferior mesenteric artery should make this unnecessary.

103. **(A) (T), (B) (T), (C) (T), (D) (T), (E) (T)**
All the statements are correct.

104. **(A) (T), (B) (T), (C) (T), (D) (T), (E) (T)**
All the statements are true.

105. **(A) (F), (B) (F), (C) (F), (D) (T), (E) (T)**
In 90% of patients, the adenoma is unilateral. The adrenal glands usually are normal in size, although 15% of patients have bilateral adrenal hyperplasia. The aldosterone hypersecretion is renin-independent, and the plasma renin level is low. Hyperaldosteronism leads to hypokalemic alkalosis, which, if prolonged, leads to hypokalemic nephropathy.

106. **(A) (T), (B) (F), (C) (T), (D) (F), (E) (F)**
When the fistula is first created, peripheral vascular resistance is lowered, and this decreases both systolic and diastolic blood pressure. Later, blood volume increases, and systolic blood pressure increases. Occlusion of the fistula increases peripheral vascular resistance with reflex slowing of the heart rate. Usually there is no severe arterial insufficiency of the extremity. Ligature of the artery proximal to the fistula can be disastrous.

107. **(A) (F), (B) (F), (C) (F), (D) (T), (E) (T)**
Most of the damage leading to Volkmann's ischemic contracture occurs within a few hours; treatment is always urgent. Both active and passive finger extension usually causes severe pain. Check active and passive finger extension in every patient with an elbow or forearm injury. The greatest damage usually is to the deepest muscles lying in close relation to the anterior interosseus artery—the flexor digitorum profundus and the flexor pollices longus. Either median or ulnar nerve may be involved, but the ulnar nerve is involved in only the most severe cases.

108. **(A) (F), (B) (T), (C) (F), (D) (T), (E) (T)**
Stress fractures may occur in any age group, and the location depends on the type of occupation or activity causing the repeated stress. They are most commonly found in the younger person who, voluntarily or otherwise, repeatedly stresses his lower extremities without proper conditioning. The second and third metatarsals, the proximal tibia, and the distal fibula are common sites. A fracture may not be evident on the x-ray films when first symptomatic. Early in the course, they may show only subtle osteoporosis of the stressed

site. Later, new periosteal bone formation is seen along with a complete or incomplete fracture.

109. **(A) (F), (B) (F), (C) (F), (D) (T), (E) (T)**
Open or compound fractures are less common in children, and nonunion is extremely rare. Open reduction of shaft fractures is avoided to prevent epiphyseal growth disturbance and deformity. Younger patients heal their fractures more rapidly than do older patients.

110. **(A) (T), (B) (T), (C) (F), (D) (T), (E) (F)**
A thyroid nodule is more likely to be cancer in men than it is in women. A solitary cold thyroid nodule in a child is cancerous in nearly 50% of patients. Therefore, thyroidectomy usually is indicated.

111. **(A) (T), (B) (T), (C) (T), (D) (T), (E) (T)**
Keep this lesion in mind when your gynecologist calls you to the operating room because on exploration he has found a small, submucosal lesion of the sigmoid colon. (Clever radiologists can diagnose this lesion preoperatively.) It is of interest that large lesions may be asymptomatic and small ones are at times responsible for very severe pain. Symptoms usually develop in the 20s and 30s, not before or at the onset of menstruation. Abnormal bleeding during the menstrual flow or abnormal periodicity of the menstrual cycle should lead you to suspect endometrial polyps or leiomyomas rather than endometriosis alone. In the majority of cases, endometriosis does not interfere with ovarian function.

112. **(A) (T), (B) (T), (C) (T), (D) (F), (E) (F)**
There is no effective method of treating a hyperacute rejection. During rejection, the kidney becomes enlarged and tender to palpation, the tenderness being caused by peritransplant inflammation and stretching of host tissues.

113. **(A) (T), (B) (T), (C) (T), (D) (T), (E) (T)**
All statements are true. It is of interest that Kaposi's sarcoma in patients with a renal transplant has been noted to regress when immunosuppressive agents are withdrawn.

114. **(A) (T), (B) (T), (C) (F), (D) (F), (E) (F)**
Morphine depresses intestinal activity. It is usually given intramuscularly. An intravenous injection requires a nurse to be in attendance during the 10 to 15 minute period of administration. The intravenous route is, therefore, practical only in the recovery room or intensive care unit. On

a regular floor, it is usually given intramuscularly, when the peak effect occurs at 1 to 2 hours. It can be given intravenously without a nurse in attendance if the dose rate is at 2 to 3 mg per hour or less.

115. **(A) (T), (B) (T), (C) (T), (D) (T), (E) (T)**
In the capillaries, several factors combine to encourage oxygen unloading. These include heat (including the heat produced by working tissues), hypoxic acidosis, carbon dioxide from cellular metabolism, and red cell DPG.

116. **(A) (T), (B) (T), (C) (T), (D) (T), (E) (F)**
On occasion, a patient receiving palliation develops urethral obstruction, but this is not common.

117. **(A) (T), (B) (T), (C) (T), (D) (F), (E) (F)**
Although biopsy of the fibrotic mass is the only way to be certain of the diagnosis, medial displacement of one or both ureters is a helpful sign. Retroperitoneal tumors displace the ureters laterally. Urinary signs and symptoms are much more common than vascular symptoms, which may, however, constitute the main problem. The fibrotic process compresses but does not invade the tubular, retroperitoneal structures. Hydronephrosis develops even without complete ureteral obstruction because peristalsis ceases in the involved segment.

118. **(A) (T), (B) (T), (C) (F), (D) (T), (E) (T)**
A minority not a majority of patients develop an interesting syndrome consisting of passage of watery mucoid stools rich in electrolytes. This may produce severe hypokalemia, hypochloremia, and often hyponatremia and uremia.

119. **(A) (T), (B) (T), (C) (F), (D) (T), (E) (T)**
Cardiac cachexia is characteristic of mitral stenosis. Mitral stenosis may cause a rise in pulmonary venous pressure, and some patients also develop an increase in pulmonary vascular resistance. These patients develop early right ventricular enlargement, tricuspid annulus dilatation and insufficiency, hepatomegaly, cardiac cirrhosis, and, ultimately, anasarca. Atrial fibrillation is common, probably secondary to atrial dilatation. Fibrillation decreases cardiac output by 20% and increases ventricular rate, decreasing filling time. Both mechanisms compound the problem of retarded pulmonary venous outflow. Systemic embolization from atrial mural thrombus is a common problem.

120. **(A) (F), (B) (T), (C) (F), (D) (T), (E) (F)**
Most of the protein loss after injury is from the storage protein in muscle. Debilitated or starved patients may lose little protein following trauma. The muscle protein catabolism following trauma is far in excess of that needed to supply energy. It may be related to the need for carbohydrate intermediates via gluconeogenesis rather than to the total energy need. Carbohydrate intermediates are used for the synthesis of nonessential amino acids, glycogen, glucose, and tricarboxylic acid cycle intermediates.

121. **(A) (T), (B) (T), (C) (T), (D) (F), (E) (F)**
Carcinomas of the kidney, breast, and lung are the most likely to metastasize to the thyroid gland, but they rarely do so as solitary nodules. For papillary carcinomas, total or nearly total thyroidectomy is an acceptable operation. Partial or subtotal thyroidectomy is contraindicated because of the shorter survival time.

122. **(A) (T), (B) (T), (C) (F), (D) (F), (E) (T)**
The infection in most cases of bacterial cholangitis can be controlled with intravenous antibiotics. In moderate cases, a cephalosporin should be used, and in severe cases, both an aminoglycoside and clindamycin should be added. Direct cholangiography is dangerous during active cholangitis. The term "suppurative cholangitis" has been used for the most severe form of this disease.

123. **(A) (T), (B) (F), (C) (T), (D) (F), (E) (T)**
Combined ultrasound scanning and AFP measurement is used to detect liver cancer in high-risk areas, such as East Asia. The AFP level can be used as an index of the success of hepatectomy. There is no place for palliative resection in patients with primary liver cancer.

124. **(A) (T), (B) (T), (C) (T), (D) (T), (E) (T)**
The modern strong alkali solutions produce severe burns that require aggressive treatment. The important fact is that full-thickness injuries cannot be diagnosed at esophagoscopy. A laparotomy and biopsy usually are required.

125. **(A) (T), (B) (T), (C) (T), (D) (F), (E) (T)**
The 5-year survival after resection for a lesion of less than 2 cm is 70%. This means that in good-risk patients, surgical resection is warrented when cancer cannot be excluded.

126. **(A) (T), (B) (T), (C) (T), (D) (T), (E) (T)**
All of these factors are of importance in determining how rapidly treatment can progress without incapacitating the patient.

127. **(A) (T), (B) (T), (C) (T), (D) (T), (E) (T)**
In most tumors of the gastrointestinal tract, urinary tract, endocrine glands, and central nervous system, the cure rate is higher with surgery than with radiation therapy.

128. **(A) (T), (B) (T), (C) (T), (D) (F), (E) (F)**
It is likely that chemotherapy or chemotherapy plus radiation will prove to be the treatment of choice for inflammatory breast cancer. Usually surgery rather than radiation therapy is advised for radiation-induced (actinic) skin cancer.

129. **(A) (T), (B) (T), (C) (F), (D) (F), (E) (T)**
Abdominal packs either moist or dry should be used sparingly because they produce abrasive serosal tears. Reperitonealization of the pelvic floor under tension has been shown to promote rather than reduce adhesion formation.

130. **(A) (F), (B) (T), (C) (F), (D) (T), (E) (F)**
Indications for renal transplantation vary from center to center, and the contraindications have become fewer in recent years. In some patients with high risks of infection following immunosuppression (severe emphysema), transplantation is not considered, whereas in others (diabetes), it is successful. The use of age as a contraindication is quite variable. Uncontrollable infections and malignancies are absolute contraindications. In Goodpasture's syndrome, nephrectomy precedes transplantation by 6 to 12 months, and transplantation is delayed until the antiglomerular basement membrane antibody has reached a low level.

131. **(A) (F), (B) (F), (C) (F), (D) (T), (E) (T)**
The hyperacute rejection that becomes apparent at the time of transplantation is likely mediated by humoral antibody, and its definite diagnosis is indication for immediate nephrectomy. It occurs most commonly in patients who have received many transfusions or who have rejected a previous transplant.

132. **(A) (T), (B) (T), (C) (T), (D) (T), (E) (T)**
All of these and a number of other complications are side effects of immunosuppression.

133. **(A) (F), (B) (T), (C) (F), (D) (T), (E) (F)**
Although halothane is one of the safest anesthetic agents when used by experienced personnel, it would be a very unsafe agent for use by the inexperienced. It is so potent that it can be given with oxygen concentration in excess of 98%. The toxic concentration is only about two times that necessary to produce surgical anesthesia. Its hypotensive effect is decreased by combining it with nitrous oxide.

134. **(A) (F), (B) (T), (C) (F), (D) (T), (E) (T)**
The most common fracture of the proximal humerus is a fracture of the surgical neck, which is prevalent in older people but may occur at any age. A similar injury in children results in a fracture of the anatomic neck. To preserve normal function if there is a fracture of the greater tuberosity, it should be reduced anatomically by open reduction and screw fixation, if necessary. Early shoulder motion is begun as soon as the fracture site is stable. In the young, it need not be started before 3 or 4 weeks, but in the elderly, to minimize shoulder stiffness, gentle exercises of the shoulder are started as early as 7 to 10 days.

135. **(A) (F), (B) (F), (C) (F), (D) (T), (E) (F)**
This is a disease of diagnostic surprises. Often the symptoms and findings do not fit the so-called classic findings of ruptured ectopic pregnancy, but even in the classic picture, crampy lower abdominal pain followed by steady pain precedes syncope. Ruptured ectopic pregnancies can occur with no history of one or two missed periods, and they occur in the face of seemingly successful contraception with the pill or with intrauterine devices. Unfortunately, one does not always find an enlarged uterus with tubal pregnancy. It is a helpful sign if present, but its absence should not cause you to rule out the possibility. The tubal pregnancy, even at rupture, does not always enlarge the tube sufficiently to produce a mass that can be found during a careful examination under anesthesia. Culdocentesis will almost always yield nonclotting blood and will lead to the correct diagnosis. When this examination fails, only laparoscopy may help to make the correct preoperative diagnosis.

136. **(A) (T), (B) (T), (C) (T), (D) (T), (E) (T)**
Patients who survive massive transfusion are not at high risk from subsequent transfusion reactions. During massive transfusion, however, they are at risk from incompatible blood transfusion, which can be prevented only by careful cross-matching, and each unit given increases the risk of homologous serum hepatitis. Warming the blood reduces the chance of hypothermic-induced cardiac arrhythmia. Excess citrate may result in skeletal and cardiac muscle conduction defects by depressing the level of ionized calcium, but reduced ionized calcium is exceedingly unlikely to result in bleeding in this circumstance.

137. **(A) (T), (B) (T), (C) (F), (D) (F), (E) (F)**
Alcoholics do better than postnecrotic patients, particularly if the alcoholic has reformed. Preoperative thrombosis of the portal vein allows the patient to adapt to diversion of the portal blood away from the liver. Constipation is harmful because it gives more time for bacterial action on the colon contents.

138. **(A) (T), (B) (T), (C) (T), (D) (T), (E) (T)**
All statements are correct.

139. **(A) (T), (B) (F), (C) (T), (D) (F), (E) (T)**
Simple hypothermia provides good preservation for a maximum of 30 hours, preferably less. The kidney may be removed up to 1 hour after cardiac arrest provided that intraaortic flush with iced solution is used for in situ cooling of the kidneys.

140. **(A) (T), (B) (F), (C) (T), (D) (F), (E) (T)**
Pulmonary arteriovenous fistulas often are multiple when polycythemia, cyanosis, and a low pulmonary venous pressure develop. These lesions are opacified by pulmonary—not aortic—arch angiography.

141. **(A) (F), (B) (T), (C) (F), (D) (T), (E) (T)**
The pain referred from under the diaphragm travels via the phrenic nerve to the area on the tip of the shoulder supplied by the C4 segment, not to the tip of the shoulder blade. The pain from cholecystitis is felt over the inferior angle of the scapula, not at the tip of the shoulder.

142. **(A) (T), (B) (T), (C) (T), (D) (T), (E) (F)**
The use of intravenous alcohol in the treatment of fat embolism is at best debatable.

143. **(A) (T), (B) (T), (C) (T), (D) (F), (E) (T)**
Fat embolism may produce a sudden drop in the hematocrit. It does not cause hemoconcentration.

144. **(A) (F), (B) (T), (C) (F), (D) (T), (E) (F)**
Simple contamination of a wound by *Clostridium* is common. In the absence of dead tissue, the

condition is not serious. Drainage of the wound and appropriate antibiotics are indicated.

145. **(A) (T), (B) (T), (C) (T), (D) (F), (E) (T)**
Tetanus toxoid is widely used in the prophylaxis of tetanus. It is not used in the treatment of this disease.

146. **(A) (T), (B) (T), (C) (T), (D) (F), (E) (F)**
Bronchogenic cysts usually are located posterior and inferior to the carcinoma. Small cell anaplastic carcinomas usually are central in location, having arisen from a proximal bronchus.

147. **(A) (T), (B) (F), (C) (T), (D) (F), (E) (F)**
In such a patient, the spleen should be preserved. Satisfactory results follow either distal pancreatectomy and oversewing the proximal severed end or anastomosis of both the ends proximal and distal to the jejunum.

148. **(A) (T), (B) (T), (C) (T), (D) (F), (E) (T)**
DIC occurs in patients with carcinoma of the prostate and in patients having prostatic operations. On rare occasions, heparin may be used to stop the pathologic clotting.

149. **(A) (T), (B) (T), (C) (F), (D) (F), (E) (F)**
Intracavity blood used during intraoperative autotransfusion does not coagulate. It has virtually no fibrinogen. Systemic anticoagulation is not required during intraoperative autotransfusion. Emboli are entirely preventable when the intraoperative autotransfusion is used properly.

150. **(A) (T), (B) (F), (C) (T), (D) (T), (E) (F)**
The cirrhotic liver has little capacity for regeneration. Most elective hepatectomies can be performed through an abdominal incision; the key to technical success is hemostasis.

151. **(A) (T), (B) (F), (C) (F), (D) (T), (E) (T)**
In acute appendicitis, perforation is a major risk, and an emergency is present. In acute cholecystitis, free perforation occurs in less than 2% of patients. The decision to perform a cholecystostomy should be made before operation because its use depends on factors apparent during the preoperative evaluation.

152. **(A) (F), (B) (F), (C) (T), (D) (F), (E) (F)**
The mean age at diagnosis is 65, and it is twice as common in men as in women. An upper gastrointestinal series has an overall false negative rate of about 20%. Endoscopy and biopsy

are the most accurate diagnostic tools. Only 25% of tumors occur at the cardia, but the frequency has changed so that proximal tumors are more common than they used to be.

153. **(A) (F), (B) (T), (C) (T), (D) (F), (E) (F)**
Pneumothorax is quite common in low birth weight infants. Tube thoracostomy drainage is safer than aspiration for these infants.

154. **(A) (T), (B) (F), (C) (F), (D) (T), (E) (T)**
Overdistention of a single lobe of the lung may cause respiratory distress in an infant. There is an increased radiolucency of the affected lobe. The diaphragm is depressed on the affected side.

155. **(A) (F), (B) (T), (C) (T), (D) (T), (E) (F)**
Myasthenia gravis occurs with tumors of any cell type but most commonly with lymphocytic tumors. The type of cancer cannot be determined by a histologic study of the thymus. The most reliable sign of malignancy is the extent of local spread.

156. **(A) (F), (B) (F), (C) (F), (D) (T), (E) (F)**
Initial treatment of TEF consists of catheter decompression of the proximal esophagus and efforts to minimize the complications from aspiration. The timing of operation depends on the infant's condition and the presence of other abnormalities. The ends of the esophagus are anastomosed at the time of the first operation.

157. **(A) (F), (B) (T), (C) (T), (D) (F), (E) (F)**
Cyclosporine is not an alkylating, antimitotic, or lympholytic agent. It inhibits the production of cytotoxic T cells, and it should be given in combination with moderate doses of prednisone. There is some evidence that it has a greater propensity to induce lymphoma than other immunosuppressive agents.

158. **(A) (F), (B) (F), (C) (T), (D) (F), (E) (T)**
Increased hemolysis may result from transfusion of incompatible blood but more often reflects destruction of fragile transfused red blood cells. Posttransfusion hepatitis occasionally occurs in the third postoperative week but usually occurs much later. Liver function tests are not helpful in determining either the cause or the severity of posthepatic bilary obstruction after an operation. Liver biopsy, ultrasound and CT scans, and transhepatic or retrograde endoscopic cholangiograms are the tests most likely to sort out the diagnostic possibilities.

159. (A) (T), (B) (T), (C) (T), (D) (F), (E) (T)
The most common organism to cause this prob-lem is *S. aureus,* and the level most commonly affected is the lumbar not the thoracic spine.

160. (A) (T), (B) (F), (C) (T), (D) (T), (E) (F)
Peritoneal lavage is positive for injury to an abdominal organ if the fluid recovered has more than 50,000 RBC/mm³. It is not usual for the amylase to be estimated.

161. (A) (F), (B) (T), (C) (F), (D) (T), (E) (T)
The principal indications for parenteral nutrition are found in severely ill patients suffering from malnutrition, sepsis, and surgical or accidental trauma who cannot be fed via the alimentary tract. This does not include a decerebrate adult or preoperative preparation for elective colec-tomy.

162. (A) (T), (B) (T), (C) (T), (D) (T), (E) (T)
There is general agreement that penetrating wounds of this region with overt evidence of deep injuries require urgent operation. A differ-ence of opinion exists regarding the necessity for operative exploration of patients without such evidence.

163. (A) (T), (B) (T), (C) (F), (D) (F), (E) (T)
Even in favorable cases, such as streptococcal empyema in young men, hospitalization is almost 2 weeks longer when needle aspiration rather than closed drainage is used. Metastatic brain abscesses are unusual when antibiotic coverage is adequate.

164. (A) (T), (B) (T), (C) (T), (D) (T), (E) (T)
Generally, bleeding at the time of or soon after a surgical operation is usually due to inadequate hemostasis. The other factors listed are less com-mon causes:

- ineffective hemostasis
- complications of blood transfusion
- a previous unsuspected hemostatic defect
- sepsis
- induced fibrinolysis or defibrination

165. (A) (T), (B) (F), (C) (T), (D) (T), (E) (T)
Steam sterilization under pressure is very effec-tive. The temperature approaches 121°C. Boiling water has a temperature of 100°C. Two percent aqueous glutaraldehyde provides effective steri-lization of catheters and similar items.

166. (A) (F), (B) (T), (C) (F), (D) (T), (E) (T)
Carbuncles are rare. Incision is usually inade-quate treatment. Excision with the cautery well beyond the apparent edge of the supuration is required. On the back of the neck, the loose skin permits the large wound to contract to a small scar.

167. (A) (T), (B) (T), (C) (T), (D) (F), (E) (F)
Copious irrigation with a hypotonic solution (not sodium hypochlorite) may destroy cells that could become implanted. Early ligature of the venous drainage not the arterial supply may prevent spread by the bloodstream.

168. (A) (T), (B) (T), (C) (T), (D) (T), (E) (T)
All are correct statements.

169. (C) Clubbing of the digits or hypertrophic pul-monary osteoarthropathy has no adverse prog-nostic significance. On the other hand, manifes-tations caused by oat cell carcinomas have a poor prognosis because of the tumor being of the oat cell type.

170. (A) The inferior pancreaticoduodenal artery is a branch of the superior mesenteric artery.

171. (C) A meal with a high fat content may remain in the stomach 6 to 12 hours. A low fat meal leaves the stomach in less than 3 hours.

172. (A) The practice of operating on symptomatic patients and not operating on patients with asymptomatic gallstones is appropriate. Possible exceptions are the special features given in the other answers to this question.

173. (A) The portal vein is formed by the junction of the superior mesenteric and splenic veins. Sudden occlusion of the portal vein causes the hepatic artery flow to rise, and occlusion of the hepatic artery causes the portal venous pressure to fall. The left gastric vein drains into the portal vein.

174. (E) The patient should take nothing by mouth until the diarrhea has subsided to less than 2.5 L per day. In a patient with this amount of residual intestine, this should occur in 2 to 3 months, when an oral diet can be gradually started.

175. (B) Prevention of serious sequelae depends on early recognition and fasciotomy.

176. **(B)** Adenocarcinoma of the rectum is much more common than all anal tumors combined. It does not arise from the epithelial surface distal to the mucocutaneous junction.

177. **(C)** Since component wear can be expected and loosening may occur due to the high demands of younger patients, it is wise to limit this procedure to older patients or those with a reduced life expectancy or diminished physical activity.

178. **(A)** The term spondylolisthesis is used to describe the condition of forward subluxation of one vertebra upon another.

179. **(E)** Megestrol acetate (Megace) is a progestational agent that offers effective palliation in premenopausal women with metastatic breast cancer. It is possibly the most popular secondary management option because it is more easily administered than aminoglutethimide.

180. **(C)** There is a 10% incidence of pseudomembranous enterocolitis following use of clindamycin. The most common causative organisms are staphylococci and *Clostridium difficile*. Treatment consists of stopping the clindamycin and giving vancomycin.

Fourth Examination
Questions

DIRECTIONS (Questions 1 through 146): Each of the numbered items or incomplete statements in this section is followed by answers or by completions of the statement. Select the ONE lettered answer or completion that is BEST in each case.

1. In striving for a well-functioning ileostomy stoma

    (A) place the stoma as far from the umbilicus as possible
    (B) do not bring the stoma through the rectus muscle
    (C) evert the nipple so that the stoma protrudes 2 cm above the adjacent skin
    (D) do not excise skin
    (E) do not suture the stomal mucosa to the skin   (3:1019)

2. An emergency operation, rather than an urgent operation, for inflammatory large bowel disease is required in many patients for which complication of the disease?

    (A) pyoderma gangrenosum
    (B) toxic megacolon
    (C) carcinoma
    (D) bleeding
    (E) liver dysfunction   (2:1178)

3. The following statements concern the management of a patient with the sudden onset of an obvious hematemesis or melena. One is FALSE.

    (A) handle the patient as if exsanguination were imminent
    (B) admit the patient to hospital
    (C) over 50% of patients with cirrhosis of the liver are bleeding from gastritis or peptic ulcer and not varices
    (D) most patients with melena—passage of black or tarry stools—are bleeding from the colon or rectum

    (E) once the patient has been stabilized, endoscopy usually is the first study (1:441)

4. The mortality of a perforated peptic ulcer is still in excess of 10% depending on the patient's age and the fact that gastric ulcers do less well than duodenal after perforation. Which statement is INCORRECT?

    (A) perforation causes sudden severe upper abdominal pain. The moment of onset can be recalled precisely
    (B) pain in the back is frequent
    (C) boardlike abdominal rigidity is present
    (D) peristaltic sounds are reduced or absent
    (E) there is no fever at the start   (1:447)

5. Which of the following is NOT a common symptom in patients with regional enteritis (Crohn's disease)?

    (A) diarrhea
    (B) constipation
    (C) abdominal pain and palpable mass
    (D) fever, lassitude, weight loss
    (E) anemia   (1:573–575)

6. A diabetic patient has peripheral neuritis and a neuropathic foot. Which of the following would NOT be expected to occur?

    (A) Charcot-type joints
    (B) dry gangrene of the toes
    (C) sinus tracts opening on the foot
    (D) thick calluses
    (E) stiffness of the metatarsophalangeal joints
                    (2:917)

7. A patient has severe atherosclerotic occlusive disease of the lower limbs. All of the following symptoms or signs indicate impending loss of the extremity EXCEPT

(A) dependent rubor
(B) night cramps in the leg
(C) ischemic ulceration of the heel
(D) pain at rest, which is improved by dependency
(E) delayed venous filling time   (4:551)

8. You are operating on a patient who has carcinoma of the head of the pancreas. You have confirmed the diagnosis with a frozen section. Which of the following does NOT render this tumor unsuitable for resection?

(A) adherence to the hepatic artery near to the origin of the gastroduodenal artery
(B) adherence to the duodenum
(C) adherence to the portal vein
(D) adherence to the superior mesenteric vein
(E) adherence to the superior mesenteric artery   (1:535)

9. The disappearance of the dorsalis pedis and posterior tibial pulses after exercise is most likely to be due to

(A) arterial spasm in an ischemic leg and foot
(B) the shunting of blood to the muscles
(C) reduction of the output of the heart
(D) increased resistance in the collateral circulation
(E) a fall in blood pressure distal to sites of arterial stenosis or thrombosis   (2:900)

10. In a patient with an arteriovenous fistula of an extremity, which of the following is generally known as Branham's sign?

(A) a thrill felt over the fistula
(B) a slowing of the pulse rate when the fistula is occluded by digital pressure
(C) an increased blood volume when the fistula is large
(D) increased limb length if the fistula forms before the epiphyses fuse
(E) a bruit heard over the fistula   (2:933)

11. A 60-year-old woman has a cholecystectomy and a choledochostomy. Five days later, a T tube cholangiogram demonstrates a residual bile duct stone. The treatment will consist of all of the following EXCEPT

(A) the stone should be removed immediately
(B) the patient should be observed for 4 to 6 weeks, since some stones will be passed
(C) use of a Dormia basket under fluoroscopic control succeeds in removing the stone in most cases
(D) endoscopic sphincterotomy succeeds if the stone is not large
(E) stones in the intrahepatic branches of the bile ducts usually can be removed during common bile duct exploration   (1:507)

12. All of the following are complications of acute cholecystitis. Which one usually does NOT cause additional symptoms?

(A) empyema of the gallbladder (suppurative cholecystitis)
(B) cholecystenteric fistula
(C) associated acute pancreatitis
(D) free perforation
(E) pericholecystic abscess   (1:500)

13. Fibromuscular hyperplasia of the renal arteries is an important cause of hypertension in

(A) young adult males
(B) young adult females
(C) middle-aged males
(D) middled-aged females
(E) females of all ages   (2:1008)

14. An extra-anatomic arterial bypass graft is of special value in which of the following situations?

(A) thrombosis of the aorta and iliac arteries in a poor-risk patient
(B) infection of an aortic prosthetic graft
(C) thrombosis of one iliac artery in an elderly patient
(D) leaking from an aortic aneuryism in a patient who is recovering from a myocardial infarction
(E) all of the above   (2:904)

15. Which of the following is out of order when the presentations of lung cancer are listed by frequency of occurrence.

(A) cough
(B) chest pain
(C) dyspnea
(D) hemoptysis
(E) asymptomatic; found on routine chest x-ray   (1:310)

16. A 15-year-old child swallows a dime. It causes no symptoms, but 2 weeks later an x-ray shows that it is still in the stomach. The best treatment is

    (A) under general anesthesia, pass a flexible gastroscope and attempt to remove the foreign body with the biopsy attachment. If this fails, open the abdomen immediately
    (B) give a cathartic
    (C) if the dime cannot be removed through the gastroscope, continue observation
    (D) give an emetic
    (E) no further observation or treatment *(2:1136)*

17. Thrombosis of the axillary-subclavian vein is frequently associated with the following predisposing factors EXCEPT

    (A) indwelling venous catheters
    (B) some unusual activity
    (C) the thoracic outlet compression syndrome
    (D) an infection of the hand
    (E) a metastasis in the axilla *(3:1728)*

18. In the control of hospital infections, the following procedures should be mandatory EXCEPT

    (A) personnel with active staphylococcal infections should be excluded from patient contact
    (B) personnel carrying staphylococci in their nasal passages should be removed from duty until they are no longer carriers
    (C) isolation of every patient with a source of communicable bacteria
    (D) prophylactic use of antibiotics should have strict indications
    (E) all open wounds should be aseptically dressed *(2:166)*

19. The following statements concern the prognosis of patients with breast cancer. All are correct EXCEPT

    (A) the histologic type of tumor is important in assessing the prognosis
    (B) the stage of breast cancer is the single most reliable indicator of the prognosis
    (C) patients with negative axillary nodes and an estrogen receptor-positive tumor have a much better prognosis than those with estrogen receptor-negative tumors and negative nodes
    (D) the mortality rate of breast cancer exceeds that of age-matched controls for 20 years

    (E) patients with an estrogen receptor-positive tumor and negative axillary nodes have a clinical cure rate of 75 to 90% *(1:267-268)*

20. Bronchiectasis formerly was considered irreversible. This is now known to be false. Which statement is INCORRECT?

    (A) 50% of patients develop bronchiectasis before the age of 3, secondary to childhood diseases, such as pertussis
    (B) bronchiectasis may be secondary to bronchial obstruction
    (C) medical treatment consists of postural drainage, cessation of smoking, antibiotics, bronchodilators, humidification, and expectorants
    (D) symptoms include cough, sputum, hemoptysis, dyspnea, and clubbing of the fingers
    (E) surgical resection often is required when medical care fails *(1:302-303)*

21. The most common of all postoperative complications is

    (A) wound infection
    (B) atelectasis
    (C) wound hematoma
    (D) pulmonary embolism
    (E) urinary tract infection *(1:25-27)*

22. The treatment of a patient with a venomous snake bite may include all of the following, but one is of special value unless only scratch marks are present.

    (A) suction and small incisions through skin and fascia
    (B) antivenom
    (C) immobilization of the part
    (D) a tourniquet to occlude veins and lymphatics
    (E) debridement of fascia and subcutaneous tissue *(2:218)*

23. All of the following are associated with an increased risk of breast cancer EXCEPT

    (A) an artificial menopause
    (B) breast cancer in a mother or sister
    (C) cancer in the other breast
    (D) cancer of the body of the uterus
    (E) first pregnancy after the age of 35 *(1:258)*

24. The most common type of diaphragmatic hernia is

(A) the sliding esophageal hiatal hernia
(B) the paraesophageal hiatal hernia
(C) the posterolateral hernia of Bochdalek
(D) a defect following traumatic rupture of the diaphragm
(E) eventration of the diaphragm   *(2:1078)*

25. Reflux of acid and pepsin from the stomach occurs in patients with a sliding hiatal hernia and produces esophagitis in most cases. Which of the following statements is true?

(A) reflux of gastric contents into the esophagus does not occur in normal people
(B) reflux during sleep is frequent in normal people
(C) the gastroesophageal junction normally is located at the level of the esophageal hiatus in the diaphragm
(D) prolonged pH monitoring has demonstrated that reflux in patients with esophagitis occurs predominantly during the day
(E) at least 50% of hiatal hernias are asymptomatic and require no treatment
     (1:387)

26. A man aged 60 has acute upper gastrointestinal bleeding. He has a history of some pain after meals for several years. He has lost no weight, and this is the first episode of bleeding. The likely cause of the bleeding is

(A) esophagitis
(B) gastric ulcer
(C) gastric carcinoma
(D) gastritis
(E) duodenal ulcer   *(2:1125)*

27. A male patient aged 45 has severe chest pain and shortness of breath. A chest film shows a large pleural effusion. A diagnostic closed-needle pleural biopsy is positive for mesothelioma of the pleura. The most likely history of this patient's previous employment would be one of a

(A) radiology technician
(B) worker at nuclear bomb test sites
(C) smoker and shipyard worker
(D) smoker and coal miner
(E) smoker, an alcoholic, and a businessman
     (2:658)

28. A man aged 35 has a mass on the chest wall. It is at the level of the seventh rib, below and lateral to the nipple. Films show a lobulated mass 4 cm × 6 cm. It has destroyed cortical bone. The radiologist considers it to be a chondrosarcoma without evidence of metastases. The best action is

(A) perform a needle biopsy before initiating treatment
(B) perform an open biopsy to determine the exact diagnosis
(C) radiation therapy after biopsy confirms the diagnosis
(D) excise widely
(E) chemotherapy and radiation therapy after biopsy establishes diagnosis   *(2:647-648)*

29. A woman aged 50 has symptoms considered to be due to thoracic outlet compression. She has bilateral cervical ribs. Which of the following symptoms is most likely to be relieved by operation?

(A) two fingers of the right hand are quite ischemic
(B) both hands become swollen and cyanotic
(C) both hands and arms become numb and tingle
(D) intermittent discomfort in the shoulders and arms
(E) mild wasting of the muscles supplied by the first thoracic nerve   *(2:642-645)*

30. A businessman and weekend farmer is crushed when his tractor rolls over onto his lower chest. Examination shows him to be in respiratory distress. There is guarding in the left upper quadrant. He is in mild shock. There are no other injuries. Films show a rupture of the left diaphragm. The best treatment would be to

(A) perform a thoracotomy and repair the diaphragm
(B) treat conservatively and repair the diaphragm in 3 months
(C) insert a prosthetic patch through a thoracotomy
(D) pass a nasogastric tube, continue resuscitation, and repair the diaphragm in 1 week
(E) repair the diaphragm through the abdomen   *(2:634-635)*

31. Which of the following statements about Pancoast's syndrome is INCORRECT?

    (A) pain and loss of strength of the upper arm develop
    (B) the bones of the upper ribs and nearby vertebrae may be destroyed
    (C) Horner's syndrome may develop
    (D) the recurrent laryngeal nerve may be paralyzed
    (E) there is a higher survival rate with Pancoast's tumor than with isolated pulmonary nodules   *(1:310)*

32. A woman aged 30 has an indurated, suppurating, painful, diffuse mass in the skin and subcutaneous tissues of both axillae and the left groin. The likely diagnosis is

    (A) carbuncles
    (B) mycosis fungoides
    (C) hidradenitis suppurativa
    (D) infected epidermoid cysts
    (E) actinomycosis   *(2:510)*

33. A 75-year-old black woman who lives alone falls and breaks her hip. This is treated with the insertion of a prosthesis. One week later, the patient feels severe pain on the right side of the face and has a fever. Her white blood cell count is 25,000. The most likely diagnosis is

    (A) an apical abscess of a tooth
    (B) an unnoticed fracture of the mandible
    (C) acute parotitis
    (D) benign postoperative parotid enlargement
    (E) mumps   *(2:458)*

34. The following statements concern the treatment of patients with carcinoma of the esophagus. Which one is NOT true?

    (A) tumors of the lower third are best treated by esophagogastrectomy and an esophagogastric anastomosis. A pyloroplasty also is performed
    (B) when possible, at least 10 cm of uninvolved esophagus should be resected proximal to the tumor
    (C) blunt esophagectomy followed by a cervical esophagogastric anastomosis is reported to give satisfactory survival rates
    (D) patients who have lost 10% or more of their body weight should receive total parenteral nutrition before surgery
    (E) palliation is better with a celestin tube than with partial removal of an

obstructing lesion using a neodymium: YAG laser   *(1:384)*

35. The central venous pressure is monitored in a patient in shock following very severe trauma to the chest and abdomen. An elevated central venous pressure is most likely to be due to

    (A) inadequate myocardial perfusion
    (B) tension pneumothorax
    (C) cardiac tamponade
    (D) a massive venous injury
    (E) increased intracranial pressure   *(2:495–496)*

36. Surgical operations may be necessary for a patient receiving long-term anticoagulant therapy. In which of the following situations should the anticoagulant therapy NOT be stopped or reversed before the operation?

    (A) an operation on the brain
    (B) an ophthalmic operation
    (C) a needle biopsy of an abdominal mass
    (D) a prostatectomy
    (E) an arterial embolectomy   *(2:918–922)*

37. Lung cancer is a leading cause of death and disability in the developed countries of the world. Which of the following statements is NOT correct?

    (A) cigarette smoking is related causally to all forms of lung cancer
    (B) since 1970, the incidence has decreased in males and increased in females
    (C) various materials (asbestos, radioactive substances) in industry and mining have been associated with lung cancer
    (D) air pollution may contribute to the development of lung cancer
    (E) cigarette smoking is related causally to squamous and oat cell types of lung cancer   *(1:309)*

38. Possible causes of the adult respiratory distress syndrome include all of the following EXCEPT

    (A) hemorrhagic shock
    (B) carcinomatosis
    (C) fat embolism
    (D) sepsis
    (E) microembolization   *(2:132)*

39. Carcinoma of the lip is characterized by which of the following?

  (A) it occurs frequently in factory workers
  (B) it is usually a well-differentiated lesion
  (C) it occurs most commonly in women
  (D) surgery is more effective than is radiation therapy
  (E) metastases occur via both the lymphatics and the bloodstream   *(2:564)*

40. A 35-year-old woman enters the hospital with a history of nervousness, swelling of the neck, weight loss, and tremor of the hands. Exophthalmos is present in only one eye, but it is quite prominent. The likely cause of unilateral exophthalmos is

  (A) orbital tumor
  (B) thyrotoxicosis
  (C) carotid cavernous arteriovenous fistula
  (D) myasthenia gravis
  (E) pituitary adenoma   *(2:1557–1558)*

41. A man aged 30 develops sudden generalized epigastric pain. He has no history of previous abdominal pain or indigestion. Films show free air in the peritoneal cavity. Your choice of treatment of the perforated duodenal ulcer 4 hours after onset of symptoms is

  (A) closure of the perforation
  (B) vagotomy, pyloroplasty, and closure of the perforation
  (C) vagotomy and antrectomy to include the area of perforation in the duodenum
  (D) subtotal gastrectomy
  (E) nasogastric suction and antibiotics   *(2:1125)*

42. The open drainage of intraperitoneal abscesses is still required in about 25% of cases. Which of these statements is INCORRECT?

  (A) satisfactory improvement is evident within 3 days if drainage has been adequate
  (B) if improvement does not follow drainage, the patient should be watched carefully and new antibiotics tried
  (C) pelvic abscesses that point into the rectum or vagina are best opened into the rectum or vagina
  (D) in all cases of pelvic abscess, direct digital exploration should be employed after open drainage to open all loculations
  (E) transperitoneal exploration is indicated if the abscess cannot be located preoperatively   *(1:412)*

43. Which of the following statements concerning bronchial adenoma is NOT correct?

  (A) they occur more frequently in women than men
  (B) bronchial adenomas are benign
  (C) cylindromas resemble salivary gland tumors
  (D) surgical cure is possible in most cases
  (E) bronchial adenomas grow slowly   *(1:309)*

44. The most common first symptom in many patients with thromboangiitis obliterans (Burger's disease) is

  (A) recurrent episodes of superficial thrombophlebitis
  (B) necrosis of the tips of the toes
  (C) claudication of the calf
  (D) sensitivity to cold
  (E) instep claudication of the foot   *(4:693)*

45. The following statements about carcinoma of the male breast all are correct EXCEPT

  (A) usually occurs as a painless lump beneath the nipple in a man aged over 50
  (B) nipple discharge is uncommon but when present indicates a 75% chance of carcinoma
  (C) blood-borne metastases are common
  (D) hormone manipulation is not useful in male patients with cancer of the breast
  (E) when operable the best treatment is modified radical mastectomy   *(1:271)*

46. A patient with the recent onset of the symptoms of Raynaud's phenomenon is best managed by the following therapeutic measures EXCEPT

  (A) stopping tobacco smoking
  (B) avoidance of cold
  (C) medication with drugs that decrease sympathetic neuromuscular transmission
  (D) protection of the extremity against injury
  (E) sympathectomy   *(4:727)*

47. The most frequent complication of lumbar sympathectomy is

  (A) impotence
  (B) postsympathectomy neuralgia
  (C) paradoxical gangrene
  (D) injury to the ureter
  (E) pulmonary embolism   *(4:656)*

48. Mammary dysplasia (fibrocystic disease or chronic mastitis) is commonly present in women aged 30 to 50. Which of the following statements concerning this problem is NOT correct?

    (A) it is rare in postmenopausal women
    (B) estrogen therapy is a causative factor
    (C) the lumps are usually painful and fluctuate in size
    (D) it is advisable to perform a biopsy when there is any suspicion of cancer
    (E) hormone therapy can cure this condition
    (1:272-273)

49. In a patient with a thoracic outlet syndrome, the symptoms are most usually

    (A) neural
    (B) venous
    (C) arterial
    (D) psychosomatic
    (E) vasomotor   *(4:710)*

50. Bench surgery is the removal of an organ such as the kidney from the body, correction of the problem, and the return of the organ to the body by autotransplantation. What is the main indication for ex vivo renal vascular surgery?

    (A) aneurysm of the renal arteries
    (B) atheromata of the renal arteries
    (C) fibromuscular dysplasia of the renal arteries
    (D) thrombosis of the renal veins
    (E) trauma to the kidney and its blood vessels
    (4:1163-1170)

51. Chemotherapy is used in the management of metastatic breast carcinoma. Which of the following statements is NOT correct?

    (A) combination therapy using multiple agents is the most effective
    (B) cytotoxic drugs are the best treatment for visceral metastasis, especially in the lungs or brain
    (C) the response is decreased considerably when cytotoxic drugs are used after a relapse from chemotherapy
    (D) cytotoxic drugs used include doxorubicin, cyclophosphamide, vincristine, methotrexate, and fluorouracil
    (E) new drugs or combinations of drugs have not received wide acceptance   *(1:270)*

52. The following statements concern the treatment of a patient with achalasia of the esophagus.

Which is INCORRECT?

    (A) calcium channel blockers decrease pressure in the lower esophageal sphincter and are of value in the management of this problem
    (B) esophagoscopy should always be performed
    (C) forceful dilatation with an inflatable bag is successful in about 75% of patients
    (D) if dilatation fails, the Heller operation is the best treatment
    (E) many surgeons recommend performance of the Nissen operation when they perform an extramucosal cardiomyotomy (Heller operation)   *(1:373)*

53. The blue toe syndrome is caused by

    (A) thrombosis of the inferior vena cava
    (B) thrombosis of the femoral vein
    (C) thrombophlebitis of the saphenous vein
    (D) embolization of the digital arteries
    (E) thrombosis of the digital arteries *(4:536-545)*

54. The best treatment for an aneurysm of the femoral or popliteal artery is

    (A) ligature of the artery proximally
    (B) excision and grafting
    (C) endoaneurysmorrhaphy
    (D) proximal and distal ligature with bypass graft
    (E) to operate only if the aneurysm enlarges or complications occur   *(4:817)*

55. Pelvic and rectal examinations are part of the clinical examination of a patient with acute abdominal disease. Which of the following statements is NOT true?

    (A) "rectal examination deferred" is an acceptable entry in the chart of a patient with an acute abdomen
    (B) diffuse tenderness on rectal examinations is nonspecific
    (C) localized or one-sided tenderness is indicative of irritation or a pelvic abscess
    (D) a pelvic examination routinely performed might help to correct the fact that the acute abdomen is more often incorrectly diagnosed in women than it is in men
    (E) a useful finding may be a pelvic or rectal tumor   *(1:398)*

56. Acute thrombophlebitis of a superficial vein is recognized by

(A) cyanosis of the extremity
(B) tenderness and cordlike appearance of the vein
(C) a high fever
(D) edema of the limb
(E) pallor of the extremity   *(2:976)*

57. Which of the following histologic types of breast cancer is seen most frequently?

(A) invasive lobular
(B) lobular in situ
(C) infiltrating and invasive ductal
(D) noninvasive intraductal
(E) lobular invasive   *(1:263)*

58. The following statements concern the differential diagnosis of acute abdomen. Which one is NOT true?

(A) any patient whose acute abdominal pain persists for more than 6 hours should be evaluated in hospital
(B) constipation is a feature of pelvic appendicitis
(C) appendectomy is well tolerated during pregnancy
(D) intestinal obstruction in an elderly woman who has not had a previous abdominal operation is often due to an incarcerated femoral hernia or gallstone ileus
(E) mesenteric adenitis may mimic acute appendicitis in children   *(1:401)*

59. Which of these arteries is an important collateral from the extracranial cerebral arteries to the intracranial circulation?

(A) common carotid artery
(B) ophthalmic artery
(C) innominate artery
(D) subclavian artery
(E) internal carotid artery   *(4:1230)*

60. Which of the following types of pain does NOT suggest arterial insufficiency?

(A) a 50-year-old man develops left chest pain radiating to the arm after exertion
(B) a 50-year-old man plays the first tennis match of a vacation. The next morning he has severe pain in the medial, upper aspect of his right thigh

(C) a patient has a coronary arteriogram via the right brachial artery. The right hand becomes cold and numb
(D) a patient recovering from a myocardial infarction suddenly develops severe pain in the left forearm and hand
(E) following resuscitation from cardiogenic shock, a patient has a bloody stool   *(4:6)*

61. The treatment of acute ischemia of the foot includes only one of the following measures. The others are without benefit or are harmful. Which is the correct treatment?

(A) apply hot packs
(B) elevate the foot
(C) bedrest with the foot dependent
(D) apply an elastic stocking
(E) operate at once   *(4:446)*

62. The following statements concern primary hyperaldosteronism. Which one is INCORRECT?

(A) a site of action is in the distal nephron, where sodium is retained and potassium is lost
(B) in about 85% of patients, the cause is an adrenal adenoma
(C) the primary treatment after preparation is surgical excision of the adenoma if present
(D) a CT scan can locate a 0.5 cm adrenal adenoma
(E) carpopedal spasm can occur from hypokalemic alkalosis   *(1:663)*

63. Pyloric obstruction is usually due to a duodenal ulcer. Which one of the following statements concerning pyloric stenosis is true?

(A) the usual cause is a prepyloric ulcer
(B) gastroscopy is rarely indicated
(C) prolonged vomiting leads to metabolic alkalosis with dehydration
(D) the vomitus contains bile
(E) an upper abdominal barium x-ray should be performed at once to establish the diagnosis   *(1:445–446)*

64. The Gott shunt is usually placed between the ascending thoracic aorta and the common femoral artery. It is not required in one of the following situations.

(A) ruptured abdominal aortic aneurysm

(B) dissecting aneurysm of the thoracoabdominal aorta
(C) aneurysm of the thoracic aorta
(D) traumatic rupture of the thoracic aorta
(E) saccular aneurysm of the thoracoabdominal aorta   *(2:879, 881, 891)*

65. The Zollinger-Ellison syndrome results from gastric acid hypersecretion caused by a gastrin-producing tumor. The management of this problem does NOT include

(A) initial treatment consisting of cimetidine 300 to 600 mg and ranitidine 300 to 450 mg four times a day
(B) resection of the gastrinoma, the ideal treatment, which is possible in about 20% of patients
(C) a Whipple operation if the gastrinoma cannot be resected
(D) parietal cell vagotomy, which facilitates control of acid secretion by H_2 blocking agents
(E) when the gastrinoma cannot be resected and acid control by drugs is unsatisfactory, total gastectomy may be indicated   *(1:438)*

66. These statements concern carcinoma of the breast. Which one is NOT correct?

(A) breast carcinoma is the most common cancer among women in the USA
(B) virtually all women over the age of 35 should be screened for breast cancer
(C) screening includes self-examination, physical examination, and mammography
(D) proliferative changes, such as papillomatosis or atypical epithelial hyperplasia, are associated with an increased risk of cancer
(E) most women who develop breast cancer do not have identifiable risk factors *(1:258)*

67. Volume overload may occur, especially during the postoperative period. All of the following statements concerning this problem are correct EXCEPT

(A) antidiuretic hormone is released during anesthesia and surgical stress
(B) water intoxication can follow the excessive intravenous administration of sodium-free fluid in the postoperative period
(C) the problem may be associated with

cardiac failure, when digitalis should be given
(D) the jugular veins become distended
(E) diuretics, such as furosemide, are required in the majority of cases   *(1:131)*

68. A patient has cancer of the rectum. Which of the following symptoms is the most likely to be present?

(A) rectal bleeding
(B) anemia
(C) intestinal obstruction
(D) constipation
(E) diarrhea   *(1:597)*

69. Paraesophageal hiatal hernia consists of part of the stomach herniating into the thorax adjacent to the undisplaced gastroesophageal junction. Which of the following statements concerning this problem is true?

(A) heartburn is a common symptom
(B) complications are uncommon
(C) viscera other than the stomach cannot herniate
(D) surgical repair is indicated rarely
(E) the usual surgical repair consists of reducing the hernia, closing the enlarged hiatus around the esophagus, and suturing the stomach to the posterior rectus sheath—anterior gastropexy   *(1:386)*

70. Which of the following does NOT increase the incidence of carcinoma of the colon?

(A) being economically poor
(B) familial polyposis
(C) hereditary site-specific colon cancer
(D) ulcerative colitis
(E) exposure to radiation   *(1:595)*

71. Chronic ischemia of the intestine without bowel necrosis causes all of the following EXCEPT

(A) decreased appetite
(B) decreased peristalsis
(C) constipation
(D) postprandial pain
(E) weight loss   *(2:1436–1438)*

72. The object of adjuvant therapy for breast cancer is to eliminate occult metastases when they are still microscopic because they may be responsible for late recurrence. Which of the following statements is NOT correct?

    (A) single drugs are superior to combinations of drugs
    (B) a trial of CMF (cyclophosphamide, methotrexate, and 5-fluorouracil) has shown that this regimen benefits premenopausal women with positive axillary nodes
    (C) the addition of hormones may improve the results of adjuvant therapy
    (D) postmenopausal women with positive nodes and positive hormone receptor levels should receive tamoxifen
    (E) the length of time adjuvant therapy must be administered remains uncertain. Several studies suggest that shorter treatment periods may be as effective as longer ones   *(1:266)*

73. Which of the following is out of order as a cause of obstruction of the large intestine?

    (A) carcinoma of the colon
    (B) volvulus
    (C) diverticulitis
    (D) inflammatory bowel disease
    (E) fecal impaction   *(1:592)*

74. The postoperative care of a patient after surgery for breast cancer includes all of the following EXCEPT

    (A) suction drainage to reduce the incidence of hematoma or seroma
    (B) the use of estrogens when a patient whose tumor was estrogen receptor positive reaches menopause
    (C) a discussion of breast reconstruction before mastectomy
    (D) reconstruction is not an obstacle to the diagnosis of recurrent cancer and should be encouraged if the patient is interested
    (E) postoperative radiotherapy increases the incidence of edema of the arm   *(1:266-267)*

75. Fluid loss in a third degree burn occurs chiefly through

    (A) cellular hemolysis
    (B) seepage from the wound
    (C) loss into the interstitial space
    (D) loss from increased respiration
    (E) loss into the alimentary tract   *(2:270)*

76. The initial rapid bolus of fluid resuscitation for the traumatized adult should be approximately

    (A) half the estimated blood loss
    (B) one quarter of the estimated blood loss
    (C) up to 1 L
    (D) 1 to 2 L
    (E) enough to achieve a normal central venous pressure (CVP)   *(9:184)*

77. A patient has a myxoma of the left atrium that mimics mitral stenosis. It is NOT true that the

    (A) patient has a continuous murmur over the apex
    (B) left atrium is enlarged
    (C) patient has pulmonary congestion
    (D) electrocardiogram is normal
    (E) tumor blocks the mitral valve intermittently   *(2:850)*

78. Which of the following findings is NOT characteristic of mitral stenosis?

    (A) left atrial enlargement
    (B) left ventricular hypertrophy
    (C) elevated pulmonary wedge pressure
    (D) lowered cardiac output
    (E) prominent pulmonary veins   *(2:822)*

79. A 3-year-old child developed a mild upper respiratory infection and became cyanotic with moderate exercise. The chest x-ray showed a dilated pulmonary artery, diminished lung markings, and an enlarged right ventricle. The right ventricular pressure was 90 mm Hg, and the right atrial pressure was 20 mm Hg. The diagnosis would be

    (A) patent ductus arteriosus
    (B) tetrology of Fallot
    (C) atrial septal defect
    (D) ventricular septal defect
    (E) pulmonary stenosis with patent foramen ovale   *(2:742)*

80. Which one of the following nerves is most likely to be injured during the excision of the submandibular salivary gland?

    (A) lingual nerve
    (B) mandibular branch of the facial nerve
    (C) hypoglossal nerve

(D) glossopharyngeal nerve
(E) spinal accessory nerve   *(2:584)*

81. Hodgkin's disease most commonly occurs

    (A) with constitutional symptoms, such as fluctuating fever, night sweats, pruritis, and weight loss
    (B) with asymptomatic splenomegaly
    (C) as isolated inguinal lymphadenopathy
    (D) around an average age of 40
    (E) as isolated cervical adenopathy   *(3:1215)*

82. The fistula tract of a second branchial cleft cyst passes

    (A) posterior to the sternocleidomastoid muscle
    (B) through the hyoid bone
    (C) between the internal and external carotid arteries
    (D) deep to the glossopharyngeal (IX) nerve
    (E) superficial to the hypoglossal (XII) nerve   *(2:2135)*

83. In a patient with an acute extradural hematoma, which one of the following statements is FALSE?

    (A) results from temporal bone fracture
    (B) conservative management produces good results
    (C) urgent operation is required
    (D) a lucid interval may have occurred
    (E) results from injury to the middle meningeal vessels   *(2:1793)*

84. Volkmann's ischemic contracture most likely follows

    (A) supracondylar fracture with anterior displacement
    (B) supracondylar fracture with posterior displacement
    (C) fracture of the shaft of the humerus
    (D) fracture of the olecranon with anterior displacement
    (E) fracture of the radius   *(2:1970)*

85. A 1-year-old child is brought to the hospital with a history of paralysis of the right leg. On physical examination, he is found to have an elevated white blood cell count. The most likely diagnosis is

    (A) abdominal peritonitis
    (B) meningitis
    (C) osteomyelitis

(D) poliomyelitis
(E) encephalitis   *(2:2011)*

86. Which of the following is the mechanism by which a Monteggia fracture is caused?

    (A) arm extended and pronated, fall on outstretched hand
    (B) arm extended and supinated, fall on outstetched hand
    (C) arm flexed, fall on the elbow
    (D) direct blow on the medial side of the forearm followed by forced pronation
    (E) direct blow on the medial side of the forearm followed by forced supination   *(2:1973)*

87. A 70-year-old man suffers a compression fracture of the seventh thoracic vertebra. The neurologic system is intact. The best treatment is

    (A) hyperextension on a Foster frame
    (B) open reduction and spinal fusion
    (C) Crutchfield tongs
    (D) Minerva-type spinal plaster jacket and ambulation
    (E) bedrest until pain subsides, then exercises, physiotherapy, and ambulation *(2:2001-2003)*

88. The main side effects of chemotherapeutic agents occur because of effects on

    (A) cells with abnormal RNA
    (B) cells with abnormal DNA
    (C) cells that are rapidly proliferating
    (D) tissues of ectodermal origin
    (E) tissues of mesodermal origin   *(2:346)*

89. Which of the following was NOT a component of the classic description of the tetralogy of Fallot?

    (A) pulmonary valvular stenosis
    (B) dextroposition of the aorta
    (C) right ventricular hypertrophy
    (D) ventricular septal defect
    (E) pulmonary artery stenosis   *(3:2223)*

90. The most common aortic arch developmental anomaly is

    (A) right-sided arch
    (B) double arch
    (C) anomalous innominate artery
    (D) anomalous carotid artery
    (E) aberrant right subclavian   *(3:2186)*

91. The most common congenital cardiac defect is

   (A) patent ductus arteriosus
   (B) aortopulmonary window
   (C) coarctation of the aorta
   (D) atrial septal defect
   (E) ventricular septal defect   (3:2212)

92. Total anomalous pulmonary venous connection is a severe congenital anomaly that appears within the first month of life. The pulmonary-systemic connection is most commonly to the

   (A) left innominate vein
   (B) ductus venosus
   (C) coronary sinus
   (D) superior vena cava
   (E) right atrium   (3:2206)

93. Vertebral basilar arterial insufficiency is suggested by all of the following EXCEPT

   (A) episodes of numbness around the mouth
   (B) drop attacks
   (C) vertigo
   (D) slurring of speech
   (E) blurring of vision   (2:944)

Questions 94 and 95

A 21-year-old college student is injured when his automobile strikes a tree at a speed of about 20 miles per hour. He has lacerations of the forehead and face. He complains of chest pain and dyspnea, and he is diagnosed as suffering from fractures of the ribs. A chest x-ray confirms the presence of fractures of the ribs and also shows widening of the mediastinum.

94. The correct management would be to

   (A) suture the lacerations and admit the patient to the hospital for observation
   (B) perform an emergency aortogram
   (C) repeat the chest film after 1 hour
   (D) take an electrocardiogram
   (E) tap the pericardium   (2:201)

95. The aortogram shows a traumatic rupture of the thoracic aorta just distal to the origin of the left subclavian artery. The correct management of the patient would be to

   (A) operate and establish a bypass before repairing the ruptured aorta
   (B) operate and repair the aortic rupture by direct suture
   (C) operate and repair the ruptured aorta with a Dacron graft

   (D) induce hypotension and treat conservatively
   (E) bypass the lesion and ligate the aorta above and below the site of rupture (3:1814)

96. When medical therapy for alkaline reflux gastritis fails, the procedure of choice to correct the problem is

   (A) cholecystojejunostomy
   (B) choledochojejunostomy
   (C) jejunal loop interposition
   (D) subtotal gastrectomy
   (E) roux-en-Y gastrojejunostomy   (3:867)

97. Stimulation of the carotid sinus nerve causes

   (A) increase in the venous return
   (B) decrease in the pulse rate
   (C) increase in the respiratory rate
   (D) increase in blood pressure
   (E) increase in cardiac output   (4:1303-1304)

98. A patient has a lesion of one cerebellar hemisphere. All of the following occur EXCEPT

   (A) hemiparesis
   (B) syncope
   (C) hypotonia
   (D) incoordination
   (E) tremor   (4:1199-1200)

99. Which of the following is a side effect of the use of anesthetic doses of narcotics?

   (A) hypertension
   (B) hypertonus
   (C) pulmonary edema
   (D) psychic disturbances on recovery
   (E) increased cardiac oxygen consumption   (3:163)

100. The best way to follow the progress of a patient with choriocarcinoma is by measurement of urinary

   (A) 17-ketosteroids
   (B) 17-hydroxysteroids
   (C) estrogen
   (D) follicular stimulating hormones
   (E) chorionic gonadotropin   (2:1753-1754)

101. Which of the following is the best treatment for a laceration of the cheek in which the parotid duct (Stenson's duct) is severed?

   (A) meticulous closure with internal drainage
   (B) suture over a catheter splint

(C) suture with external drainage
(D) pressure dressing
(E) leave open and close by delayed primary suture after 4 or 5 days   *(2:2140)*

102. The first cells active in the inflammatory response to bacterial invasion are

(A) lymphocytes
(B) monocytes
(C) granulocytes
(D) eosinophils
(E) mast cells   *(3:260)*

103. Radiation injury to bowel results from

(A) release of free radicals in mucosal cells
(B) injury to radiation-sensitive parasympathetic nerves
(C) submucosal fibrosis
(D) genetic damage to the rapidly dividing mucosal cells
(E) endarteritis and thrombosis of small vessels   *(3:1001)*

104. A patient has a high bifurcation of the brachial artery, and the ulnar artery is superficial at the elbow. This is not recognized, and the patient, who is to have a submucous resection of the nasal septum, receives by mistake an injection of thiopental into the artery. You should

(A) leave the needle in the artery and inject 5000 units of heparin into the artery
(B) start an intravenous infusion at a new site
(C) complete the operation when the patient is stable
(D) place a tourniquet above the site of arterial injection
(E) perform a brachial plexus block after heparinization   *(4:501-510)*

105. Excision of a local recurrence of a malignancy is recommended in all of the following circumstances EXCEPT

(A) soft tissue sarcoma
(B) anastomotic recurrences of colon cancer
(C) squamous carcinoma of the skin
(D) basal cell carcinoma of the skin
(E) adrenal carcinoma   *(2:340)*

106. The most reliable preoperative indicator of ampullary obstruction in a patient with chronic pancreatitis is

(A) endoscopic retrograde cholangiopancreatography
(B) ultrasound
(C) CT scan
(D) endoscopic manometry
(E) percutaneous transhepatic cholangiopancreatography (PTCP)   *(3:1187)*

107. Which of the following is a CONTRAINDICATION to treating a thrombosis of the superficial femoral artery with a saphenous vein bypass graft?

(A) atherosclerotic heart disease
(B) diabetes mellitus
(C) gangrene of the toes
(D) occluded distal arterial tree
(E) bilateral disease   *(2:911)*

Questions 108 and 109

A 17-year-old girl with a history of irregular menses had a 24-hour history of lower abdominal pain of sudden onset. The abdomen was silent, slightly distended, and tender on the right as well as the left. Her pulse rate was 84, blood pressure 90/60, hemoglobin 8.6, white blood cell count 11,000, temperature 98.4°F. Cervical smear was negative for gonococci. On rectal examination, a boggy mass was palpable in the cul de sac.

108. The most likely diagnosis is

(A) acute appendicitis
(B) acute salpingitis
(C) ruptured ectopic pregnancy
(D) torsion of an ovarian cyst
(E) ruptured ovarian cyst   *(2:1250)*

109. The surgeon, although suspicious that the patient has a ruptured ectopic pregnancy, wants confirmatory evidence before he operates. Which of the following studies would be most useful?

(A) abdominal x-ray films
(B) culdoscopy or laparoscopy
(C) pregnancy test
(D) barium enema
(E) blood culture   *(2:1774-1775)*

110. A 28-year-old white male complains of pain 2 weeks after a fall on the outstretched hand. X-rays at the time of injury were negative. The most likely diagnosis is

(A) Colles' fracture
(B) fractured navicular
(C) dislocation of the lunate
(D) sprained wrist
(E) fracture of the radial styloid   *(2:1976-1977)*

Questions 111 through 114

A 60-year-old man is making good progress 5 days after an acute myocardial infarction. He is still in the cardiac intensive care unit, and he is scheduled to be transferred to a regular floor, but he develops quite severe colicky abdominal pain. He becomes pale, and his pulse rate rises to 110. He vomits, and the vomitus contains some blood. He also has a bowel movement and this too contains mucus and blood. His abdomen is tender and moderately distended and his colicky pain has become a dull, generalized, abdominal pain. His electrocardiogram has not changed, and his blood pressure is 100/60.

111. Which of the following investigations would be the most rewarding?

(A) upper gastrointestinal series
(B) barium enema
(C) intravenous pyelogram
(D) catheter arteriogram of the abdominal aorta and its branches
(E) intravenous cholangiogram   *(2:1433)*

112. The most likely diagnosis is

(A) dissecting aneurysm of the aorta
(B) embolus of the superior mesenteric artery
(C) paralytic ileus
(D) acute cholecystitis
(E) renal infarction   *(2:1433)*

113. The best initial treatment would be

(A) conservative management
(B) immediate laparotomy
(C) resuscitation for a few hours, followed by laparotomy
(D) heparin plus conservative management
(E) immediate thoracotomy   *(2:1433-1435)*

114. A laparotomy is performed on the patient. The surgeon finds an embolus of the superior mesenteric artery with severe ischemia, but not per-

foration of the midgut. The procedure of choice would be

(A) resection of the ischemic intestine and restoration of continuity with an end-to-end anastomosis
(B) perform a mesenteric embolectomy and resect that portion of the intestine that is still ischemic after 30 minutes' observation under warm saline packs
(C) resect the intestine and exteriorize each stoma as an enterostomy
(D) perform mesenteric embolectomy, close the abdomen, and observe carefully; reoperate at the first sign of perforation or peritonitis
(E) perform a mesenteric embolectomy, close the abdomen, and open it for a second look 12 hours later   *(2:1433-1435)*

115. A 35-year-old man has a history of ulcerative colitis of at least 15 years' duration. He has had episodes of activity and remission of his disease. During the past year, the remissions have decreased greatly in length, and the symptoms during the active phases have become more severe. The diagnosis has been confirmed radiologically and histologically. In the left colon there are two segments of well-marked pseudopolyposis. The best operation would be

(A) total coloproctectomy with an ileostomy or mucosal proctectomy with endorectal ileoanal anastomosis
(B) ileostomy
(C) resection of the left colon and coloproctostomy
(D) transverse colostomy
(E) total colectomy followed by ileoproctostomy if the rectal disease heals   *(2:1175)*

116. An elderly, edentulous woman with atrophic oral mucosa and brittle spatulate fingernails is most likely to have which of the following esophageal lesions?

(A) Schatzki ring
(B) esophageal web
(C) pulsion epiphrenic diverticulum
(D) traction diverticulum
(E) Zenker's diverticulum   *(3:729)*

117. Pseudomyxoma peritonei is associated with

(A) mucocele of the appendix and cystadenoma of the ovary

(B) carcinoma of the stomach and colon
(C) omphaloenteric cysts
(D) mucocele of the appendix and carcinoma of the colon
(E) mucocele of the appendix and carcinoma of the stomach   *(2:1769)*

Questions 118 and 119

A 25-year-old white male has right lower quadrant abdominal pain, fever, and diarrhea. On abdominal exploration, his appendix is found to be normal, with the distal end of the ileum red, inflamed, and edematous. The cecum at the base of the appendix is mildly inflamed.

118. The treatment would be

    (A) remove the appendix
    (B) close the abdomen
    (C) right hemicolectomy
    (D) ileum-to-transverse colon bypass
    (E) resect the terminal ileum and the appendix   *(2:1152)*

119. Which of the following is the most likely subsequent course?

    (A) enterocutaneous fistula
    (B) disease regresses and never recurs
    (C) the patient will develop appendicitis
    (D) the patient will have severe difficulty, requiring a second operation
    (E) the patient may continue to have abdominal problems that can be treated without another operation   *(2:1152)*

120. Which one of the following is NOT a toxic side effect of the local anesthetics?

    (A) anxiety
    (B) tinnitus
    (C) myocardial irritability
    (D) convulsions
    (E) respiratory failure   *(3:165)*

121. Which of the following studies would NOT aid in the diagnosis of myeloma?

    (A) plasma proteins
    (B) Bence Jones proteins
    (C) serum calcium
    (D) x-rays of the skeleton
    (E) bone marrow biopsy   *(2:1918)*

122. A child age 2 years has a painful, punched-out lesion of the frontal bone and a palpable mass in the abdomen. Which of the following is the most likely diagnosis?

    (A) neuroblastoma
    (B) Wilms' tumor
    (C) adenocarcinoma of the gastrointestinal tract
    (D) osteosarcoma
    (E) Ewing's tumor   *(2:1533)*

123. In which of the following ways does liver disease interfere with coagulation?

    (A) decreased production of prothrombin-related factors
    (B) decreased production of fibrinogen
    (C) release of tissue thromboplastin
    (D) results in platelet destruction
    (E) decreased metabolism of fibrinolytic products   *(3:102)*

124. Which of the following muscles is innervated by the femoral nerve?

    (A) adductor magnus
    (B) adductor brevis
    (C) gracilis
    (D) semitendinosis
    (E) rectus femoris   *(15:1233)*

125. Which of the following penicillins is ineffective against all *Pseudomonas?*

    (A) carbenicillin
    (B) ampicillin
    (C) mezlocillin
    (D) azlocillin
    (E) piperacillin   *(18:820)*

126. A Mallory-Weiss mucosal tear at the gastroesophageal junction may be associated with

    (A) alcoholism
    (B) pregnancy
    (C) peptic ulcer disease
    (D) weight lifting
    (E) bowel obstruction   *(3:730)*

127. Hypophysectomy decreases the output of all of the following EXCEPT

    (A) estrin
    (B) aldosterone
    (C) hydrocortisone
    (D) thyroxine
    (E) progesterone   *(2:1475–1486)*

128. The most common cause of spontaneous pneumothorax in the developed countries of the western world is

 (A) tuberculosis
 (B) emphysematous blebs
 (C) congenital lung cysts
 (D) carcinoma of the bronchus
 (E) pneumonia   (2:675)

129. A 6-month-old infant has two 1.0-cm abscesses in the lower lobe of the right lung. In addition to appropriate antibiotic therapy, the treatment of choice would be

 (A) tube drainage
 (B) supportive therapy
 (C) needle aspirations repeated as necessary
 (D) resection of appropriate bronchial segments
 (E) right lower lobectomy   (2:678)

Questions 130 through 133

A 35-year-old woman has a 3-year history of intermittent hemoptysis and intermittent yellow sputum. X-ray shows a 2-cm density in the region of the hilum of the lower lobe of the right lung.

130. The most likely diagnosis is

 (A) tuberculosis
 (B) bronchiectasis
 (C) foreign body
 (D) tumor of bronchial gland origin
 (E) bronchogenic carcinoma   (2:707–710)

131. The most helpful diagnostic procedure would be

 (A) sputum cytology
 (B) sputum culture
 (C) bronchography
 (D) bronchoscopy
 (E) tomogram   (2:707–710)

132. The best treatment for this lesion would be

 (A) pneumonectomy
 (B) lobectomy
 (C) antituberculosis drug therapy
 (D) postural drainage and antibiotics
 (E) physiotherapy and observation   (2:707–710)

133. The most likely outcome after correct treatment would be

 (A) no further trouble
 (B) death from metastases

 (C) continued problems but improved
 (D) recurrence in the other lung
 (E) lung abscess and empyema   (2:707–710)

Questions 134 and 135

A 60-year-old asbestos worker has hemoptysis and cough. His chest film shows an enlarged mediastinal shadow with opacification of the left upper lobe. He has a palpable mass in the left supraclavicular region.

134. The most likely diagnosis is

 (A) pulmonary hamartoma
 (B) tuberculosis
 (C) silicosis
 (D) histoplasmosis
 (E) carcinoma of the lung   (2:694)

135. The cytologic examination of the sputum for malignant cells is negative, and the bronchoscopic examination is indeterminant. The next step toward establishing the diagnosis would be

 (A) right scalene node biopsy
 (B) left scalene node biopsy
 (C) repeat bronchoscopy
 (D) thoracotomy
 (E) tomography   (2:699)

136. The major mechanism terminating the action of the thiobarbiturates is

 (A) metabolism in the liver
 (B) metabolism in the kidney
 (C) excretion by the kidney
 (D) excretion by the lungs
 (E) redistribution   (3:162)

Questions 137 through 139

A 50-year-old woman was esophagoscoped because of a history of dysphagia and weight loss. The distal esophagus was inflamed, but the esophagoscope passed easily into the stomach. Six hours later, the patient began to complain of back, chest, and epigastric pain. The upper abdomen was rigid, and bowel sounds were hypoactive. The pain became worse, and her respiratory rate was increased.

137. The most likely additional physical finding would be

 (A) cervical emphysema
 (B) an abnormal electrocardiogram
 (C) abdominal rebound tenderness

(D) blood from a pleural tap
(E) blood from an abdominal tap   *(2:1097–1101)*

138. The most definitive diagnostic procedure would be

(A) bronchoscopy
(B) esophagoscopy
(C) plain abdominal films
(D) electrocardiogram
(E) water-soluble contrast swallow *(2:1097–1101)*

139. The best treatment would be

(A) immediate laparotomy
(B) thoracotomy
(C) observation
(D) antibiotics and nasogastric aspiration
(E) catheter drainage of the chest *(2:1097–1101)*

140. A 45-year-old woman has an apparently uncomplicated cholecystectomy for gallstones. Twenty-four hours later, her temperature is 102°F, and her pulse rate is 110. The most likely cause is

(A) urinary infection
(B) cholangitis
(C) wound infection
(D) subphrenic abscess
(E) atelectasis   *(2:461–462)*

141. The most common cause of spontaneous chylothorax is

(A) a congenital lymphatic malformation
(B) spontaneous rupture of the thoracic duct
(C) thrombosis of the subclavian vein
(D) mediastinal malignancy
(E) tuberculous lymphadenitis   *(3:2027–2028)*

142. The earliest sign of esophageal perforation is

(A) mediastinal crunch
(B) subcutaneous emphysema
(C) dyspnea
(D) shock
(E) tachycardia   *(3:750)*

143. A healthy high school student has a chest film. This shows a well-defined, rounded mass 4 cm in diameter in the anterior mediastinum just above the heart. There appears to be some calcium in the periphery of the lesion. The most likely diagnosis is

(A) neuroblastoma
(B) lymphoma
(C) reduplication of the esophagus

(D) pleuropericardial cyst
(E) dermoid cyst   *(2:721)*

144. Which of the following cephalosporins provides the most long-lasting high serum levels, making it the best agent for surgical prophylaxis?

(A) cephalothin
(B) cefazolin
(C) cefoxitin
(D) moxalactam
(E) imipenem   *(18:821–834)*

145. A child inhales a bean, and it produces complete obstruction of the right mainstem bronchus. Which of the following will be the primary pathologic change produced?

(A) emphysema of the right lung
(B) emphysema of the left lung
(C) atelectasis of the right lung
(D) atelectasis of the left lung
(E) pneumonia of the right lung   *(2:1643)*

146. A patient with a recent full-thickness circumferential burn of the arm begins to complain of numbness and tingling in the hand and fingers. The best treatment for this problem is

(A) escharotomy
(B) fasciotomy
(C) sedation and elevation of the limb
(D) active exercises of shoulder and elbow joints
(E) changing dressing from silver nitrate to Sulfamylon   *(2:273–274)*

DIRECTIONS (Questions 147 through 180): Each question consists of an introduction followed by five statements. Mark T (true) or F (false) after each statement.

147. Fecal impaction after surgery commonly occurs in association with

(A) old age
(B) diarrhea
(C) dehydration
(D) a gastrointestinal series
(E) prolonged, severe pain   *(2:1214)*

148. All of the following statements concern tetanus.

(A) the first symptom is usually limitation of movement of the jaws
(B) the infected site must be debrided as soon as possible
(C) tracheostomy is often required
(D) the injection of human immune globulin should precede surgery
(E) an attack of tetanus confers lasting immunity   (2:186–188)

149. The following statements are in regard to the bite of a black widow spider.

(A) the spider that bites has a shiny black body with a red hourglass design on the ventral abdomen
(B) the male spider is dangerous; the female does not bite
(C) pain begins after 48 hours from the time of the bite
(D) boardlike abdominal rigidity develops
(E) a specific antivenom is not available (2:220)

150. The increase in drug abuse has resulted in a number of atypical infections. The following statements concern this problem.

(A) the problem occurs from the intravascular or extravascular injection of irritating and even necrotizing substances that are infected
(B) a typical problem is a grossly swollen, tense, immobile forearm that is acutely tender but shows no localizing signs of infection
(C) if an abscess is suspected, sonograms and CT scan may be used to localize it
(D) tetanus is prevalent among drug adicts
(E) acquired immunodeficiency syndrome (AIDS) should be suspected whenever the response to treatment is inadequate   (1:12)

151. It is advisable to obtain an estrogen receptor assay for every breast cancer at the time of initial diagnosis by biopsy.

(A) the presence or absence of estrogen and progesterone receptors in the cytoplasm of tumor cells is very important when managing patients with recurrent or metastatic disease
(B) more than 50% of patients with metastic breast cancer respond to hormone manipulation if the tumor was estrogenic receptor negative

(C) progesterone receptors may be a more sensitive indicator than estrogen receptors of a patient's response to hormonal manipulation
(D) patients whose primary tumor is receptor positive have a more favorable course after mastectomy than those whose tumor is receptor negative
(E) receptors are also an indicator of the response to chemotherapy   (1:263)

152. Classic hemophilia (factor VIII deficiency)

(A) occurs chiefly in males
(B) seldom causes hemarthrosis
(C) is associated with contractures of the elbows and knees
(D) is inherited as a sex-linked dominant
(E) results in a high incidence of peptic ulcer   (2:91)

153. Acute gastric mucosal erosions with hemorrhage occur with

(A) bony trauma
(B) burns
(C) sepsis
(D) stress
(E) steroid therapy   (2:1129–1131)

154. Hyperparathyroidism historically was diagnosed in patients with bone pain and deformity (osteitis fibrosa cystica) and later nephrolithiasis and nephrocalcinosis. Today, most patients are detected by routine screening often before symptoms develop.

(A) after successful surgery, many patients thought to be asymptomatic become aware of improvement in unrecognized symptoms
(B) symptoms of hyperparathyroidism include muscle fatigability, weakness, psychiatric disturbances, polydipsia, polyuria, and constipation
(C) squamous cell lung cancer may cause ectopic hyperparathyroidism
(D) a high serum calcium and low phosphate level suggest hyperparathyroidism, but half of the patients with hyperparathyroidism have a normal serum phosphate
(E) the serum parathyroid hormone level is low or zero in patients with hypercalcemia due to all causes other than primary or ectopic hyperparathyroidism   (1:249–251)

155. You would advise radiation rather than operative removal for most patients with which of the following tumors?

(A) nasopharynx
(B) oat cell carcinoma of the lung
(C) Hodgkin's disease
(D) actinic skin cancer
(E) renal cell carcinoma   (2:345)

156. Torsion of the testicle

(A) causes abdominal pain, nausea, and vomiting
(B) should be operated on as an emergency
(C) when treated, operation includes exploring the contralateral scrotum
(D) often occurs spontaneously, even during sleep
(E) causes testicular atrophy   (2:1685)

157. Which of the following tumors has a familial tendency?

(A) medullary carcinoma of the thyroid
(B) pheochromocytoma
(C) carcinoma of the colon
(D) osteogenic sarcoma
(E) breast cancer   (2:530,1197,1527,1571,1935)

158. Which of the following is/are associated with Meigs' syndrome?

(A) lymphedema of the leg
(B) fibroma of the ovary
(C) liver metastases
(D) ascites and hydrothorax
(E) ovarian carcinoma   (2:1771)

159. Crohn's colitis

(A) is more common than ulcerative colitis
(B) is increasing in incidence
(C) rarely poses the hazard of colonic malignancy
(D) when successfully operated, does not recur
(E) if treated with steroids, recurrence is less likely than if steroids are not used
                            (2:1179–1180)

160. A middle-aged man dines and drinks well. Soon after, he vomits and notices the sudden onset of severe pain in the chest. The diagnosis is spontaneous perforation of the esophagus (Boerhaave syndrome). The following statements concern this problem.

(A) the perforation occurs most frequently at the gastroesophageal junction
(B) the overlying pleura is not torn at the time of perforation
(C) an esophagogram using water-soluble contrast medium should be performed
(D) early surgery with closure of the perforation and external drainage is the best treatment
(E) resection should be performed if an associated resectable carcinoma of the esophagis is found   (1:377)

161. The following statements are in regard to gas gangrene (diffuse clostridial myonecrosis).

(A) there is marked tachycardia
(B) the wound is not painful
(C) give penicillin in large doses
(D) give antitoxin in large doses
(E) the patient is hypothermic   (2:185)

162. Which of the following statements is/are true of carcinoma of the oral cavity?

(A) carcinoma of the oral cavity is more differentiated and less aggressive than is carcinoma of the oropharynx
(B) the symptoms are minimal in the early stages
(C) carcinoma of the tongue metastasizes to the cervical lymph nodes only after many years
(D) the most common malignancy of the lower lip is a basal cell carcinoma
(E) the so-called verrucous carcinoma of the buccal mucosa is highly malignant
                            (2:570–574)

163. The conservative management of a patient with thrombosis of the superficial femoral artery should include

(A) stopping smoking
(B) treating anemia if present
(C) weight reduction in the obese
(D) control of diabetes
(E) no alcoholic beverages   (2:911)

164. An astrocytoma has the following characteristics.

(A) in adults, often occurs in the cerebrum
(B) in children, often occurs in the cerebellum
(C) may be cystic
(D) rarely reaches a large size
(E) is the most common brain tumor   (2:1800)

165. Villous adenoma accounts for 4 to 8% of all colon lesions and is usually found in the older population. These lesions

    (A) are diagnosed easily on rectal examination
    (B) can almost all be found with a 25-cm sigmoidoscope
    (C) have a high malignant potential
    (D) are more likely malignant when firm areas and ulceration are noted
    (E) are more likely malignant when they hypersecrete fluid and electrolytes   *(3:1003)*

166. There has been much controversy about the nature of Schatzki's rings. At present, the evidence indicates that Schatzki's rings are

    (A) similar to esophageal webs
    (B) secondary to esophageal reflux
    (C) located at the junction of squamous and columnar epithelium
    (D) congenital anomalies
    (E) premalignant   *(3:728)*

167. Of the following coagulation factors, which is/are present in banked blood?

    (A) factor IX (Christmas factor)
    (B) factor V (proaccelerin)
    (C) fibrinogen
    (D) factor VIII (antihemophilic factor A)
    (E) prothrombin   *(2:104)*

168. A patient has suffered a massive pulmonary embolus with reflex bronchial constriction. Which of the following statements concerning heparin therapy is/are true?

    (A) a large dose of heparin should be given initially
    (B) subcutaneous heparinization is preferable to intravenous heparinization
    (C) a large total dose of heparin should be given in the first 24 hours
    (D) heparinization is contraindicated
    (E) heparin is not given after completion of treatment with streptokinase   *(3:1740)*

169. During transfusion for hemorrhagic hypotension, a severe transfusion reaction occurs. You would

    (A) transfuse with compatible blood
    (B) use vasopressors if necessary to combat hypotension
    (C) give sodium bicarbonate
    (D) remove the venous catheter through which the incompatible blood is running
    (E) discard the incompatible blood   *(3:111)*

170. When positive end-expiratory pressure (PEEP) ventilation is working to the benefit of the patient, it

    (A) decreases the functional residual capacity (FRC)
    (B) increases the compliance
    (C) decreases venous return
    (D) increases arterial oxygen tension
    (E) decreases atelectasis   *(2:137)*

171. Which of the following statements is/are true concerning a patient who is undergoing anticoagulation therapy?

    (A) the prothrombin time should be determined before beginning heparin therapy
    (B) the one-stage prothrombin time is the preferred method of controlling anticoagulation with coumarins
    (C) the partial thromboplastin time can be used as the method of controlling anticoagulation with heparin
    (D) an accurate prothrombin time cannot be carried out in a patient who has received heparin 3 hours earlier
    (E) the coumarins keep the prothrombin time five times normal   *(3:1740)*

172. Which of the following statements about Wilms' tumor is/are correct?

    (A) the prognosis is better in younger patients
    (B) treatment is a combination of surgery, radiotherapy, and chemotherapy
    (C) bilateral lesions occur in 5% of patients
    (D) usually occurs as a flank mass
    (E) may contain calcium   *(2:1668–1669)*

173. Which of the following statements about myelomeningocele is/are true?

    (A) they are most common in the lumbosacral region
    (B) operative intervention rarely is indicated during the first year of life
    (C) the birth of a child with meningomyelocele increases the risk of another child of the same parents being born with an anomaly of the nervous system
    (D) the incidence of hydrocephalus is about 15%
    (E) operate early if the meningocele is open and there is motor function in the legs   *(2:1824)*

174. The following statements concern the problem of bilateral breast carcinoma.

(A) in patients with breast cancer, mammography should be performed on both breasts before treatment and at regular intervals thereafter on the opposite breast

(B) bilateral breast cancer is most common in women over 50

(C) the longer a patient lives, the greater the likelihood of cancer in the second breast

(D) bilateral breast carcinoma is most common when the primary breast tumor was of the lobular type

(E) routine biopsy is mandatory   *(1:261)*

175. The following statements are in regard to ulcerative colitis.

(A) when the operation for ulcerative colitis is an emergency or even urgent, the rectum must be removed

(B) the rectum is more likely to be removed in operations for ulcerative colitis than for Crohn's disease

(C) if the operation is urgent and the patient is in poor condition, an ileostomy alone may be the first stage of operative treatment

(D) the age of onset affects the likelihood of developing a malignancy

(E) patients operated successfully for ulcerative colitis before developing a malignancy still do not have a normal life expectancy   *(2:1170–1176)*

176. In tubal pregnancy

(A) the first symptom is shock in 70 to 80% of patients because of exsanguinating hemorrhage that occurs at the time of rupture

(B) the patient usually has the symptoms and signs of early pregnancy and always has a history of recent menstrual irregularity

(C) the uterus will be enlarged and soft even if there is no history of menstrual irregularity

(D) a tubal mass may not be palpable even if the patient is symptomatic from a tubal pregnancy

(E) a test for pregnancy will be positive   *(2:1753)*

177. The first signs of the malignant hyperthermia syndrome during anesthesia include

(A) respiratory acidosis

(B) metabolic acidosis

(C) bradycardia

(D) sustained muscle contracture after succinylcholine

(E) dark venous blood in the operative field   *(1:172)*

178. The following are features of acute cholecystitis.

(A) the cause is usually obstruction of the cystic duct by a small gallstone

(B) the cause in the vast majority of cases is obstruction of the cystic duct by a stone in Hartmann's pouch

(C) most attacks progress to generalized peritonitis

(D) jaundice develops in most patients

(E) an oral cholecystogram is a valuable study   *(1:488)*

179. The following statements concern treatment of carcinoma of the stomach.

(A) palliative resection is indicated if the stomach is still removable

(B) proximal submucosal spread should be suspected at operation. A frozen section of the proximal margin can be useful

(C) adjuvant chemotherapy should follow curative surgery

(D) total gastrectomy and splenectomy is required for tumors of the proximal half of the stomach

(E) for tumors of the antrum, the best reconstruction is a Billroth I gastroduodenal anastomosis   *(1:452)*

180. Protein loss after injury

(A) is due to impaired protein synthesis

(B) occurs primarily from muscle

(C) is commensurate with the protein catabolism needed to supply energy

(D) is greater in healthy young men than in debilitated, elderly men

(E) is greater in the malnourished than in the well nourished   *(2:26–28)*

Answers and Explanations

1. **(C)** Before 1950, the stoma was not everted and sutured to the surrounding skin routinely. The older technique resulted in serositis of the stoma and subsequent stricture in more than half of the patients. Problems are minimized by preoperative marking of the stoma site with the patient standing and by constructing an everted, protruding stoma.

2. **(B)** Toxic megacolon is near to the end-stage of disintegrative colitis, and it may be reversible but an emergency operation is often required. Patients whose disease is progressive under treatment should be operated on before they reach this end-stage, since it has a very high mortality rate.

3. **(D)** Most patients with melena are bleeding from the upper gastrointestinal tract.

4. **(B)** Back pain is uncommon in patients with a perforated peptic ulcer.

5. **(B)** Constipation is not a symptom commonly seen in patients with Crohn's disease.

6. **(B)** Dry gangrene is due to poor blood supply, not neuropathy. In the neuropathic foot, painless ulcers often lead to neglected infections and osteomyelitis.

7. **(B)** Night cramps are not the result of ischemia of the limb.

8. **(B)** The duodenum is resected in a Whipple operation.

9. **(E)** With exercise, blood is shunted to supply the muscles. If there is a proximal arterial obstruction, the peripheral pulses may disappear with exercise and return after rest.

10. **(B)** Bradycardia with occlusion of an arteriovenous fistula is usually referred to as the bradycardia phenomenon, but it is sometimes called Branham's sign.

11. **(B)** There are several methods for removing retained bile duct stones; none should be tried until 4 to 6 weeks have elapsed.

12. **(B)** If an acutely inflamed gallbladder perforates into the intestine, the gallbladder is decompressed and the acute disease resolves. The clinical situation then improves, and the cholecystentric fistula is unsuspected.

13. **(B)** Fibromuscular hyperplasia of the renal arteries is rare, but when hypertension occurs in young adult women, it is a common cause of the elevated blood pressure.

14. **(E)** Operations for extra-anatomic bypass grafts usually are much less stressful to the patient than are anatomic graft procedures. The extra-anatomic graft is used when an anatomic graft becomes infected.

15. **(E)** Between 10 and 20% of patients are asymptomatic when lung cancer is first diagnosed, usually by a chest x-ray. Cough is the only presentation that is more frequent.

16. **(C)** It is often possible to remove such a foreign body with the biopsy attachment of a flexible gastroscope. Prolonged failure of a foreign body, even a blunt one, to progress through the gastrointestinal tract is an indication for operation if the object cannot be retrieved in another way. Arrested pointed and blunt foreign bodies do erode through the wall of the gastrointestinal tract.

17. **(D)** Infections of the hand do not cause axillary-subclavian venous thrombosis.

18. **(B)** Many people carry staphylococci in their nasal passages. These people do not need to be treated and are not removed from duty except in extraordinary circumstances. The proper use of prophylactic antibiotics when indicated does reduce infection, but the indiscriminate use of prophylactic antibiotics increases the infection rate.

19. **(A)** The histologic type of breast tumor, medullary, lobular, or comedo, is of little prognostic significance.

20. **(E)** Surgical therapy is now rarely necessary, although it was the standard treatment before the introduction of antibiotics. Today, antibiotic therapy not only has made surgery a rarity but also has largely prevented this disease.

21. **(B)** Atelectasis may follow any operation, even those performed under local anesthesia, and it is the most common postoperative complication.

22. **(B)** Antivenom of the right type can be lifesaving.

23. **(A)** An early menarche or late menopause is associated with an increased incidence of breast cancer. Patients with a late menarche or artificial menopause have a lower rate of breast cancer.

24. **(A)** Esophageal hiatal hernia is the most common type of diaphragmatic hernia, and the sliding hernia is the most common esophageal hiatal hernia.

25. **(B)** Reflux occurs in normal people but is uncommon in such individuals during sleep. The gastroesophageal junction is normally located in the abdomen, and reflux in those with esophagitis occurs mostly at night.

26. **(E)** Duodenal ulcer is the most probable cause of this man's bleeding.

27. **(C)** The combination of smoking and exposure to asbestos dust (shipyard workers may be exposed to asbestos dust) is associated with mesothelioma.

28. **(D)** A biopsy in these tumors often fails to provide proof of malignancy. The proper treatment for patients with a well-localized chondrosarcoma of this type is wide excision as the initial operative procedure. In the patient described, one would remove at least the rib above and the rib below the lesion.

29. **(A)** Neural symptoms are much more common than vascular symptoms in patients with the thoracic outlet syndrome, but surgery is more likely to relieve the vascular symptoms.

30. **(E)** The patient may have a ruptured spleen or other undetected intraabdominal injury. Laparotomy with repair of the diaphragm from below allows examination of the abdominal viscera.

31. **(D)** The recurrent laryngeal nerve usually is not paralyzed in patients with Pancoast's tumor.

32. **(C)** The patient described almost certainly has infected and inflamed apocrine glands, and this is termed hidradenitis suppurativa.

33. **(C)** Older patients after an injury or operation and patients with severely debilitating illnesses may develop parotitis if they become dehydrated or if they have improper care of the oral cavity. Preventive measures have markedly reduced the incidence.

34. **(E)** When technically possible, endoscopic laser therapy is preferable to the use of a celestine tube.

35. **(C)** A raised central venous pressure after trauma leading to shock raises the possibility of cardiac tamponade.

36. **(E)** Continued anticoagulation during operation to perform arterial embolectomy may prevent further emboli or propagation of the thrombus. There is a high risk of dangerous bleeding in the other procedures listed.

37. **(A)** Cigarette smoking is related causally to lung cancer of the squamous cell and oat cell types but not to adenocarcinoma or alveolar cell carcinoma.

38. **(B)** Control of ventilation in patients at high risk of developing the adult respiratory distress syndrome has improved the survival of such patients. Carcinomatosis alone does not cause the syndrome.

39. **(B)** Carcinoma of the lip is usually well differentiated and often responds well to radiation therapy. Such lesions metastasize via the lymphatics and most commonly occur in men.

40. **(B)** The most common cause of exophthalmos, unilateral or bilateral, is thyrotoxicosis.

41. **(A)** A young patient with no previous history of ulcer disease should have simple closure of the ulcer. A definitive operation at the time of operation for perforation should be reserved for patients in good condition who have a history of chronic or recurrent ulcer disease.

42. **(B)** Failure to improve indicates inadequate drainage. Additional studies to locate the problem followed by repeated percutaneous or open drainage should be undertaken urgently.

43. **(B)** Bronchial adenomas are sometimes benign, but metastasis will occur if the tumor is not resected.

44. **(E)** In Burger's disease, peripheral arterial occlusions often produce instep (arch) claudication before other symptoms are manifest.

45. **(D)** Since breast cancer in men is frequently a disseminated disease, hormone manipulation is of considerable importance in its management. Castration in advanced cases is the best palliative measure.

46. **(E)** Sympathectomy is not particularly effective in Raynaud's phenomenon, and even a good effect may be short-lived. The operation is not considered for the initial management of a newly diagnosed patient.

47. **(B)** Postsympathectomy neuralgia is a distressing and common complication. Fortunately, it subsides in 6 weeks to 3 months.

48. **(E)** Hormone therapy is not advisable because it does not cure mammary dysplasia and has side effects. Danazol, a synthetic androgen, suppresses pituitary gonadotropins and may be used for rare patients who have severe pain.

49. **(A)** In the true thoracic outlet syndrome, the most common symptoms are related to nerve compression.

50. **(E)** Renal injuries that are impossible to correct in vivo may be salvaged by bench surgery.

51. **(C)** Prior adjuvant chemotherapy does not appear to alter the response rate in patients who have relapses.

52. **(A)** Calcium channel blockers decrease pressure in the lower esophagus and improve swallowing, but they are of no value because of the side effects.

53. **(D)** Microemboli are the common cause of the blue toe syndrome.

54. **(D)** Ligature of the artery proximal and distal to the aneurysm with insertion of a vein bypass graft is a good treatment. The aneurysm need not be excised if this technique is used.

55. **(A)** A rectal examination should never be omitted in a patient with an acute abdomen.

56. **(B)** Superficial thrombophlebitis is recognized by examination of the thrombosed (hard, tender) vein. There is local erythema initially and often mild, local edema.

57. **(C)** Most cancers of the breast are infiltrating and invasive ductal. Subtypes include modullary, colloid, tubular, and papillary.

58. **(B)** Pelvic appendicitis causes mild abdominal pain, vomiting, and loose stools. It does not cause constipation.

59. **(B)** The ophthalmic artery is a very important collateral from the extracranial to the intracranial circulation.

60. **(B)** Muscle strain is the likely cause of the patient's severe upper thigh pain following unaccustomed exercise.

61. **(C)** Local heat, elevation of the part, and compression all harm an ischemic extremity. Bed rest with mild dependency is helpful. Resuscitation and fluid replacement should precede operation.

62. **(C)** The excision of an adenoma is curative, but there is little urgency about the operation. In mild cases, the disease can be managed indefinitely by spironolactone or amiloride if side effects do not develop.

63. **(C)** Prolonged vomiting leads to a depletion of chloride and excess of sodium and potassium. Dehydration occurs, and in advanced cases tetany may appear. Gastroscopy should precede operation if cancer is suspected.

64. **(A)** A shunt is not required for the repair of an abdominal aortic aneurysm.

65. **(C)** If the gastrinoma cannot be enucleated, a distal pancreatectomy may be indicated, but a Whipple operation usually can be avoided.

66. **(A)** Breast cancer is second only to lung cancer among women as a cause of death from cancer in the USA.

67. **(E)** In most cases, restriction of water intake will be sufficient to correct the problem. Occasionally, a diuretic, such as furosemide, should be given and isotonic saline should be infused intravenously at a rate equal to the urine output.

68. **(A)** Rectal bleeding, even in a patient with an obviously benign lesion such as hemorrhoids, must be considered to be due to cancer until it is ruled out.

69. **(E)** Heartburn does not occur. Such complications as hemorrhage, incarceration, obstruction, and strangulation are common. Other viscera, such as the intestine or spleen, can herniate. Surgical repair is indicated because complications are common. The usual surgical repair is described in **E.**

70. **(A)** Being economically prosperous increases the risk of colon cancer probably because the diet of the rich segment of society contains more fat and less fiber.

71. **(B)** Chronic ischemia of the intestine does not decrease peristalsis. It increases peristalsis unless necrosis occurs.

72. **(A)** Combinations of drugs are clearly superior to single drugs, and tamoxifen has been shown to enhance the beneficial effects of melphalan and fluorouracil in women whose tumors were estrogen receptor positive.

73. **(B)** Diverticulitis is a much more frequent cause of large bowel obstruction than is volvulus.

74. **(B)** The use of estrogens or progesterone agents is inadvisable after treatment of breast cancer, particularly in those patients who are estrogen receptor positive.

75. **(C)** Loss of fluid from the vascular compartment into the interstitial space is due to increased capillary permeability.

76. **(D)** The initial rapid bolus of isotonic salt solution (Ringer's lactate is the first choice) is usually 1 to 2 L. This is 20 to 40% of the normal 5-L blood volume of a 70-kg patient. In the pediatric patient, the bolus is 20 ml/kg. This bolus is given as rapidly as possible, and the response is carefully monitored as a guide to further therapy. The ultimate amount of fluid administered roughly follows a 3 for 1 rule—3 times the volume of blood lost will need to be replaced as crystalloid. The CVP is a crude measure of volume status and is subject to error from vasoconstriction, catheter malposition, cardiac dysfunction, and pneumothorax. It is not a good endpoint for assessing the effect of the bolus. The ultimate goal of organ perfusion is better reflected by a urine output of 50 ml/hour in the adult and 1 ml/kg/hour in the child (2 ml/kg/hour under 1 year of age).

77. **(A)** A patient with a myxoma of the left atrium may have a diastolic murmur suggesting mitral stenosis, or a systolic murmur. He does not have a continuous systolic and diastolic murmur.

78. **(B)** In pure mitral stenosis, the left ventricle does not hypertrophy. A heaving left ventricular impulse suggests associated mitral insufficiency or aortic valvular disease.

79. **(E)** Many children with pulmonary stenosis and an intact interventricular septum have no symptoms and develop normally, but most patients with pulmonary stenosis have a patent foramen ovale. Cyanosis and symptoms develop due to right ventricular failure.

80. **(B)** The mandibular or lowest branch of the facial nerve passes over the upper part of the submandibular salivary gland and is most likely to be injured. The lingual nerve may also be injured during the division of Wharton's duct.

81. **(E)** Asymptomatic cervical adenopathy is the most common presentation of Hodgkin's disease (65 to 80%), followed by axillary and inguinal presentations (15 and 12%, respectively). Sys-

temic symptoms indicate advanced disease with diffuse spread and put the patient in the B classification, which carries a worse prognosis. The spleen is rarely palpable. Hodgkin's disease has a binodal age distribution, with peaks in the late 20s and mid-40s. Biopsy of the most central of a cluster of enlarged nodes is most likely to demonstrate the multinucleated Reed-Sternberg giant cell, which establishes the diagnosis.

82. **(C)** The majority of branchial anomalies represent remnants of the second branchial cleft. The artery of the second branchial arch is the external carotid artery, and the internal carotid artery is the artery of the third branchial arch. The track of a second branchial cleft fistula, therefore, passes between the internal and external carotid arteries.

83. **(B)** The optimum treatment of acute extradural hematoma is urgent operation. The high mortality is due to irreversible changes occurring before surgical relief.

84. **(B)** Volkmann's ischemic contracture follows injuries around the elbow joint, particularly supracondylar fractures with compression of the brachial artery.

85. **(C)** Voluntary movement may be inhibited in acute osteomyelitis, resulting in an apparent paralysis.

86. **(D)** The Monteggia deformity consists of a fracture of the proximal third of the shaft of the ulna and a dislocation of the head of the radius. The fracture is produced by a blow on the medial or ulnar side of the forearm followed by forced pronation and dislocation of the head of the radius.

87. **(E)** Compression fractures of the thoracic spine are usually stable, and there is no way of satisfactorily reducing these fractures. At age 70, treatment is designed to prevent chest complications or ileus.

88. **(C)** The basic goal of cancer chemotherapy is the development of agents with selective toxicity against replicating tumor cells that at the same time spare the replicating host tissues.

89. **(A)** Pulmonary valvular stenosis was not included in the original description of tetralogy of Fallot, although it occurs in 20% of cases. The key feature of the anomaly is pulmonary infundibular outflow obstruction, which creates resistance to right ventricular emptying, forcing blood from right to left through the ventricular septal defect, which equalizes the pressures in the ventricles. Postnatally, the patent ductus arteriosus prevents cyanosis, and in most cases, the patient remains hemodynamically stable until surgical correction can be performed around age 3 to 5.

90. **(B)** A double arch accounts for 40% of aortic arch anomalies. When this anomaly causes symptoms of tracheal or esophageal compression, it may become necessary to divide one arch. Otherwise, these generally are benign conditions.

91. **(E)** Ventricular septal defect is the most common congenital cardiac lesion, comprising 30 to 40%. Only 10 to 20% of these patients have a defect large enough to cause serious problems.

92. **(A)** Rather than draining into the left atrium, the pulmonary veins most often join the left innominate vein (26%). Almost as frequently, the connection is to the ductus venosus (24%). The coronary sinus, superior vena cava, and right atrium are the remaining common connections in decreasing order of frequency. The majority of these infants are in distress, with congestive heart failure and cyanosis in the perinatal period. Early restoration of drainage into the left atrium is the only hope of salvage and is meeting with increasing success.

93. **(E)** The characteristic visual disturbance of vertebral-basilar arterial insufficiency is diplopia, not blurring of vision.

94. **(B)** A widened mediastinum after a deceleration injury may be due to a hematoma of which an important cause is rupture of the thoracic aorta. An emergency aortogram is the only way to establish the diagnosis of this potentially lethal lesion.

95. **(A)** Good results sometimes follow aortic repair without bypass, but it is safer to establish either an aorta-to-aorta bypass or an aorta-to-femoral artery bypass before clamping and repairing the aortic rupture.

96. **(E)** Alkaline reflux gastritis most commonly occurs in patients who have had pylorus-disrupting gastric surgery. In patients who have failed ther-

apy with aluminum hydroxide, bland diet, and cholestyramine, the preferred treatment is Roux-en-Y gastrojejunostomy with 40 to 60 cm separation between the flow of bile and the stomach. Isoperistaltic jejunal loop interposition has been tried in the past and found to be unreliable. Biliay–enteric anastomoses and gastric resection are not indicated.

97. **(B)** Stimulation of the carotid sinus nerve slows the pulse, lowers the blood pressure, decreases the cardiac output, and reduces the venous return.

98. **(A)** Hemiparesis is caused by a lesion of the cerebrum, not the cerebellum.

99. **(B)** Hypertonus, particularly truncal rigidity in young muscular individuals, is a side effect of narcotic anesthesia, which is counteracted with muscle relaxants. Narcotics are noteworthy for not altering cardiovascular dynamics and are used for relief of pulmonary edema.

100. **(E)** The persistence of chorionic gonadotropin in the serum or urine 4 to 6 weeks after a hydratidiform molar pregnancy is presumptive evidence of active trophoblastic tissue.

101. **(B)** Repair of the parotid duct with fine sutures over a plastic catheter represents the optimal treatment of an injury to the superficial portion of the parotid duct.

102. **(C)** Granulocytes predominate in the first phase of the cellular response of inflammation. During the humorally mediated (endotoxin, histamine, kinins, prostaglandins) first phase, early microvascular alterations occur (sphincter contraction, venular and capillary dilatation), endothelial cells separate and granulocytes marginate and diapedese into the interstitial space. The more numerous but short-lived (24 hours) granulocytes move randomly until within range of a chemoattractant, at which time they move in a directed way to phagocytize invading organisms. As the first wave of granulocytes dwindles, the monocytes and macrophages become relatively more numerous and continue the phagocytosis.

103. **(E)** Radiation endarteritis is the primary lesion resulting in bowel injury. Most such injuries occur in the high rectum (10 to 14 cm) after radiation for cervical and uterine cancer (although only 1 to 2% of women so treated develop

the complication). The pain, bleeding, and diarrhea of radiation proctitis are treated conservatively and usually subside when the radiotherapy is stopped. A small number go on to rectal stenosis 6 to 18 months after radiation, and these patients may require resection.

104. **(B)** This disastrous event is now also seen in drug abusers. Heparin (15,000 units) should be given and an intravenous infusion set up at a new site. Because of the need for heparin anticoagulation, the submucous resection of the nasal septum should be deferred. A tourniquet would make matters much worse. A nerve block should not be performed in the presence of full heparinization.

105. **(E)** Whether the treatment of choice for a recurrent basal cell carcinoma would be irradiation or reexcision would depend on such factors as size, location, previous therapy, and the facilities available. Additional surgery is not likely to be effective in controlling recurrent adrenal carcinomas.

106. **(D)** Ultrasound and CT will demonstrate a dilated pancreatic duct but give little information about the ampulla. ERCP demonstrates the ductal architecture, as does PTCP, but yields no functional information about the ampulla. Only manometry demonstrates functional abnormality, such as spasm.

107. **(D)** An essential factor in the success of an arterial bypass graft is at least a partially patent distal arterial tree.

108. **(C)** The history of irregular menses, sudden lower abdominal pain, and the signs of intraabdominal bleeding are diagnostic of a ruptured ectopic pregnancy.

109. **(B)** When a pathologic condition of the tube or ovary is suspected, direct vision with culdoscopy or laparoscopy can provide an accurate diagnosis.

110. **(B)** Young adults who fall on the outstretched hand frequently fracture the navicular. The fracture line may not be seen on films taken at the time of injury.

111. **(D)** It is probable that this patient has suffered an embolus of the superior mesenteric artery and that the source of this embolus is the wall of the left ventricle where a thrombus has formed

at the site of the myocardial infarction. This is a difficult diagnosis to make on purely clinical grounds, and it is important to avoid an unnecessary abdominal operation in a patient who recently has had an acute myocardial infarction. Catheter arteriography of the abdominal aorta with lateral views will provide definite evidence of the presence or absence of obstruction to the mesenteric arteries. This investigation has definite risks, but the gains would outweigh the risks in a patient of this type.

112. **(B)** An essential part of the diagnosis of an embolus of any vessel in the body is to have a source for the embolus. In this patient, the recent myocardial infarction is a clear source because of mural thrombus that may form at this site. It has long been recognized that ischemia of the intestine can occur in the absence of arterial occlusion, but these patients are often very ill and are not recovering satisfactorily from the myocardial infarction.

113. **(C)** Reported series (Oltinger and Austen, 1967) suggest that operative relief of an acute obstruction of the superior mesenteric artery is always indicated and that conservative management has little place. It is true that persistent infarction of the midgut is not compatible with life, but conservative care for a short period is of great value. It consists of fluid replacement, anticoagulation, antibiotics, and correction of acidosis plus continued treatment of the cardiac problem. If resuscitation is satisfactory and the diagnosis is established, laparotomy is justified because without it the mortality is, for practical purposes, 100%.

114. **(E)** After a successful embolectomy of the superior mesenteric artery and the restoration of blood flow to the midgut, it is usually impossible to predict the degree of recovery of the intestine. The best way out of this dilemma is to close the abdomen and perform a second-look procedure 12 to 24 hours later. At this time, any ischemic areas can be resected, but recovery may be complete and none of the intestine will have to be sacrificed.

115. **(A)** The goals of operative treatment are cure of the symptoms and prevention of carcinoma. This is only achieved by total coloproctectomy. The rectum or the mucosa of the rectum must be removed. Ileoproctostomy is unsatisfactory

because symptoms persist, and carcinoma may develop in the rectum.

116. **(B)** Sideropenic dysphagia (Plummer-Vinson syndrome) consists of cervical dysphagia, usually due to an esophageal web in anemic, edentulous women over the age of 40. With a high incidence in Great Britain and Scandinavia, this condition is associated with a 10% rate of cancer in the oral cavity, hypopharynx, and esophagus. The diverticula cited are not part of this syndrome. A Schatzki ring or distal esophageal web is a circular shelf of mucosa and submucosa at the squamocolumnar junction in some patients with a sliding hiatal hernia. The etiology is unclear.

117. **(A)** Pseudomyxoma peritonei usually results from rupture of a pseudomucinous cystadenoma of the ovary or, rarely, a mucocele of the appendix.

118. **(B)** A difficult problem occurs when regional enteritis is found at operation for suspected acute appendicitis. Should the appendix be removed? About one quarter of patients with regional enteritis and an enterocutaneous fistula have had recent appendectomy, but if the appendix is not removed, a later attack of real appendicitis may be allowed to perforate because it is considered to be a further exacerbation of the regional enteritis. A good rule is to remove the appendix if the cecum near to the base of the appendix is not involved by the enteritis.

119. **(E)** The patient may continue to have abdominal problems that often can be controlled without another operation.

120. **(C)** The local anesthetics cause decreased myocardial excitability and are used for suppressing ectopic foci. Anxiety, tinnitus, and CNS toxicity, which can lead to convulsions, may result from excessive dosage, rapid absorption, or accidental intravenous injection.

121. **(C)** The serum calcium level is normal in a patient with multiple myeloma.

122. **(A)** A neuroblastoma is a common tumor in childhood. Except in infancy, metastases to bone are frequent.

123. **(A)** The liver is the sole source of the prothrombin-related factors (II, VII, IX, X) and fibrinogen (factor I). Hepatic dysfunction commonly affects the former but only causes a drop in fibrinogen

when severely diseased. The liver also metabolizes fibrin split products produced by the fibrinolytic system. These products can act as antithrombins, interfere with platelet function, and damage capillary endothelium. When cirrhosis causes portal hypertension, splenomegaly, and hypersplenism, platelets are consumed in the spleen.

124. **(E)** The femoral nerve supplies the quadriceps femoris muscle group, of which the rectus femoris is a part.

125. **(B)** Ampicillin, a third-generation, extended-spectrum penicillin, is ineffective against all *Pseudomonas* species. Carbenicillin, a third-generation carboxypenicillin, is effective against *Pseudomonas,* as are all the fourth-generation, broad-spectrum penicillins, mezlocillin, azlocillin, and piperacillin. The latter are also particularly effective against *Klebsiella.* The first-generation natural penicillins G and V have a limited, predominantly gram-positive spectrum. The second-generation penicillins were designed for penicillinase resistance.

126. **(A)** Violent emesis against a closed glottis is the presumed mechanism in a Mallory–Weiss tear. Increased intracavitary pressure, as with the strain of weightlifting, is not reported to cause this condition. The wide variety of conditions that can cause forceful vomiting often distract attention from the diagnosis. In most cases, the bleeding stops spontaneously with conservative measures. Rarely is transgastric oversewing necessary.

127. **(B)** Although aldosterone secretion is slightly influenced by ACTH, it depends primarily on the secretion of renin and angiotensin for its regulation. Hypophysectomy leads to atrophy of the adrenal cortex, but the glomerular zone is only partially under pituitary control and aldosterone continues to be elaborated and secreted.

128. **(B)** In young patients, emphysematous blebs, and in older patients, blebs associated with generalized emphysema are the most common cause of spontaneous pneumothorax.

129. **(B)** In infants, lung abscesses usually resolve with antibiotics and supportive therapy.

130. **(D)** Bronchial tumors were formerly considered to be one of three types of bronchial adenomas.

They show a spectrum of behavior from benign to malignant.

131. **(D)** Bronchoscopy is the most important procedure in the diagnosis of bronchial carcinoid tumors.

132. **(B)** This patient is producing yellow sputum. This means that secondary infection has caused bronchiectasis. Therefore, lobectomy is the best treatment.

133. **(A)** The prognosis after adequate excision is good, with a long-term survival of close to 90%.

134. **(E)** Carcinoma of the lung is a common lesion, particularly if the patient has suffered from chronic irritation for many years.

135. **(B)** This patient has a palpable mass in the left supraclavicular area. Biopsy of this should confirm the diagnosis of carcinoma of the lung.

136. **(E)** The ultrashort-acting thiobarbiturates, such as thiopental, lose their CNS anesthetic effects when they are rapidly redistributed to other tissues. The primary degradation of these drugs is in the liver, and the products are excreted in the urine, but this process proceeds slowly, long after reversal of CNS effects.

137. **(A)** Crepitus in the neck, although sometimes minimal, is a common finding in patients with a perforation of the esophagus.

138. **(E)** Water-soluble contrast swallow with fluoroscopy is an important diagnostic procedure in such patients.

139. **(B)** This patient suffered from both abdominal and chest pain. The likely site for the perforation is, therefore, the thoracic esophagus.

140. **(E)** Atelectasis usually occurs during the first 24 hours after an operation. Occurrence after 48 hours is rare.

141. **(D)** The most common causes of chylothorax are trauma and malignancy. The most common malignancy causing chylothorax is lymphosarcoma, but metastatic carcinoma is also an important cause.

142. **(E)** Tachycardia is usually the earliest sign of

esophageal perforation and reflects early mediastinitis from spillage of esophageal contents. There follows a progression from tachypnea to hypotension and shock. Signs of mediastinal and subcutaneous air occur later than changes in vital signs, although the progression is often rapid and catastrophic. Dyspnea often represents rupture into a pleural cavity. Because the pain and other signs of rupture can mimic cardiovascular and gastrointestinal emergencies, it is important to have a high index of suspicion and watch for the early signs after esophageal instrumentation.

143. **(E)** Dermoid cysts are well defined on the x-ray and show calcification in the wall.

144. **(B)** Cefazolin (Ancef), a first-generation cephalosporin, provides the most long-lasting high serum levels, making it the best agent for surgical prophylaxis. Ideally, the first dose is given just before surgery to establish optimal blood levels. The second-generation cephalosporins, such as cefoxitin, extended the spectrum against gram-negative bacilli and anaerobes, although they are less effective against staphylococci and streptococci. The third-generation agents, such as mox-alactam, have increased effectiveness against *Enterobacter, Serratia,* and *Pseudomonas.* The carbapenems, such as imipenem, could be considered the fourth-generation cephalosporins and have the widest spectrum of any antibiotic.

145. **(C)** Complete obstruction of a bronchus is followed by absorption of the air trapped behind the obstruction, followed by atelectasis, and then suppuration, if not treated.

146. **(A)** A circumferential full-thickness burn may produce increasing constriction with venous stasis, and then arterial obstruction with gangrene. The treatment is splitting of the eschar.

147. **(A) (T), (B) (T), (C) (T), (D) (T), (E) (T)** Fecal impaction is the arrest and accumulation of feces in the rectum that are progressively dehydrated by the colonic mucosa.

148. **(A) (T), (B) (T), (C) (T), (D) (T), (E) (F)** An attack of tetanus does not confer immunity. Unless immunized, the patient is susceptible to a second attack.

149. **(A) (T), (B) (F), (C) (F), (D) (T), (E) (F)** The female spider is dangerous. The pain comes on immediately. A specific antivenom is available.

150. **(A) (T), (B) (T), (C) (T), (D) (T), (E) (T)** All statements are true.

151. **(A) (T), (B) (F), (C) (T), (D) (T), (E) (F)** Up to 60% of patients with metastatic breast cancer respond to hormone manipulation if the tumor contains estrogen receptors. Receptors probably have no relationship to the response to chemotherapy.

152. **(A) (T), (B) (F), (C) (T), (D) (F), (E) (F)** Hemophilia often causes a hemarthrosis. It is inherited as a sex-linked recessive. There is not an increased incidence of peptic ulcer.

153. **(A) (T), (B) (T), (C) (T), (D) (T), (E) (T)** All of the conditions are associated with acute gastric erosions.

154. **(A) (T), (B) (T), (C) (T), (D) (T), (E) (T)** All statements are true.

155. **(A) (T), (B) (T), (C) (T), (D) (F), (E) (F)** The cure rate for actinic skin cancer is about equal with surgery or radiotherapy. Renal cell carcinoma is best treated by surgery.

156. **(A) (T), (B) (T), (C) (T), (D) (T), (E) (T)** Torsion of the testicle requires urgent surgery if testicular function is to be preserved. Because of the high incidence of bilateral abnormalities, both sides should be treated surgically.

157. **(A) (T), (B) (T), (C) (T), (D) (F), (E) (T)** Sarcoma of bone does not have a familial tendency; the other tumors do.

158. **(A) (F), (B) (T), (C) (T), (D) (T), (E) (T)** Meigs' syndrome pertains to ascites and hydrothorax associated with ovarian fibromas. Other ovarian tumors are often present, particularly ovarian carcinoma. Lymphedema of the leg is not part of this syndrome.

159. **(A) (F), (B) (T), (C) (T), (D) (F), (E) (F)** The incidence of Crohn's colitis is increasing, and malignant change rarely occurs.

160. **(A) (F), (B) (F), (C) (T), (D) (T), (E) (T)** The perforation is usually a linear tear in the left posterolateral aspect of the esophagus 3 to 5 cm above the gastroesophageal junction.

161. **(A) (T), (B) (F), (C) (T), (D) (F), (E) (F)** Clostridial myonecrosis is painful, increases the pulse rate, and may respond to penicillin, and

antitoxin is of no value therapeutically. The patient has a fever.

162. **(A) (T), (B) (T), (C) (F), (D) (F), (E) (F)**
Carcinoma of the tongue spreads to the cervical nodes early in many patients. Squamous cell carcinoma is the most common in the lip. Verrucous carcinoma in older tobacco chewers progresses slowly.

163. **(A) (T), (B) (T), (C) (T), (D) (T), (E) (F)**
Thrombosis of the superficial femoral artery is usually treated medically. Alcohol in moderation is a vasodilator.

164. **(A) (T), (B) (T), (C) (T), (D) (T), (E) (T)**
There are four grades of astrocytoma. Grades III and IV are known as glioblastomas and are the most malignant and the most common.

165. **(A) (F), (B) (T), (C) (T), (D) (T), (E) (F)**
Villous adenomas usually have a thick mucous covering and are easy to identify visually but are soft and difficult to identify by palpation. One third of lesions are within reach of the finger, and 80 to 90% are found below 25 cm. Ulceration and induration are signs of malignancy, and the malignant potential of these lesions is high (12 to 40% harbor invasive carcinoma at diagnosis). The uncommon hypersecreting lesions usually are large but rarely malignant.

166. **(A) (T), (B) (T), (C) (T), (D) (F), (E) (F)**
The cause of Schatzki's rings has not been determined. Although the results of therapy have been disappointing, the condition is not premalignant.

167. **(A) (T), (B) (F), (C) (T), (D) (F), (E) (T)**
Factor V is not stable in banked blood. Factor VII rapidly deteriorates during storage.

168. **(A) (T), (B) (F), (C) (T), (D) (F), (E) (T)**
Anticoagulants form the primary basis for therapy in most patients with pulmonary embolization. Heparin is usually employed, and its effect when administered intravenously is almost immediate.

169. **(A) (T), (B) (T), (C) (T), (D) (F), (E) (T)**
It is not necessary to remove the catheter through which incompatible blood is given. It can be used for further transfusions with compatible blood.

170. **(A) (F), (B) (T), (C) (F), (D) (T), (E) (T)**
PEEP decreases venous return and hence the cardiac output. This means that fluids are needed to ensure an adequate intravascular volume. The FRC is high in patients with chronic obstructive pulmonary disease. For these patients a decrease of the FRC is detrimental.

171. **(A) (T), (B) (T), (C) (T), (D) (T), (E) (F)**
Coumadin (warfarin sodium) is usually given in sufficient dosage to keep the prothrombin time 2 to 2½ times the normal level.

172. **(A) (T), (B) (T), (C) (T), (D) (T), (E) (T)**
Wilms' tumor usually occurs as an asymptomatic mass in the upper abdomen.

173. **(A) (T), (B) (F), (C) (T), (D) (F), (E) (T)**
Today in North America operative treatment is usually carried out early in life. About 85% of patients also have hydrocephalus. Unfortunately, closure of the defect in the back does not improve lower extremity function, but it does protect the nervous system from mechanical trauma.

174. **(A) (T), (B) (F), (C) (T), (D) (T), (E) (F)**
Bilateral breast cancer occurs more commonly in women under 50 than over 50. Routine biopsy of the other breast is not usually warranted; regular mammography is.

175. **(A) (F), (B) (T), (C) (F), (D) (F), (E) (F)**
The definitive treatment is proctocolectomy for ulcerative colitis. This is preferably done in one stage, though some surgeons prefer to remove the rectum at a second stage. An ileostomy alone is not effective. The long-term results of proctocolectomy are favorable.

176. **(A) (F), (B) (F), (C) (F), (D) (T), (E) (F)**
This is a disease of surprises. Cramps are often the first symptom. Symptoms of pregnancy are often not present. A tubal mass is palpable in about 50% of patients, and a pregnancy test is negative in half the patients.

177. **(A) (T), (B) (T), (C) (F), (D) (T), (E) (T)**
Malignant hyperpyrexia is a rare life-threatening complication of general anesthesia. The temperature may rise above 41.5°C. The pulse rate rises too.

178. **(A) (F), (B) (T), (C) (F), (D) (F), (E) (F)**
In 95% of patients, the cause is a stone in Hartmann's pouch. Free perforation is uncommon and occurs in less than 2% of patients. Jaundice is not a feature. An oral cholecystogram cannot be relied on during an attack of acute cholecystitis.

179. **(A) (T), (B) (T), (C) (F), (D) (T), (E) (F)**
Adjuvant chemotherapy after curative surgery has not been of value with the regimens tested to date. A Billroth I reconstruction has the disadvantage that postoperative growth of residual tumor may obstruct the anstomosis.

180. **(A) (F), (B) (T), (C) (F), (D) (T), (E) (F)**
An increase in urinary nitrogen excretion occurs rapidly after an injury and reaches a peak after 1 week. It may persist for 3 to 7 weeks.

Fifth Examination
Questions

DIRECTIONS (Questions 1 through 180): Each of the numbered items or incomplete statements in this section is followed by answers or by completions of the statement. Select the ONE lettered answer or completion that is BEST in each case.

1. A newborn child is found to have an imperforate anus. A membrane is palpable by the tip of the finger in the anus. The best operation is

   (A) simple resection of the intervening structures in the perineum
   (B) colostomy
   (C) combined abdominoperineal resection
   (D) anterior abdominal approach with repair
   (E) pull through operation   (2:1658-1659)

2. When penicillin and the cephalosporins cannot be used against resistant staphylococci, the drug of choice is

   (A) erythromycin
   (B) tetracycline
   (C) doxycycline
   (D) vancomycin
   (E) amikacin   (18:794-795)

3. A child who sustains a burn covering most of the head and one upper extremity has approximately what percentage of body surface area involved?

   (A) 9%
   (B) 14%
   (C) 18%
   (D) 27%
   (E) 36%   (9:289)

4. The exact etiology of the dumping syndrome is not known, but which of the following probably plays NO ROLE in the causation?

   (A) decrease in the blood volume
   (B) changes in the pulse rate and blood pressure
   (C) decrease in the extracellular fluid
   (D) hemoconcentration
   (E) hypomotility   (2:1123)

5. The percentage of patients with perforated duodenal ulcer who have free air demonstrated by abdominal x-ray is approximately

   (A) 15%
   (B) 35%
   (C) 55%
   (D) 75%
   (E) 95%   (3:829)

6. A woman, age 74, had for 18 years suffered from indigestion. It had not been severe and consisted of occasional mild and brief attacks of crampy abdominal pain. She had not been in the hospital before. One week before admission, she had complained of epigastric fullness and nausea after a large meal. Vomiting started the next day and persisted intermittently with colicky abdominal pain until admission. The admission x-ray of the abdomen was diagnostic of obstruction of the small intestine. The likely cause of this problem is

   (A) metastatic intraperitoneal carcinoma
   (B) abdominal adhesion
   (C) gallstone ileus
   (D) carcinoma of the right colon
   (E) abdominal lymphosarcoma   (2:1323)

7. In dislocation of the shoulder joint, which of the following is the LEAST likely to be true?

(A) it is the result of abduction
(B) it is usually through the anterior capsule
(C) the head of the humerus usually lies anterior and inferior
(D) the coracoid process is often fractured
(E) it is likely to become recurrent   *(2:1965)*

8. Which of the following does NOT pertain to a patient with an intracapsular fracture of the neck of the femur?

(A) is more common in an elderly patient
(B) the lower limb is abducted and externally rotated
(C) often leads to nonunion
(D) avascular necrosis is common
(E) the fracture is usually comminuted *(2:1980)*

Questions 9 through 11

A 56-year-old man has suffered from mild intermittent claudication for 8 years. Six months before the present hospital admission, he began to complain of mild, upper abdominal crampy pains. These pains gradually became worse and more frequent. They were made worse by eating a large meal. He has lost 15 pounds. He has suffered from both diarrhea and constipation, and a bruit can be heard in the epigastrium.

9. The most likely diagnosis is

(A) chronic pancreatitis
(B) peptic ulcer
(C) chronic cholecystitis
(D) carcinoma of the colon
(E) chronic intestinal ischemia   *(2:1436-1438)*

10. The patient is fully investigated. Which of the following studies would be positive?

(A) upper gastrointestinal series
(B) barium enema
(C) mesenteric and celiac arteriogram
(D) cholecystogram
(E) tests for pancreatic function   *(2:1436-1438)*

11. A laparotomy is performed that confirms the radiologic findings of a thrombosis of the celiac artery, a severe stenosis of the superior mesenteric artery near its origin from the aorta, and a somewhat enlarged inferior mesenteric artery. The best operative procedure would be

(A) bypass grafts from the aorta to the celiac and superior mesenteric arteries
(B) vein graft bypass from aorta to the superior mesenteric artery
(C) bypass graft from the aorta to the celiac artery using the splenic artery
(D) thromboendarterectomy of the celiac and superior mesenteric arteries
(E) division of the splanchnic nerve with resection of the celiac ganglion   *(2:1437)*

Questions 12 through 14

A 28-year-old male with a history of previous emotional disturbances enters the hospital with a history of weight loss and regurgitation of food, which has been getting worse for the past 9 months. The regurgitation is worse when he lies down.

12. The most likely diagnosis is

(A) hiatal hernia
(B) peptic esophagitis
(C) achalasia of the esophagus
(D) pyloric stenosis
(E) duodenal ulcer   *(2:1069)*

13. The best initial treatment would be

(A) forceful pneumatic dilatation
(B) Heller procedure
(C) antispasmodic drugs
(D) repair of the hiatal hernia
(E) vagotomy and pyloroplasty   *(21:349)*

14. The response to dilatation has been unsatisfactory. The most acceptable treatment would now be

(A) resection of the distal esophagus and jejunal interposition
(B) resection of the distal esophagus and esophagogastrostomy
(C) Heller myotomy
(D) esophagogastrostomy
(E) vagotomy   *(21:392)*

15. Among the following factors, the one absolute CONTRAINDICATION to the use of the pneumatic antishock garment is

(A) pelvic fracture
(B) myocardial dysfunction
(C) head injury
(D) intrathoracic bleeding
(E) diaphragmatic rupture   *(9:189)*

16. Bleeding from Meckel's diverticulum in the male is most commonly due to

    (A) aberrant gastric mucosa and ileal ulcer
    (B) inflammatory ulceration
    (C) aberrant pancreatic tissue
    (D) strangulation
    (E) ulcer in the diverticulum   *(2:1159)*

17. Septic shock is most commonly associated with

    (A) staphylococcal septicemia
    (B) subphrenic abscess
    (C) pneumococcal pneumonia
    (D) gram-negative septicemia
    (E) meningococcal meningitis   *(2:154)*

Questions 18 and 19

A 15-year-old boy sustains a valgus injury to the right arm and is brought to the hospital 1 hour later with swelling and tenderness over the medial epicondyle and numbness and tingling in the fourth and fifth fingers of the right hand. X-ray reveals a small fragment of bone near the olecranon.

18. The most likely diagnosis is

    (A) dislocation of the elbow joint
    (B) fracture of the medial epicondyle of the humerus
    (C) fracture of the olecranon
    (D) rupture of the annular ligament
    (E) a supracondylar fracture of the humerus
    (2:1971)

19. The treatment of choice would be

    (A) suture of the annular ligament
    (B) closed reduction and Kirschner wire traction
    (C) reduction in extension and pronation
    (D) open reduction of the fracture and repair of the flexor origin
    (E) application of a sling and active motion within the range of pain tolerance *(2:1971)*

20. Considering all age groups, open operation is most frequently required in which of the following fractures?

    (A) femoral neck
    (B) head of radius
    (C) neck of humerus
    (D) shaft of femur
    (E) shaft of tibia   *(2:1980)*

21. A patient has a full leg cast applied with 5° of knee flexion after a fracture-dislocation of the knee joint has been reduced. Soon after, it is noted that the pedal pulses are absent. The treatment should be

    (A) hot cradle
    (B) inject intraarterial papaverine
    (C) arteriogram of popliteal artery
    (D) paravertebral block
    (E) elevation of the limb   *(3:1479)*

22. A 10-year-old boy has headache and is found to have a solitary lesion of the right frontal bone. It is tender. There is a palpable defect, and x-ray reveals a radiolucent area. The most likely diagnosis is

    (A) osteogenic sarcoma
    (B) osteoid osteoma
    (C) monostotic fibrous dysplasia
    (D) eosinophilic granuloma
    (E) Ewing's tumor   *(2:1928)*

23. An 8-year-old boy has sudden onset of pain in the thigh radiating to the knee. He keeps the hip joint of that side extended, and he limps. The most likely diagnosis is

    (A) coxa valga
    (B) coxa plana (Legg-Calve-Perthes disease)
    (C) Osgood-Schlatter's disease
    (D) epiphyseal coxa vara
    (E) tuberculosis of the hip joint   *(2:1874–1875)*

Questions 24 through 26

A black male, age 62, who is known to be hypertensive, is admitted with severe pain of sudden origin in the back, chest, and upper abdomen. He has been in good health apart from the high blood pressure.

24. The most likely diagnosis is

    (A) myocardial infarction
    (B) dissecting aneurysm of the aorta
    (C) ruptured aortic aneurysm
    (D) perforated peptic ulcer
    (E) spontaneous rupture of the esophagus
    (2:885–887)

25. The most useful investigation would be

   (A) an electrocardiogram
   (B) a lumbar puncture
   (C) an angiocardiogram
   (D) an aortogram with a percutaneous femoral catheter
   (E) an abdominal paracentesis   *(2:885-887)*

26. The best treatment would be

   (A) thoracotomy and immediate repair
   (B) lower the blood pressure to 100 to 120 systolic and operate as a semiemergency in 24 to 48 hours
   (C) lower the blood pressure and treat conservatively
   (D) insert bilateral axillary-to-femoral bypass grafts
   (E) immediate laparatomy   *(2:885-887)*

27. A man is involved in an automobile accident, sustaining a facial fracture and closed head injury. He develops rhinorrhea. Which of the following should NOT be done during the first 48 hours?

   (A) obtain glucose determination on the fluid
   (B) repair the meningeal defect through a transfrontal exposure
   (C) place on antibiotics
   (D) observe the patient carefully
   (E) reduce the facial fracture   *(3:1311)*

28. Aortic insufficiency from acquired aortic valvular disease becomes clinically significant when what percentage of ejected blood regurgitates?

   (A) 10%
   (B) 30%
   (C) 50%
   (D) 70%
   (E) 90%   *(3:2336)*

29. The preferred primary therapy of gastric lymphoma is

   (A) wedge resection
   (B) subtotal gastrectomy
   (C) total gastrectomy
   (D) radiotherapy
   (E) chemotherapy   *(3:861)*

30. Squamous carcinoma of the esophagus, which constitutes over 95% of esophageal cancers, occurs

   (A) with equal frequency throughout the esophagus
   (B) most often in the cervical esophagus
   (C) most often in the upper two thirds of the thoracic esophagus
   (D) most often in the lower third of the thoracic esophagus
   (E) most often in Barrett's mucosa   *(3:738)*

31. The goal of resuscitation for hemorrhagic shock is

   (A) replacement of estimated blood loss
   (B) replacement of three times the estimated blood loss
   (C) maintenance of central venous pressure (CVP) between 5 and 10 cm of water
   (D) maintenance of CVP between 10 and 15 cm of water
   (E) restoration of organ perfusion   *(9:190)*

32. Splenic artery aneurysm

   (A) should be observed closely for enlargement
   (B) commonly results from medial dysplasia in men
   (C) commonly results from atherosclerosis in women
   (D) is at increased risk for rupture during pregnancy
   (E) can only be identified by angiogram   *(3:1228)*

33. The classic triad of symptoms seen in chronic pancreatitis is

   (A) weight loss, diabetes, diarrhea
   (B) weight gain, confusion, diabetes
   (C) weight loss, diabetes, steatorrhea
   (D) anorexia, nausea, epigastric pain
   (E) diaphoresis, weight loss, steatorrhea *(3:1186)*

34. The most accurate diagnostic test for acute cholecystitis is

   (A) supine and upright abdominal x-rays
   (B) oral cholecystogram
   (C) intravenous cholangiogram
   (D) ultrasound
   (E) technetium scan   *(3:1139)*

35. The majority of bile duct strictures result from

   (A) congenital anomaly
   (B) pancreatitis
   (C) calculus impaction

(D) iatrogenic injury

(E) abdominal trauma *(3:1134)*

36. The minimum blood loss a healthy person must suffer in order to show a drop in systolic pressure is

(A) 5% of blood volume

(B) 15%

(C) 15 to 30%

(D) 30 to 40%

(E) >40% *(9:181)*

37. In the international system of tumor classification (TNM system), which of the following tumors has the best prognosis?

(A) T1, N0, M1

(B) T0, N0, M0

(C) T1, N2, M0

(D) T3, N0, M3

(E) T1, N0, M0 *(2:335)*

38. When renal ischemia is unilateral, the ischemic kidney would produce urine (when compared with the normal kidney's urine) with which characteristics?

(A) greater volume, lower sodium concentration

(B) greater renin concentration

(C) less volume, greater sodium concentration

(D) less volume, less creatinine concentration

(E) less sodium concentration, greater insulin concentration *(6:890)*

39. A patient has the carcinoid syndrome. The primary tumor was in the small intestine and has been resected. The patient now has hepatic metastases. What percentage of such patients may be expected to survive for 5 years or longer?

(A) none

(B) 20%

(C) 40%

(D) 60%

(E) 80% *(2:1156)*

40. Pure neurogenic shock is associated with all the following EXCEPT

(A) hypotension

(B) normal blood volume

(C) isolated head injury

(D) normal pulse rate

(E) cutaneous vasodilatation *(9:183)*

41. A woman age 52 develops an enlarged cervical node 2 years after surgery for carcinoma of the breast. The original tumor was estogen receptor positive. The initial treatment of this patient should consist of

(A) oophorectomy

(B) adrenalectomy

(C) oophorectomy and adrenalectomy

(D) hypophysectory

(E) tamoxifen *(2:550)*

42. A 35-year-old alcoholic man is admitted with a lung abscess in the lower lobe of the right lung. Following intensive treatment with antibiotics and postural drainage, he has chills and fever. The chest x-ray reveals a residual density in the right lower lobe with a fluid level. The treatment of choice would be

(A) repeated aspiration of the pus

(B) thoracotomy and drainage of the abscess

(C) lobectomy

(D) pneumonectomy

(E) change to broad-spectrum antibiotics *(2:679)*

Questions 43 through 45

During a football game, a young man suffered acute pain in his right knee. Following the game, the acute pain subsided fairly rapidly, but a joint effusion occurred, associated with discomfort and stiffness. At a later examination, he reported episodes when his knee gave way, and when, for a period of time it locked, he could not fully extend his knee.

43. The injury you suspect he has sustained is

(A) an isolated rupture of the anterior cruciate ligament

(B) rupture of the lateral collateral ligament

(C) a medial meniscus tear

(D) an undisplaced fracture of the patella

(E) a combined medial meniscus tear with complete rupture of the medial collateral ligament *(2:1986–1988)*

44. This injury would likely occur under which circumstance?

(A) knee rotated while flexed

(B) varus force applied to extended knee

(C) direct blow on anterior surface of flexed knee

(D) hyperextension of knee

(E) forced flexion of an actively contracting quadriceps *(2:1986–1988)*

45. If the patient had been examined the day after injury and had a large, painful joint effusion, what treatment would you advise?

    (A) immediate operation
    (B) immobilization in plaster with the knee in 30° of flexion
    (C) bedrest with elevation of the leg
    (D) aspiration of the knee effusion
    (E) compression bandage with the knee in 30° of flexion   (2:1986–1988)

46. While working in a stable, a patient suffers a puncture wound of the hand from a nail in an old board. He does not report the incident, and he has not been immunized against tetanus. Which of the following is the most characteristic EARLY presenting symptoms of tetanus?

    (A) fever
    (B) headache
    (C) stiffness of the jaw
    (D) convulsions
    (E) suppuration in the wound   (2:187)

47. A patient has lived for many years in southern Argentina. He has a cystic mass in the right lobe of the liver. A complement-fixation test and Casoni's skin test are both positive for infestation with *T. echinococcus*. In the life cycle of this small tapeworm, which of the following mammals plays a similar role to humans?

    (A) cow
    (B) horse
    (C) dog
    (D) sheep
    (E) goat   (2:1269)

48. Primary hyperaldosteronism is associated with all of the following EXCEPT

    (A) adrenal cortical adenoma
    (B) arterial hypertension
    (C) hypokalemia
    (D) polyuria
    (E) serum sodium in the range of 120 mEq per 100 ml   (2:1510)

49. A young man, 4 hours before admission, was shot in the abdomen. The entry wound is in the left lower quadrant; there is a laceration of the colon about 2 cm above the peritoneal reflection. There are no other major injuries. Which of the following procedures should be carried out?

    (A) exteriorize the injured colon

(B) debridement and closure of the colon wound with proximal diverting colostomy and drainage
(C) Hartmann's operation and drainage
(D) debridement and closure of the colon with drainage and careful observation
(E) debridement and closure of the colon wound with drainage and tube cecostomy   (2:242)

50. Which of the following is uniquely associated with septic shock?

    (A) hypotension
    (B) tachycardia
    (C) cutaneous vasoconstriction
    (D) wide pulse pressure
    (E) mental status changes   (9:183)

Questions 51 through 53

A 55-year-old man enters the hospital with a 3-week history of dysphagia. He can swallow liquids but not solid food. He has lost 15 pounds.

51. The most likely diagnosis is

    (A) carcinoma of the esophagus
    (B) achalasia of the esophagus
    (C) esophageal diverticulum
    (D) hiatal hernia
    (E) peptic esophagitis   (2:1093)

52. The investigative procedure of LEAST value would be

    (A) gastric analysis
    (B) esophagoscopy
    (C) cytology of esophageal washings
    (D) upper gastrointestinal series with fluoroscopy
    (E) chest x-ray   (2:1093)

53. The best treatment would be

    (A) esophagectomy
    (B) esophageal dilatation
    (C) gastrostomy
    (D) repair of the hiatal hernia
    (E) indwelling Celestin tube   (2:1094)

54. A 60-year-old right-handed man is demonstrated on arteriography to have a thrombosis of the left internal carotid artery, probably of long duration. He also has moderate stenosis of the bifurcation of the right common carotid artery.

Which of the following symptoms is UNLIKELY to be associated with these arterial lesion?

(A) almost complete recovery from a right hemiplegia
(B) some continuing speech difficulty
(C) dizzy spells
(D) transient weakness of the left hand
(E) transient weakness of the left leg and foot

(2:944)

55. A small girl has an ulcerated mass in the region of the foramen cecum of the tongue. The mass bleeds occasionally and is about 2 × 3 cm in size. Before excising a lesion of this type, it is most important to perform

(A) an arteriogram
(B) scanning with ^{123}I
(C) a tracheostomy
(D) ligature of the lingual arteries
(E) a biopsy

(2:1547)

56. The rotator cuff of the shoulder consists of the common tendinous insertion of all of the following muscles EXCEPT

(A) supraspinatus
(B) infraspinatus
(C) teres minor
(D) teres major
(E) subscapularis

(2:2038)

57. Which of the following statements correctly applies to increased calcification of the proximal fragment in a fractured neck of the femur? It

(A) is due to an inflammatory reaction
(B) signifies Paget's disease of bone
(C) indicates satisfactory bone repair
(D) indicates aseptic necrosis
(E) is probably a pathologic fracture

(3:1473)

58. Which of the following statements is true of fractures of the surgical neck of the humerus?

(A) occurs usually in young individuals
(B) can often be treated with a sling and protection of the shoulder
(C) nonunion commonly occurs
(D) internal fixation is frequently required
(E) impaction rarely occurs

(2:1967)

59. Which of the following platelet-related substances causes platelet deaggregation?

(A) thromboxane
(B) prostacyclin

(C) serotonin
(D) thrombosthenin
(E) platelet factor III

(3:99)

60. Which statement about pancreatic ascites is true?

(A) it is usually cured rapidly with the use of diuretics
(B) it occurs only in association with a pseudocyst
(C) drainage is the surgical treatment of choice
(D) it is indicative of the presence of both cirrhosis and pancreatitis
(E) it is indicative of the presence of both congestive heart failure and pancreatitis

(20:668–676)

61. Which of the following substances has as one of its functions the lysis of fibrin?

(A) kallikrein
(B) plasmin
(C) kinin
(D) thromboxane
(E) prostacyclin

(3:100)

62. In constrictive pericarditis, which of the following is NOT found?

(A) elevated right ventricular end-diastolic pressure
(B) venous pressure elevated to 20 to 40 cm of water
(C) elevated pulmonary wedge pressure
(D) bradycardia
(E) enlargement of the liver

(2:861)

63. A 4-year-old child is known to have had a cardiac murmur since birth. He is acyanotic and has a loud systolic murmur at the level of the third and fourth intercostal spaces to the left of the sternum. A palpable thrill is present. There is a history of exercise intolerance. On x-ray, there is mild enlargement of the heart with an enlarged pulmonary artery and prominent vascular markings in the lung fields. The diagnosis is

(A) atrial septal defect
(B) ventricular septal defect
(C) pulmonary stenosis
(D) patent ductus arteriosus
(E) tetralogy of Fallot

(2:768–769)

64. Which two of the following conditions require immediate operation?

 (A) diaphragmatic hernia of Bochdalek and torsion of the testicle
 (B) ventricular septal defect and torsion of the testicle
 (C) torsion of the testicle and cleft palate
 (D) cleft palate and ventricular septal defect
 (E) none of the above   *(2:1083–1084)*

65. Which of the following types of carcinoma of the thyroid has the best prognosis?

 (A) papillary carcinoma
 (B) follicular adenocarcinoma
 (C) medullary carcinoma
 (D) anaplastic adenocarcinoma
 (E) metastatic carcinoma   *(2:1568–1569)*

66. The most common cause of hemobilia is

 (A) trauma
 (B) infection
 (C) gallstones
 (D) visceral artery aneurysm
 (E) tumor   *(3:1093)*

67. A patient has an infection of the flexor pollicis longus tendon and subsequently develops an infection of the flexor tendon of the fifth finger. The path this infection has followed is

 (A) through the midpalmar space
 (B) through the thenar space
 (C) through the web space
 (D) via the radial and ulnar bursa
 (E) via the lumbrical sheaths   *(2:2081)*

68. A patient lacerates the ulnar nerve just above the wrist. Which of the following physical findings is most likely to be present? Inability to

 (A) extend the wrist
 (B) flex the wrist
 (C) flex the distal phalanges of the fourth and fifth fingers
 (D) oppose the thumb and fingers
 (E) spread the fingers   *(2:2093)*

69. The most common underlying cause of acute cholangitis is

 (A) benign strictures
 (B) malignant tumors
 (C) choledocholithiasis
 (D) invasive procedures
 (E) parasites   *(3:1155–1160)*

70. In a glomus tumor, which of the following is involved?

 (A) periosteum
 (B) pulp of the distal phalanx
 (C) neurovascular shunt mechanism of the distal phalanx
 (D) the lymphatics
 (E) the matrix of the nailbed   *(2:513)*

71. The most common congenital coagulopathy has as its defect a deficiency of factor

 (A) VIII
 (B) IX
 (C) X
 (D) XI
 (E) XII   *(3:101)*

72. With abdominal trauma, the most frequent abdominal organ injury is to the

 (A) liver
 (B) spleen
 (C) colon
 (D) small bowel
 (E) pancreas   *(3:997)*

73. Colonic involvement with lymphogranuloma venereum is best treated with

 (A) systemic steroids
 (B) steroid enemas
 (C) sulfasalazine
 (D) amphotericin
 (E) tetracycline   *(3:1000)*

74. The major cause of death from pancreatic trauma is

 (A) peritonitis from leaking pancreatic enzymes
 (B) cardiac failure from myocardial depressant factor
 (C) late complications from secondary pancreatic pseudocyst
 (D) injury to surrounding vessels
 (E) duodenal rupture with leak of activated pancreatic enzymes   *(3:1192)*

75. The initial treatment of choice for bleeding esophageal varices is

 (A) emergency shunt
 (B) endoscopic sclerotherapy
 (C) tamponade
 (D) intravenous vasopressin
 (E) intraarterial vasopressin   *(3:1101)*

76. All of the following are presinusoidal causes of portal hypertension EXCEPT

(A) schistosomiasis
(B) vinylchloride injury
(C) Budd-Chiari syndrome
(D) portal vein thrombosis
(E) early primary biliary cirrhosis   *(3:1100)*

77. In recent series of pyogenic liver abscess, the most frequent route of bacterial invasion is

(A) portal vein
(B) hepatic artery
(C) biliary tract
(D) direct extension
(E) cryptogenic   *(3:1069)*

78. The acute form of disseminated intravascular coagulation (DIC) may be triggered by all of the following mechanisms EXCEPT

(A) malignancy
(B) thrombophlebitis
(C) tissue embolism
(D) hemolysis
(E) crush injury   *(3:103)*

79. Dehiscence of an abdominal wound is especially likely to occur in patients with the following EXCEPT

(A) carcinomatosis
(B) age greater than 45 years
(C) ascites
(D) a hematocrit of 35
(E) chronic obstructive pulmonary disease   *(2:456)*

80. During a cholecystectomy, the surgeon mistakenly divides the common bile duct. He immediately recognizes his error. The best way to correct this situation is

(A) insert a T tube and repair around the vertical limb
(B) repair the common bile duct with an end-to-end anastomosis over a T tube and bring the vertical limb out of the bile duct at a separate site
(C) repair with an end-to-end anastomosis and simple external drainage
(D) anastomose the proximal stump of the bile duct Roux-en-Y to the jejunum
(E) anastomose the proximal stump to the side of the duodenum   *(2:1320)*

81. A Bennett's fracture has slipped after two manipulations with plaster splintage and traction. You would now

(A) apply skeletal traction with plaster fixation
(B) reduce by manipulation and fix with a percutaneous pin across the fracture site
(C) reduce by manipulation and fix with a percutaneous pin through the metacarpal shaft and into the greater multangular
(D) perform open reduction with internal fixation
(E) excise the fragment and start early active movements   *(2:1978)*

82. A patient aged 10 had a well-defined, dark brown, slightly elevated lesion on the sole of the foot. It has been present since infancy and is diagnosed as a junctional nevus. The best management is

(A) immediate excision with a wide margin and skin graft
(B) radiation therapy
(C) reassurance
(D) regular observation and excision if there is any change in the appearance of the lesion
(E) early local excision   *(2:516)*

83. A patient has a traumatic arteriovenous fistula of the posterior tibial artery and vein. Which of the following is the LEAST likely to develop?

(A) dilatation of the artery proximal to the fistula
(B) dilatation of the vein proximal to the fistula
(C) an extensive collateral circulation
(D) dilatation of the artery distal to the fistula
(E) dilatation of the vein distal to the fistula   *(2:932-933)*

84. The most serious extracolonic manifestation of ulcerative colitis is

(A) choroiditis
(B) ankylosing spondylitis
(C) pyoderma gangrenosum
(D) sclerosing cholangitis
(E) migratory arthritis   *(3:1017)*

85. A patient underwent an operation on the heart, which was uneventful, and she made a satisfactory postoperative recovery. About 2 weeks after surgery, she developed severe anterior chest pain, a fever of 102°F, and chills. Chest films taken after surgery and after the onset of the complication did not show any abnormality. Which of the following is the most likely cause of this patient's problem?

    (A) pulmonary embolism
    (B) staphylococcal pericarditis
    (C) myocardial infarction
    (D) osteomyelitis of the sternum
    (E) postpericardiotomy syndrome   *(2:816)*

86. Which of the following is the LEAST likely to be true of eosinophilic granuloma of bone? The local lesion or lesions

    (A) may be symptomatic
    (B) are multiple
    (C) may heal spontaneously
    (D) regress(es) when treated with steroids
    (E) is/are sometimes associated with eosinophilia   *(2:1928)*

87. In a patient who has received 4 units of blood during a 6-hour abdominal operation, the most likely cause of significant intraabdominal bleeding is

    (A) dilutional coagulopathy
    (B) disseminated intravascular coagulation
    (C) a poorly ligated vessel
    (D) calcium depletion from citrated blood
    (E) platelet dysfunction   *(3:104)*

88. The storage life of platelets is

    (A) 24 hours
    (B) 48 hours
    (C) 72 hours
    (D) 4 days
    (E) 5 days   *(3:106)*

89. Vascularization of a free skin graft is indicated by the development of a pink color. This indicates a take. It occurs in which of the following time intervals?

    (A) within 24 hours
    (B) within 48 hours
    (C) between the third and fifth days
    (D) at about 1 week
    (E) between 7 and 10 days   *(2:2104)*

90. An undescended testicle is most commonly associated with

    (A) indirect inguinal hernia
    (B) direct inguinal hernia
    (C) hypospadias
    (D) paraphimosis
    (E) testicular tumor   *(2:1704)*

91. A 7-year-old boy is seen in the emergency room with a history of acute painful swelling in the right scrotum, which prevents him from sleeping. The right side of the scrotum is found to be swollen, firm, and extremely tender. The overlying skin is reddened and edematous. The most likely diagnosis is

    (A) acute hydrocele
    (B) acute epididymitis
    (C) traumatic orchitis
    (D) torsion of the spermatic cord or of a testicular appendix
    (E) testicular tumor   *(2:1685)*

92. Acute adrenal insufficiency causes all of the following findings EXCEPT

    (A) pigmentation of the skin and mucosa
    (B) hypotension
    (C) tachycardia
    (D) nausea and vomiting
    (E) low blood volume   *(2:1516–1518)*

Questions 93 through 95

A young man has recently been stabbed. He has a wound of the right shoulder and an apparently superficial stab wound of the fourth left intercostal space. The blood pressure is slightly decreased, the breath sounds are clearly heard bilaterally, the heart sounds are somewhat distant, and the neck veins are slightly distended.

93. The most likely diagnosis is

    (A) stab wound of the heart
    (B) diabetic coma
    (C) blood loss from the two wounds
    (D) pulmonary embolism
    (E) cardiac failure   *(2:201)*

94. The best way to confirm the diagnosis would be to

    (A) aspirate the pericardium
    (B) measure the central venous pressure
    (C) do a blood sugar

(D) take an electrocardiogram

(E) x-ray the chest   *(2:201)*

95. The condition of the patient begins to deteriorate. The neck veins become more distended, the blood pressure falls, and the pulse rate rises. The pericardial aspirate was blood. The correct treatment is

(A) open the chest and pericardium and repair the cardiac wound

(B) aspirate the pericardium with a large-bore needle and repeat if necessary

(C) insert a drainage tube into the pericardial sac

(D) repair the cardiac wound and perform an exploratory laparotomy

(E) aspirate the pericardium and return the blood as a transfusion   *(2:201)*

96. The factor that has the greatest impact on oxygen delivery is

(A) cellular oxygen-carrying capacity (2,3-DPG level)

(B) hematocrit

(C) perfusion

(D) patient metabolism (fever, burn, activity)

(E) acidosis or alkalosis   *(3:107–108)*

97. Cancer of the large intestine occurs with an increased incidence in all EXCEPT

(A) multiple polyposis

(B) chronic ulcerative colitis

(C) amebiasis

(D) villous adenoma

(E) previous cancer of the large intestine   *(2:1197)*

98. The most important diagnostic finding for the Zollinger-Ellison syndrome is

(A) large gastric mucosal folds

(B) multiple duodenal and jejunal ulcerations

(C) acid hypersecretion

(D) demonstration of pancreatic tumor on angiogram

(E) elevated serum gastrin   *(3:833)*

99. Which of the following lesions of squamous epithelium is NOT premalignant?

(A) leukoplakia

(B) intradermal nevus

(C) Bowen's disease

(D) chronic radiation dermatitis

(E) actinic keratosis   *(2:516)*

100. A man, aged 70 with advanced carcinoma of the prostate, develops uncontrolled bleeding after a palliative transurethral resection. The most likely cause would be

(A) intravascular hemolysis

(B) vitamin K deficiency

(C) widespread destruction of the bone marrow

(D) fibrinolysis

(E) technically poor hemostasis   *(2:85)*

101. The highest incidence of severe central nervous system disease is associated with which of the following pulmonary infections?

(A) tuberculosis

(B) actinomycosis

(C) blastomycosis

(D) aspergillosis

(E) cryptococcosis   *(2:686)*

102. A 46-year-old man is admitted with a history of massive bleeding from a duodenal ulcer 6 years before and a history of rheumatic fever in childhood. He is known to have mitral stenosis and insufficiency and some involvement of the aortic valve. He was well compensated before this admission and was not fibrillating. On admission, he is pale, cold, and sweating. His pulse rate is 90, blood pressure 85/60, and hematocrit 26. A Levine tube is passed, and blood is aspirated. After a 24-hour period of management, which includes adequate blood transfusion, he is still bleeding from the gastric tube, and he has passed several melena stools. Which of the following statements indicates the best management?

(A) he should not be operated upon because the heart disease is severe and he would be unlikely to survive the procedure

(B) iced saline gastric lavage

(C) continue blood transfusion another 24 hours

(D) discontinue blood transfusion

(E) operate before continued blood transfusion has raised the risks of surgery   *(2:1128)*

103. Following poor reduction of a Pott's fracture, which of the following is most likely?

    (A) traumatic fusion of the ankle
    (B) traumatic arthritis
    (C) osteomyelitis
    (D) fat embolism
    (E) nonunion   *(2:1991)*

104. The preferred treatment for Zollinger-Ellison syndrome is

    (A) total gastrectomy
    (B) subtotal gastrectomy
    (C) cimetidine
    (D) excision of the pancreatic tumor
    (E) debulking of the metastatic tumor   *(3:834)*

105. A 60-year-old man is found to have a transitional cell carcinoma of the left ureter. The opposite kidney and ureter are normal. The best treatment of this patient would be

    (A) left nephroureterectomy
    (B) irradiation
    (C) left nephroureterectomy and postoperative irradiation
    (D) chemotherapy
    (E) left nephroureterectomy and chemotherapy   *(2:1709)*

106. A patient complains of hallucinations of unpleasant odors. The most likely cause is a tumor located in the

    (A) internal capsule
    (B) frontal lobe
    (C) parietal lobe
    (D) temporal lobe
    (E) cerebellum   *(6:1264)*

107. What is the most important communication between the superior and inferior mesenteric arteries providing the main collateral circulation if either artery is occluded

    (A) gastroduodenal artery
    (B) inferior pancreaticoduodenal artery
    (C) middle colic artery
    (D) marginal artery of Drummond
    (E) ileocolic artery   *(2:1438)*

Questions 108 and 109

A previously healthy 9-month-old male child is admitted with a history of sudden onset of intermittent abdominal pain. The child has vomited and has bloody diarrhea.

108. The most likely diagnosis is

    (A) bleeding from a Meckel's diverticulum
    (B) staphylococcal enteritis
    (C) lymphoma of the jejunum
    (D) intussusception
    (E) Henoch-Schönlein purpura   *(2:1655)*

109. The best diagnostic procedure would be

    (A) colonoscopy
    (B) upper gastrointestinal series
    (C) barium enema
    (D) intravenous pyelogram
    (E) urinalysis   *(2:1656)*

110. Signs of fat embolism typically appear after injury at

    (A) 3 hours
    (B) 3 days
    (C) 3 weeks
    (D) immediately
    (E) unpredictable times   *(3:1768)*

111. In idiopathic thrombocytopenic purpura (ITP), the platelet count drops because

    (A) platelets and fibrin are deposited in capillaries and arterioles as hyaline
    (B) splenic vein occlusion causes splenic congestion and stasis, with increased platelet consumption
    (C) hypersplenism of unknown etiology destroys platelets
    (D) hypersplenism associated with long-standing rheumatoid arthritis destroys platelets
    (E) a circulating antiplatelet antibody binds to platelets, causing them to be destroyed by the reticuloendothelial system *(3:1210-1225)*

Questions 112 through 114

A woman, age 40, is admitted with a history of 1 year of diarrhea, steatorrhea, weight loss, abdominal pain, and peripheral neuritis. She is found to be severely anemic and gives a history of three previous abdominal operations for intestinal obstruction.

112. The most likely diagnosis is

    (A) the blind loop syndrome
    (B) ulcerative colitis

(C) regional enteritis
(D) lead poisoning
(E) chronic pancreatitis   *(2:1161)*

113. The anemia is

(A) similar to pernicious anemia
(B) microcytic
(C) sickle cell
(D) hemolytic
(E) porphyria erythropoietica   *(2:1162)*

114. The best long-term treatment is

(A) tetracyclines and vitamin B_{12}
(B) surgical correction of the abnormality
(C) splenectomy
(D) pancreatic enzymes by mouth
(E) Lomotil   *(2:1162)*

115. An adolescent girl has dyspnea on exertion. She is not cyanotic. The pulmonary vascularity is increased, there is a right bundle branch block, the right ventricle is enlarged, and a soft systolic murmur is heard over the second and third interspaces. The most likely diagnosis is

(A) pulmonary stenosis
(B) coarctation of the aorta
(C) patent ductus arteriosus
(D) atrial septal defect
(E) tetralogy of Fallot   *(2:759)*

Questions 116 through 119

A 45-year-old man was admitted to the hospital 30 minutes after an automobile accident. He was found to have bilateral fractures of the second, third, fourth, and fifth ribs, anteriorly. There was minimal paradoxical motion. The blood pressure was 130/100, and the pulse rate was 100. He was not in severe distress.

116. Which of the following would be the most helpful diagnostic procedure?

(A) an electrocardiogram
(B) central venous pressure determination
(C) blood gas studies (oxygen, carbon dioxide)
(D) blood volume estimation
(E) chest x-ray   *(2:621-625)*

117. The LEAST likely initial therapeutic procedure would be

(A) tracheostomy
(B) pericardiotomy
(C) insertion of a chest catheter

(D) blood transfusion
(E) nasal oxygen   *(2:201)*

118. Without treatment, the most likely complication of this injury would be

(A) hemorrhage and shock from the fractured ribs
(B) cardiac tamponade
(C) contusion of the heart
(D) nonunion of the rib fractures
(E) atelectasis and pneumonia   *(2:620)*

119. Large amounts of blood and intravenous fluids should NOT be administered to the patient because

(A) contused lungs are prone to develop pulmonary edema
(B) heart injury may lead to heart failure
(C) renal excretion is impaired
(D) a pericardial effusion often is present
(E) vomiting may occur secondary to gastric dilatation   *(2:632)*

120. A 62-year-old man has had a previous myocardial infarction with a satisfactory recovery. On chest x-ray, he is found to have an opacification of the right upper lobe. Bronchoscopy and biopsy show a squamous cell carcinoma of the upper lobe of the right lung. Scalene node biopsy is negative. Which is the most logical treatment for this patient?

(A) intrapleural radioactive gold
(B) x-radiation therapy
(C) chemotherapy
(D) right pneumonectomy
(E) right upper lobectomy   *(2:700)*

Questions 121 and 122

A 56-year-old white male has a long history of dyspnea and cyanosis. He is admitted to the hospital, where a chest x-ray reveals a lesion in the left upper lobe and a second lesion of the left lower lobe behind the heart. On physical examination, it is noted that there are multiple telangiectases and spider nevi over the chest and abdomen. The patient also gives a history of nosebleeds for many years.

121. The best single diagnostic test in the patient would be

(A) bronchoscopy
(B) bronchography
(C) tomography
(D) pulmonary angiography
(E) thoracotomy   *(2:688)*

122. The treatment of choice would be

(A) segmental resection of both lesions
(B) left pneumonectomy
(C) lobectomy
(D) radiotherapy
(E) nitrogen mustard and radiotherapy *(2:668)*

123. In the staging of Hodgkin's disease

(A) lymphocyte-predominant histology is more likely to be found in an advanced stage
(B) the spleen is considered a lymph node
(C) localized extranodal extension of disease makes the patient a stage IV
(D) the 5-year survival for stage II disease with treatment is 50%
(E) splenic involvement in stage III disease does not alter the prognosis for this stage
                    (3:1216)

124. The operation of highly selective vagotomy, sometimes called proximal gastric vagotomy, is best accompanied by

(A) pyloroplasty
(B) gastroenterostomy
(C) antrectomy and Billroth I anastomosis
(D) antrectomy and Billroth II anastomosis
(E) no other procedure   *(2:1128)*

125. A herniated nucleus pulposus at the L5–Sl level produces all of the following EXCEPT

(A) hypesthesia of the medial side of the foot
(B) hypesthesia of the lateral side of the foot
(C) reduced or absent ankle jerk

(D) pain in the back, posterior thigh, and calf
(E) pain aggravated by the Valsalva maneuver
                    (2:1840)

Questions 126 and 127

A 55-year-old man is found on x-ray to have an osteolytic lesion of the mandible. A biopsy is done, and this shows a brown-colored tumor with giant cells and fibrous stroma.

126. The most likely diagnosis is

(A) monostotic fibrous dysplasia
(B) actinomycosis
(C) hyperparathyroidism
(D) osteoclastoma (giant cell tumor)
(E) multiple myeloma   *(2:1594)*

127. Which preoperative laboratory investigation would be most useful?

(A) serum calcium and phosphorus
(B) serum alkaline phosphatase
(C) phosphorus clearance test
(D) Bence Jones protein
(E) culture of the biopsy material   *(2:1596)*

128. The common cause of the adrenogenital syndrome is

(A) decreased function of the adrenal cortex
(B) an adrenal tumor
(C) an ovarian tumor
(D) disordered pituitary function
(E) congenital adrenal hyperplasia   *(2:1503)*

129. A woman with difficulties from endometriosis becomes pregnant. Her problem with endometriosis will

(A) get worse during pregnancy
(B) get better during pregnancy
(C) not change during pregnancy
(D) require termination of the pregnancy
(E) require cesarean section at term *(2:1755)*

130. Carcinoma of which of the following is LEAST likely to metastasize to bone?

(A) prostate
(B) breast
(C) thyroid
(D) colon
(E) lung   *(2:1946)*

131. What is the optimum age for the repair of a cleft lip?

(A) 1 week
(B) 1 month
(C) 2 to 3 months
(D) 6 months
(E) 1 year   *(2:2128)*

132. Non-Hodgkin's lymphoma

(A) has a better prognosis than Hodgkin's disease
(B) invades and spreads in a manner similar to carcinomas
(C) is evaluated by staging laparotomy
(D) is usually localized at diagnosis
(E) has a worse prognosis in patients between 35 and 65 years of age   *(3:1217–1218)*

133. Following a black widow spider bite, the associated abdominal pain can be best controlled by

(A) epinephrine
(B) steroids
(C) aspirin
(D) potassium chloride
(E) calcium gluconate   *(2:220)*

134. A 40-year-old female has a 2-day history of a tender swelling of the entire right cheek. Examination reveals a markedly red, tender, firm induration of the right cheek with sharp, raised borders. Temperature is 101°F. White blood count is 21,000. Which of the following would be the best treatment?

(A) incision and drainage
(B) cruciate incision and raise flaps to drain
(C) warm, moist compresses and antibiotics
(D) x-ray therapy
(E) extract the infected tooth   *(2:170)*

Questions 135 through 138

A 55-year-old laborer has a firm nodule on the palm of the hand at the base of the thumb. There are also thickened areas extending onto the flexor surfaces of the middle two fingers with some flexion deformity.

135. Which of the following men first described this syndrome?

(A) deQuervain
(B) Cooper
(C) Dupuytren

(D) Billroth
(E) Cushing   *(2:1871)*

136. The etiology of the condition is

(A) chronic infection
(B) tuberculosis
(C) repeated trauma
(D) neoplastic change
(E) not known   *(2:1871)*

137. The pathologic process is

(A) stenosis of the flexor tendon sheath
(B) neoplastic infiltration
(C) thickening and fibrosis of the palmar fascia
(D) ischemic changes
(E) not known   *(2:1871–1872)*

138. The treatment of the condition is

(A) hydrocortisone injections
(B) heat and massage
(C) multiple incisions
(D) excision of the palmar fascia
(E) antituberculosis drugs   *(2:1872)*

139. The 5-year survival rate for treated stage I gastric carcinoma is

(A) 10%
(B) 30%
(C) 50%
(D) 70%
(E) 90%   *(3:885)*

140. Intestinal angina is a result of

(A) embolism from a cardiac mural thrombus
(B) atherosclerotic stenosis of major visceral vessels
(C) nonspecific colonic ischemia
(D) low flow of blood due to cardiac failure or drugs
(E) vasculitis related to collagen disease *(3:1000)*

Questions 141 through 143

A 48-year-old woman is admitted to the hospital with a history of lack of concentration, forgetfulness, episodes of weakness, sweating, and a history of unconsciousness for about half an hour. She consumes large amounts of food.

141. The most likely diagnosis is

    (A) pheochromocytoma
    (B) brain tumor
    (C) carcinoid syndrome
    (D) islet cell insulinoma
    (E) psychoneurosis   *(2:1365-1367)*

142. The most revealing diagnostic test would be

    (A) arteriography of the abdominal arteries
    (B) skull x-ray
    (C) retroperitoneal air insufflation and x-ray
    (D) cerebral arteriography
    (E) upper gastrointestinal series   *(2:1365-1367)*

143. The laboratory test most likely to be abnormal would be

    (A) fasting blood sugar
    (B) tolbutamide tolerance test
    (C) electroencephalogram
    (D) urinary catecholamines
    (E) 17-hydroxycorticosteroids   *(2:1365-1367)*

144. Which of the following statements concerning lymphogranuloma (lymphopathia) venereum is NOT true?

    (A) complement-fixation test positive
    (B) Frei's test positive
    (C) Donovan bodies are present
    (D) inguinal adenopathy occurs
    (E) rectal strictures quite common   *(2:1236)*

145. A young woman is noticed to have rapidly developed virilism and arterial hypertension. Which of the following is the most likely diagnostic possibility?

    (A) coarctation of the aorta
    (B) adrenal cortical hyperplasia
    (C) adrenal cortical carcinoma
    (D) pituitary adenoma
    (E) arrhenoblastoma   *(2:1506)*

146. In a patient with a subphrenic abscess, which of the following is NOT correct?

    (A) a pleural effusion is common

    (B) weight loss occurs
    (C) fever over 103°F often occurs
    (D) the diaphragm becomes fixed
    (E) with antibiotics, most subphrenic abscesses resolve   *(2:1413-1414)*

147. The frequency of lymph node metastases at the time of diagnosis of esophageal carcinoma is

    (A) 15%
    (B) 35%
    (C) 55%
    (D) 75%
    (E) 95%   *(3:738)*

148. Classic hemophilia is a disease of males. Which of the following statements concerning this disease is correct?

    (A) also known as von Willebrand's disease
    (B) due to hypofibrinogenemia
    (C) due to thrombocytopenia
    (D) a factor VIII deficiency
    (E) a factor IX deficiency   *(2:91-95)*

149. About one third of patients with Crohn's disease have extraintestinal manifestations. Which of the following organs or systems is NOT involved in this disease?

    (A) skin
    (B) eye
    (C) joints
    (D) central nervous system
    (E) hepatobiliary   *(3:921)*

150. A 40-year-old woman suffers from the sudden onset of severe paroxysms of stabbing pain over one side of the face. The attacks may be brought on by washing the face, brushing the hair, and cleaning the teeth. The likely diagnosis is

    (A) migraine headaches
    (B) temporal arteritis
    (C) trigeminal neuralgia
    (D) dental apical abscess
    (E) nasal sinusitis   *(1:776)*

151. The serum amylase may be elevated in all of the following conditions EXCEPT

    (A) strangulated obstruction of the small intestine
    (B) acute cholecystitis
    (C) mesenteric vascular occlusion
    (D) acute pancreatitis
    (E) serum hepatitis   *(2:1352)*

152. In a 25-year-old woman with thyrotoxicosis, which of the following might be due to hyperthyroidism?

(A) serum cholesterol of 340
(B) a sleeping pulse of over 80
(C) sodium loss in the urine
(D) polycythemia
(E) low PBI   (2:1556)

153. A 62-year-old man complains of annoying frequency of urination and nocturia. On rectal examination, he has a smooth enlargement of the prostate. He has a transurethral prostatectomy. His problems may include all of the following EXCEPT

(A) carcinoma of the residual prostate
(B) a 50% incidence of recurrent problems
(C) urethral stricture
(D) low-grade fever for 6 weeks
(E) a 10 to 25% need for further surgery in the future   (2:1716)

154. All of the following are common findings in association with early mechanical small bowel obstruction EXCEPT

(A) crampy abdominal pain that waxes and wanes
(B) abdominal distention
(C) paucity or absence of colonic gas on abdominal plain films
(D) absence of bowel sounds
(E) hypovolemia   (3:908)

155. The most common cause of mechanical intestinal obstruction in North America today is

(A) adhesions
(B) strangulated groin hernia
(C) carcinoma of the bowel
(D) volvulus of the intestines
(E) intraabdominal abscess   (2:1034)

156. Morbidity and mortality in cases of appendicitis are related most closely to

(A) constitution of the fecaliths
(B) location of the appendix
(C) presence or absence of rupture
(D) disposition of the appendiceal stump
(E) degree of antibiotic coverage   (2:1254)

157. The localization of pain to the right lower quadrant, which often occurs in individuals who have acute appendicitis, is the result of

(A) inflammation of the parietal peritoneum
(B) distention of the appendix
(C) perforation of the appendix
(D) vascular engorgement
(E) bowel infarction   (2:1023)

158. Indications for operation in acute pancreatitis include all EXCEPT

(A) deteriorating clinical picture
(B) severe pain
(C) uncertainty in diagnosis
(D) associated biliary lithiasis
(E) treatment of complications   (2:1353)

159. Cancer of the head of the pancreas is characterized by all of the following EXCEPT

(A) palpable gallbladder
(B) jaundice
(C) hemobilia
(D) abdominal and back pain
(E) weight loss   (2:1361)

160. Peritoneal lavage is reserved for those patients who have abdominal trauma and

(A) unexplained hypotension
(B) closed head injury requiring surgery
(C) ETOH/drug-induced mental status changes
(D) major orthopedic surgery requiring prolonged immediate surgical management
(E) all of the above   (2:231)

161. Adenocarcinoma of the stomach is best treated by

(A) 5-FU
(B) radiation
(C) total gastrectomy
(D) subtotal gastrectomy
(E) wedge resection   (2:1134)

162. Carcinoma of the stomach generally spreads

(A) within the gastric wall
(B) directly into adjacent organs
(C) via bloodstream
(D) by peritoneal seeding
(E) all of the above   (2:1133)

163. Which of the following is the LEAST likely to be confused with acute appendicitis?

(A) perforated peptic ulcer
(B) mesenteric cyst
(C) pneumonia
(D) cholecystitis
(E) acute pancreatitis   (2:1656)

164. Late complications of peptic ulcer surgery include all of the following EXCEPT

(A) dumping syndrome
(B) diarrhea
(C) alkaline reflux gastritis
(D) gas bloat syndrome
(E) marginal ulcer   (3:843)

165. Condyloma accuminata in the perianal area are most often associated with which of the following?

(A) poor hygiene
(B) dirty toilet seats
(C) herpes progenitalis
(D) homosexuality
(E) fungi   (2:1235)

166. A carcinoma of the rectum, two-thirds circumferential, at the 5 cm level from the anal verge, is best treated by which of the following?

(A) sphincter splitting with excision
(B) transanal excision
(C) abdomino-perineal resection
(D) 5-fluorouracil
(E) transsacral excision   (2:1203)

167. Large proximal (upper) third rectal cancers are best treated by

(A) anterior resection
(B) abdominoperineal resection
(C) transanal resection
(D) transsacral resection
(E) chemotherapy   (2:1203)

168. The cricopharyngeus muscle is associated with which esophageal abnormality?

(A) traction diverticulum
(B) Zenker's diverticula
(C) epiphrenic diverticulum
(D) achalasia
(E) none of the above   (2:1087)

169. A patient with a paraesophageal hernia is best treated by

(A) fundoplication
(B) hernia reduction, diaphragm repair, and an antireflux procedure
(C) antacids
(D) awaiting symptoms
(E) none of the above   (2:1082)

170. The seemingly important factor common to all contemporary surgery for gastroesophogeal reflux is

(A) re-creation of a lower esophageal high pressure zone
(B) closing the hiatus to prevent herniation
(C) fixing the stomach in the abdomen
(D) ensuring a length of intraabdominal esophagus
(E) all of the above   (2:1078)

171. Which of the following hernias may NOT obstruct bowel even when strangulation takes place?

(A) indirect
(B) direct
(C) Richter's
(D) Petit's
(E) femoral   (2:1463)

172. The key to defining an incarcerated hernia is its

(A) painfulness
(B) associated swelling
(C) irreducibility
(D) associated erythema
(E) all of the above   (2:1457)

173. Pain out of proportion to the physical findings is typical of

(A) appendicitis
(B) small bowel obstruction
(C) pelvic inflammatory disease
(D) infarcted bowel
(E) cholcystitis   (2:1433)

174. The line of division between the right and left lobes of the liver is best approximated by

(A) the bed of the gallbladder
(B) the falciform ligament
(C) the ligamentum teres
(D) the coronary ligament
(E) the triangular ligament   (2:1278)

175. Major portal-systemic vascular anastomoses include all EXCEPT

(A) retroperitoneal veins
(B) epigastric veins
(C) renal veins
(D) hemorrhoidal veins
(E) esophageal veins   *(2:1281)*

176. Liver tumors in women associated with oral contraceptives when noted incidentally are best treated

(A) by discontinuing oral contraceptives
(B) by transfemoral embolization
(C) radiation
(D) hepatic artery ligation
(E) expectantly   *(2:1271)*

177. The most specific marker of hepatocellular carcinoma is elevation of

(A) carcinoma embryonic antigen (CEA)
(B) alpha-fetoprotein (AFP)
(C) haptoglobin
(D) ceruloplasmin
(E) alpha-antitrypsin   *(3:1080)*

178. Humoral and cellular immunity conferred by the spleen has led to attempts at splenic preservation.

The critical mass of residual spleen necessary to confer immune protection is

(A) 10%
(B) 30%
(C) 50%
(D) 70%
(E) 90%   *(3:1208)*

179. The pre-operative diagnosis of appendicitis should be confirmed during surgery in no less than

(A) 90–95 percent of cases
(B) 80–85 percent of cases
(C) 70–75 percent of cases
(D) 60–65 percent of cases
(E) 50–55 percent of cases   *(2:1249)*

180. The recognition of appendicitis as a clinical and pathologic entity is credited to

(A) Charles McBurney
(B) Reginald Fitz
(C) William Halsted
(D) William Morton
(E) Theodor Billroth   *(2:1246)*

Answers and Explanations

1. **(A)** In low anomalies of the anus, the rectum has traversed the puborectalis portion of the levator ani muscle, and a simple perineal procedure is usually sufficient.

2. **(D)** Vancomycin is the drug of choice against gram-positive infection by methicillin-resistant organisms when penicillin and cephalosporins cannot be used. It is effective against streptococcal endocarditis, resistant gram-positive infections of prosthetic devices, and *Clostridium difficile* colitis.

3. **(D)** A child's head accounts for approximately 18% of body surface area, twice the amount represented by the adult head. The child's upper extremity contains 9% of surface area, the same as for an adult. Thus this child's burn area is approximately 27%. Both because this child's burn is greater than 20% and because of probable eye and ear involvement, he or she would require treatment in a burn unit. Besides the head, the other surface area difference between children and adults is that the child's lower extremity is a slightly smaller proportion (14% vs. 18%).

4. **(E)** Hypomotility appears to play no role, although hypermotility and rapid emptying of the stomach are factors.

5. **(D)** Approximately 75% of patients with perforated duodenal ulcer show free air on upright or decubitus abdominal x-rays. This is a confirmatory test that may increase the information available to the surgeon about what he or she is likely to find, but in the 25% without demonstrable free air, boardlike abdominal rigidity makes the necessity for surgery clear. The presence of free air does not differentiate perforated duodenal ulcer from perforation of another viscus, such as a colonic diverticulum, but the pa-

tient's history may favor one or the other. Treatment choices range from simple Graham omental patch to more definitive ulcer procedures, depending on several factors: degree of soilage, friability of tissues, chronicity of the ulcer disease, and the patient's condition.

6. **(C)** A feature of gallstone ileus is that the symptoms may be so mild that the patient does not seek medical attention until intestinal obstruction develops.

7. **(D)** The coracoid process is rarely injured when the shoulder dislocates.

8. **(E)** Fractures of the intracapsular portion of the neck of the femur are rarely comminuted.

9. **(E)** Chronic intestinal ischemia produces a symptom complex that has been termed both "mesenteric angina" and "mesenteric intermittent claudication." The cause is stenosis or thrombosis of the mesenteric or celiac arteries. Usually two of the three arteries supplying the alimentary tract are involved, and the usual cause is atherosclerosis.

10. **(C)** The diagnosis of mesenteric ischemia is often made by exclusion. Gastrointestinal series, barium enema, cholecystogram, and pancreatic function studies are all normal. After this, lateral aortogram and celiac and mesenteric arteriogram will establish the diagnosis.

11. **(A)** In patients of this type, it is sufficient to restore a pulsatile flow to either the celiac or superior mesenteric artery. But these grafts may occlude. Therefore, on the principle that two grafts are better than one, the practice today is to place grafts to both the celiac and superior mesenteric arteries.

12. **(C)** Achalasia occurs slightly more frequently in men than in women. The cause is probably neurogenic, but the patient often has a history of emotional problems.

13. **(A)** For dilatation to be successful, it must be forceful, so that the esophageal muscle is fully stretched.

14. **(C)** About 15 percent of patients with achalasia will require surgery. The Heller myotomy is now used almost exclusively for this problem.

15. **(B)** The pneumatic antishock garment raises systolic pressure, probably by a combination of shifting blood volume and increasing peripheral vascular resistance and afterload. Because of the latter effect, myocardial dysfunction manifested by pulmonary edema or circulatory instability is the absolute contraindication to the use of this garment. Stabilization and tamponade of pelvic fracture are indications for the use of the garment. Use with head injuries is controversial. Intrathoracic bleeding and diaphragmatic rupture are relative contraindications, and caution should be exercised in these situations.

16. **(A)** Heterotopic tissue is found in approximately 50 percent of all Meckel's diverticula. In 80 percent of cases, the heterotopic tissue is gastric mucosa.

17. **(D)** Septic shock is most often due to gram-negative septicemia.

18. **(B)** This child has suffered a fracture of the medial epicondyle with trauma to the ulnar nerve.

19. **(D)** The treatment of a fracture of the medial epicondyle with an ulnar nerve injury is open reduction and pinning of the fragment.

20. **(A)** Fractures of the femoral neck are usually treated by some form of internal fixation or replacement with a prosthesis.

21. **(C)** Injury of the popliteal artery at the time of dislocation of the knee is a recognized complication requiring urgent arteriography and then operation if necessary.

22. **(D)** Eosinophilic granuloma may be solitary but is often multiple. Most patients are under the age of 20 and the skull is a frequent site.

23. **(B)** Legg-Calve-Perthes' disease, or coxa plana, is a disease of boys aged 5 to 9 years.

24. **(B)** Dissecting aneurysm of the aorta is especially likely to develop in a black male over 60 years of age who has hypertension.

25. **(D)** An aortogram performed with a percutaneous catheter introduced distally is the most accurate method of diagnosing and localizing a dissecting aneurysm of the aorta.

26. **(B)** The first essential is to lower the systolic blood pressure to the range of 120 to 100. This enables the situation to stabilize, but delayed rupture 2 to 3 days later is sufficiently frequent to effect a semiemergency operation 24 to 48 hours later, with repair of the dissection the best treatment.

27. **(B)** In many patients, cerebrospinal rhinorrhea ceases spontaneously. The repair of the meningeal defect should not be performed during the first 2 weeks after the injury. If the cerebrospinal fluid discharge persists after this interval, operation through a transfrontal exposure and closure of the defect in the meninges often is indicated. Before this, the diagnosis is confirmed by determination of the glucose content of the fluid. Every effort should be exerted to prevent meningitis while awaiting spontaneous closure of the fistula. Associated facial fractures should be treated as required.

28. **(C)** When regurgitation through the aortic valve reaches 50% of the blood ejected from the left ventricle, symptoms occur and may progress to congestive heart failure. Left ventricular hypertrophy and dilatation may compensate for years and maintain a normal left ventricular and diastolic pressure. Coronary blood flow is maintained, but a relative ischemia may develop because of the increased muscle mass and prolonged isometric contraction. Angina and congestive failure reflect progression and indicate that surgery is warranted.

29. **(B)** The preferred treatment for primary gastric lymphoma is subtotal gastrectomy when possible. Total gastrectomy carries a significantly higher mortality. Because of the usual extent of the lesion and the indistinct margins, local resection is not practical. Radiotherapy may be a useful adjunct to surgery or may be used as primary

therapy for an unresectable lesion. Chemotherapy also may be used adjunctively or for extensive disease.

30. **(C)** The upper two thirds of the thoracic esophagus is the most frequent site of squamous carcinoma, followed by the lower third. Cervical esophagus is the least frequent site. Barrett's columnar epithelium in the distal esophagus is a metaplastic change associated with reflux esophagitis and is a site of adenocarcinoma. The high frequency of adenocarcinomas at the gastroesopageal junction represents cancers of predominantly gastric rather than esophageal origin. The other 5% of esophageal malignancies consist of leiomyosarcomas, rhabdomyosarcomas, adenoacanthomas, carcinosarcomas, and primary malignant melanomas.

31. **(E)** Restoration of organ perfusion is the primary goal of resuscitation in hemorrhagic shock. This is manifested by adequate urine output (50ml/hour in the adult), appropriate CNS function, good skin color, and restoration of pulse and blood pressure. The most common and serious complication of hemorrhagic shock is late organ failure due to periods of hypoperfusion and ischemia when volume replacement was not vigorous enough. Calculated replacement volumes and CVP measurements are not reliable endpoints.

32. **(D)** Splenic artery aneurysm most often is seen as a result of medial dysplasia in women and atherosclerosis in men. It often occurs as an incidental finding of a rim of eggshell calcification in an asymptomatic patient. When discovered, such an aneurysm should be excised if the patient is a good operative risk, especially in women of childbearing age, in whom there is an increased risk of rupture during pregnancy.

33. **(C)** Deterioration of endocrine and exocrine function is manifested by diabetes and steatorrhea (foul, bulky, floating stools from lack of lipase). Weight loss may be due to malabsorption. Hypoglycemic symptoms, such as confusion and diaphoresis, are associated with insulin-secreting beta-cell tumors.

34. **(E)** Excretion of injected ^{99m}technetium-iminodiacetic acid through the biliary system will show a failure to fill the gallbladder in virtually all cases of cholecystitis. Only 5% of patients with normal gallbladders will fail to visualize. Rarely,

plain abdominal x-rays will show findings of biliary tract disease, such as calcified calculi (15%), air in the wall of the gallbladder and lumen (emphysematous cholecystitis), or air in the biliary tree (as in a cholecystoenteric fistula). Intravenous cholangiography and oral cholecystography have been supplanted by ^{99m}Tc scan and ultrasound. Ultrasound will document stones and masses but is not specific for cholecystitis.

35. **(D)** Ninety percent of bile duct strictures result from iatrogenic injury, usually associated with cholecystectomy. Congenital atresia does not usually take the form of an isolated stricture. Pancreatitis, calculus, and trauma account for the rest of the strictures.

36. **(D)** Decrease in systolic blood pressure occurs only with blood loss major enough to overwhelm the body's cardiovascular compensatory mechanisms. A loss of 30 to 40% of blood volume is the boundary at which this takes place. For a 70-kg individual whose blood volume is 7% of ideal weight, or about 5 L, this represents about 2000 ml. With smaller amounts of blood loss, catecholamines increase peripheral resistance, which increases diastolic pressure and narrows pulse pressure. Other fluid deficits, such as dehydration, affect the patient's hemodynamic status. Vital signs, urine output, central venous pressure, and mental status reflect the volume status more accurately than estimated blood loss or hematocrit.

37. **(E)** This is a trick question that is unlikely to appear on any well-constructed written examination, but it can help you learn the meaning of the classifications. Tumors are classified in increasing order of size as T1, T2, T3, or T4. There is no T0 that, presumably, would mean no tumor. N refers to the presence or absence of regional nodes, and M to the presence or absence of distant metastases. N0—no regional nodal metastases, N1—regional nodal metastases; M0—no distant metastases; M1—distant metastases.

38. **(E)** Collection of urine from each kidney by ureteral catheterization shows less urine, decreased sodium concentration, and greater concentration of substances, such as inulin and creatinine, which are not subject to tubular resorption.

39. **(B)** Carcinoid tumors grow slowly. Even after a palliative resection, more than 20% live for 5 years or longer.

40. **(C)** Neurogenic shock is a state of decreased sympathetic tone due to brainstem dysfunction or spinal cord injury. It is not caused by isolated head injury. The patient with a head injury who is in shock must be evaluated for other etiologies. The drop in blood pressure in neuogenic shock results from loss of peripheral resistance and increased vascular capacitance. The blood volume initially is unaltered. Absence of tachycardia and absence of cutaneous vasoconstriction are the two characteristic findings differentiating neurogenic from hemorrhagic shock. Treatment proceeds as if the patient were hypovolemic, which in a relative sense is true.

41. **(E)** For postmenopausal patients with recurrent estrogen receptor-positive breast carcinoma, the choice is between additive and antiestrogen therapy. Of these, tamoxifen, an antiestrogen that acts by blocking estrogen receptor sites, is the favorite.

42. **(C)** Unless a carcinoma is present as well, only a few patients with lung abscesses require surgical treatment. Failure to respond to adequate antibiotic therapy with the persistence of the abscess over several weeks is an indication for lobectomy.

43. **(C)** Although this might describe a lateral meniscus tear also, tears of the medial meniscus are much more common in this country. The ligamentous injuries would likely result in continued pain, and isolated ligamentous and patellar injuries would not be expected to cause locking of the knee—a sign of meniscus injury.

44. **(A)** A varus force applied to the knee may rupture the lateral collateral ligament. A direct blow on the anterior surface of the flexed knee may fracture the patella or rupture the anterior cruciate ligament. Forced flexion of the actively contracting quadriceps may also fracture the patella.

45. **(D)** Aspiration of a severe effusion may afford considerable relief. Although operative treatment of complete ligamentous tears should be carried out early, the possible isolated meniscus injury should be reevaluated after acute symptoms subside. The knee is immobilized with a splint or compression bandage in maximal extension and is allowed to bear weight between crutches with the quadriceps taut.

46. **(C)** The prodromal symptoms of tetanus last from 12 to 24 hours before the tonic contractions and spasms develop. The characteristic prodromal symptom is stiffness of the jaw, which becomes true trismus, or lockjaw, when the disease is fully developed.

47. **(D)** *T. echinococcus* spends its adult life in the intestine of the dog. The ova are excreted in the feces and are then eaten by either the sheep or humans. The cystic stage is spent in the sheep or humans. The dog then eats the liver or other organs of the sheep or human and becomes infected to restart the life cycle.

48. **(E)** The serum sodium in a patient with primary hyperaldosteronism is in the high-normal or just-above-normal range. About 90% of patients have an adrenal cortical adenoma, and every patient has arterial hypertension and hypokalemia. Polyuria is a frequent symptom of primary hyperaldosteronism.

49. **(B)** The principles of management of patients with wounds of the colon are well established. It is recommended that wounds of the left colon be either exteriorized as a colostomy or repaired and returned to the peritoneal cavity, with a proximal diverting colostomy being performed at the time of the initial surgery. It is not possible to exteriorize the colon 2 cm from the peritoneal reflection. Therefore, the treatment is repair and immediate diverting colostomy.

50. **(D)** Septic shock differs from hypovolemic shock in that there is a widened rather than a narrowed pulse pressure. Instead of a catecholamine-induced vasoconstriction, which raises dyastolic pressure in hypovolemic shock, there is vasodilatation (manifested by the characteristic warm pink skin). Systolic pressure is near normal, and tachycardia may be modest.

51. **(A)** Carcinoma of the esophagus is seen most frequently in men between 50 and 60 years of age. Dysphagia and weight loss are the characteristic symptoms.

52. **(A)** The gastric analysis does not change in patients with carcinoma of the esophagus.

53. (A) Carcinoma of the esophagus is treated by surgery and by radiotherapy. Surgery is the best treatment for carcinoma of the distal esophagus.

54. (C) The symptom groups A and B indicate recovery from the effects of thrombosis of the left internal carotid artery. Symptom groups D and E are caused by the stenosis of the right internal carotid artery close to its origin from the right common carotid artery. Dizzy spells are rarely due to diseases of the carotid arteries. They are more frequently associated with the vertebral–basilar arterial disease.

55. (B) The ¹²³I scan will confirm the likely diagnosis of a lingual thyroid.

56. (D) The rotator cuff consists of a common tendinous insertion for the supraspinatus, infraspinatus, teres minor, and subscapularis muscles. This tendinous insertion is closely adherent to the underlying shoulder capsule.

57. (D) Avascular or aseptic necrosis of the head of the femur is a frequent complication of fractures of the femoral neck. The necrotic bone shows an increased density on x-ray.

58. (B) Fracture of the surgical neck is the most common fracture of the proximal humerus. It occurs most often in the elderly. Undisplaced or impacted fractures require little treatment beyond a sling and guarding of the shoulder.

59. (B) Prostacyclin, a product of prostaglandin metabolism elaborated by endothelial cells, causes platelet deaggregation and local vasodilatation. These effects are the direct opposite of the effects of thromboxane and serotonin, which are produced by platelets and released at a site of injury. Platelets aggregated on exposed collagen are compacted by a platelet-derived contractile protein, thrombosthenin. Platelet factor III is a phospholipid that promotes coagulation.

60. (C) Pancreatic ascites often requires surgical drainage. Sump catheter drainage, internal drainage of a pseudocyst, or pancreaticojejunostomy in some combination may be required depending on the operative findings. Only occasional cases respond quickly to repeated paracentesis and nasogastric suction.

61. (B) Plasmin, the end product of the fibrinolytic system, splits fibrin and provides a dynamic balance in the coagulation scheme. Plasmin is a protease that also degrades other coagulation factors (II, V, VIII) and activates factor XII, which can trigger the coagulation, complement, and kinin systems. Kallikrein is a part of the kinin system, which also can activate factor XII as well as activate the conversion of plasminogen to plasmin. Thromboxane and prostacyclin have opposing effects on platelet aggregation and vascular smooth muscle contraction.

62. (D) The stroke volume is decreased in patients with constrictive pericarditis. This results in a compensatory tachycardia, but the cardiac output is decreased.

63. (B) Small ventricular septal defects are asymptomatic. Large defects give the symptoms and clinical findings listed.

64. (A) A foramen of Bochdalek hernia often occurs as an acute respiratory emergency at or soon after birth. Torsion of the testicle must be operated on promptly in order to salvage the testis.

65. (A) Papillary carcinoma of the thyroid grows slowly.

66. (A) Trauma is the most common cause of hemobilia, and the trauma is most often a result of auto accidents. Approximately half the cases of hemobilia are accounted for by blunt and penetrating trauma. The condition may appear even weeks or months after trauma. The other etiologies listed appear in descending order of frequency. Percutaneous transhepatic manipulations now add a small percentage of cases.

67. (D) The ulnar bursa extends from the level of the distal joint of the fifth finger to incorporate all the flexor tendons of the other fingers. Behind the transverse carpal ligament, it frequently communicates with the radial bursa from the thumb.

68. (E) The interossei are the muscles that abduct and adduct the fingers. The interossei are all supplied by the ulnar nerve.

69. (C) The majority (60%) of cases of acute cholangitis are secondary to choledocholithiasis. The other conditions listed are predisposing causes occurring less frequently. Biliary-enteric fistula also is a cause of cholangitis.

70. (C) Glomus tumors are derived from the glomeric end-organ apparatus consisting of arteriovenous anastomoses, which function normally to regulate the blood flow in the extremity.

71. (A) Patients with classic hemophilia, type A, lack factor VIII. Patients with hemophilia B (Christmas disease), the second most common congenital coagulopathy, are deficient in factor IX and suffer milder effects. Patients lacking von Willebrand's factor usually have only mild bleeding from mucous membranes. Cryoprecipitate derived from a single donor contains factor VIII and von Willebrand's factor and is used periodically to maintain levels of factor VIII in hemophilia A and as needed for the less severe coagulopathies. Death in hemophilia A is usually due to intracerebral bleeding.

72. (A) The liver is the most frequently injured abdominal organ, followed by the colon. Most colon injuries are perforations resulting from a seatbelt placed too high across the abdomen. Management ranges from simple closure for right-sided injuries to exteriorization or resection with colostomy for left-sided injuries. Mortality is directly related to the number and severity of associated organ injuries.

73. (E) Early in the course of colonic involvement with the lymphogranuloma venereum bacterium, tetracycline treatment is curative. Progression of the colonic manifestations to sinus tracts and long tubular strictures causes intractable obstruction and carries a significant risk for development of carcinoma. Elective abdominoperineal resection during a quiescent period may be required.

74. (D) The intimate relationship of the great vessels, superior mesenteric and splenic vessels to the pancreas puts them at great risk of injury associated with pancreatic trauma. Since most pancreatic trauma in the urban setting results from penetrating wounds, it is understandable why major hemorrhage from these vessels is the leading cause of death in pancreatic trauma. Leakage from duodenal rupture usually remains retroperitoneal and requires a high index of suspicion to recognize before the patient is terminally septic. Pancreatic leak and late pseudocyst are less life threatening.

75. (D) Intravenous vasopressin is the initial treatment of choice for variceal bleeding. By causing splanchic vasoconstriction at the arteriolar level, it restricts the inflow of blood to the portal system and lowers portal pressure. Selective superior mesenteric infusion of vasopressin has no advantage over the intravenous route. Sclerotherapy, tamponade, and surgery are remedies to apply after failure of vasopressin. Because of its short half-life (8 to 16 minutes), a 20-unit loading dose is followed by continuous infusion of 0.4 unit per minute. The dose is slowly tapered (0.1 unit decrease every 6 to 12 hours) after control is achieved.

76. (C) Budd-Chiari syndrome causes a postsinusoidal block by occlusion of the hepatic veins. Schistosomiasis, vinylchloride poisoning, portal vein thrombosis, and early primary biliary cirrhosis are among the presinusoidal causes of portal hypertension. The distinction between the two causes is important because preserved hepatocyte function with presinusoidal obstruction lowers the risk of hepatic failure, and these patients do better with shunting.

77. (C) Bilary tract infection is the most common etiologic agent of pyogenic liver abscess in recent collected series (41.9%). The portal venous route, although significantly less common than in the preantibiotic era, still accounts for 17.9% in the same series. The gastrointestinal origin of the bacteria in this latter group is most commonly the appendix. Surprisingly, the number of liver abscesses from an unknown source has remained steady at approximately 20%. Documented hepatic artery seeding during sepsis and direct extension, as from empyema of the gallbladder, are uncommon, accounting for about 7% each. The pattern of liver abscess that develops after suppurative cholangitis is frequently one of multiple foci. In the USA, 80 to 90% of liver abscesses are pyogenic, and the rest are amebic. In both types of infection, directed laminar portal vein blood flow favors localization in the right lobe, which receives the greater portion of superior mesenteric vein drainage.

78. (B) Malignancies of organs rich in thromboplastin (pancreas, prostate, lung) can trigger DIC, as can tissue embolism, such as amniotic fluid, fat, and bone marrow. Crush injury may act through the mechanism of tissue embolization. Hemolysis releases a thromboplastic phospholipid in the stroma of red blood cells that may initiate DIC. Thrombophlebitis is not associated with DIC. The ongoing low-grade DIC associated with severe infection and hypoperfusion is more poorly understood and does not respond to heparin therapy as does the more acute form.

79. **(D)** Moderate anemia does not delay wound healing or lead to wound dehiscence, but hypovolemia does interfere with healing. Except for incisions that become severely infected, a closure carefully planned to suit the patient can almost prevent wound dehiscence completely.

80. **(B)** Early recognition of this error makes possible an end-to-end anastomosis. A T tube should be used and the vertical limb brought out at a separate site so as not to interfere with the healing of the anastomosis.

81. **(C)** This fracture is unstable and reduction without pin fixation often fails.

82. **(E)** If a lesion is considered to be a junctional nevus, excision is advisable.

83. **(D)** The artery distal to the fistula becomes smaller than normal. It does not dilate.

84. **(D)** Sclerosing cholangitis is a devastating condition associated with ulcerative colitis. Fifty percent of patients with sclerosing cholangitis have or will develop ulcerative colitis. Ophthalmic manifestations include iritis, choroiditis, and rarely panophthalmitis. Migratory arthritis usually parallels the activity of the colon disease and is reversible, whereas axial skeletal involvement, such as ankylosing spondylitis, is less prone to parallel the disease and is more likely to cause permanent deformity. Skin lesions include erythema nodosum and pyoderma gangrenosum. Most of these problems will resolve after definitive treatment by colectomy.

85. **(E)** This puzzling syndrome is quite common after an operation in which the pericardium is opened, even if extracorporeal circulation has not been employed.

86. **(D)** The lesion may regress spontaneously or may heal after curettage or after radiotherapy. Cortisone produces only temporary relief by reducing the inflammatory reaction.

87. **(C)** The most common cause of significant postoperative bleeding is failure of mechanical hemostasis. There is little evidence that dilution of clotting factors severe enough to compromise coagulation occurs except in the case of massive transfusion administered extremely rapidly (e.g., several units in a row at 5-minute intervals). Free citrate is rapidly metabolized, and calcium mobilization quickly compensates for any deficiency long before coagulation is impaired. Disseminated intravascular coagulation is an unlikely cause of postoperative bleeding.

88. **(C)** The storage life of platelets is only 72 hours, so platelet packs concentrated from several donors are prepared only when needed.

89. **(C)** The pink appearance indicating a take occurs between the third and fifth days.

90. **(A)** Nearly 90% of undescended testicles are associated with an indirect inguinal hernia.

91. **(D)** The diagnosis of torsion of the spermatic cord may be difficult. Because prompt treatment is necessary to save the testis, exploration is usually recommended if the diagnosis is in doubt and the patient is seen as early as this child was.

92. **(A)** Pigmentation is a characteristic finding of chronic but not of acute adrenal insufficiency.

93. **(A)** A stab wound in this location, combined with distended neck veins and even slight hypotension, is strongly suggestive of a cardiac stab wound.

94. **(A)** If cardiac tamponade is suspected as a possibility, the pericardium should be aspirated promptly. Such aspiration confirms the diagnosis of hemopericardium and partially relieves the tamponade.

95. **(A)** A cardiac wound with early tamponade is often in a favorable situation for repair of the heart wound.

96. **(B)** Change in hematocrit has the single most dramatic impact on oxygen delivery to tissues. However, a patient who is hypovolemic with a very low hematocrit may benefit more from volume expansion than from increased red cell mass. Such factors as coronary artery disease in the older patient must be considered when making decisions about transfusion. Red blood cells can increase their production of 2,3-DPG in response to anemia and double their oxygen-delivery capacity by reducing the affinity of hemoglobin for oxygen. Oxygen release at the tissue level is then

greatly facilitated. The limit of this compensation, logically, is at 50% hemoglobin loss.

97. **(C)** All of the choices except amebiasis are associated with an increased incidence of large intestine cancer.

98. **(E)** The demonstration of elevated serum gastrin by radioimmunoassay in the face of increased acid secretion is the critical diagnostic test for confirming Zollinger-Ellison syndrome. Mild gastrin elevations seen with pyloric obstruction and retained antral mucosa will decrease with administration of secretin, whereas gastrin levels in the Zollinger-Ellison syndrome will increase. Acid hypersecretion causes ectopic and multiple ulcers as well as diarrhea. Mucosal folds are edematous and enlarged. In about a third of patients, the nonbeta-cell pancreatic tumor may be demonstrated by angiogram.

99. **(B)** All of the choices are premalignant except the intradermal nevus, which requires no treatment except for cosmetic reasons.

100. **(D)** The plasminogen activator present in prostatic tissue is activated by urokinase. This leads to increased fibrinolysis on the raw wound surface.

101. **(E)** In cryptococcosis, central nervous system involvement is an indication for active treatment with amphotericin B.

102. **(E)** Massive and continued bleeding from a duodenal ulcer is an indication for surgery.

103. **(B)** Maintenance of a normal mortise of the ankle joint is a prerequisite for painless ankle motion.

104. **(C)** The current preferred treatment of Zollinger-Ellison syndrome is medical management with cimetidine. The earlier standard treatment of removing the target organ, the stomach, has proved effective and may still be indicated for those patients not controlled by cimetidine. If a solitary gastrinoma can be identified in the pancreas, it should be excised in hope of curing the patient. Less than total gastrectomy is not effective.

105. **(A)** Neither radiation therapy nor chemotherapy add to the survival rate of patients with carcinoma of the ureter.

106. **(D)** Temporal lobe tumors often produce uncinate fits and hallucinations of unpleasant or unusual smells or tastes.

107. **(D)** The marginal artery of Drummond may become as big as 1 cm in diameter and forms a major collateral between the superior and inferior mesenteric circulations.

108. **(D)** This is the history of a child with intussusception. Intussusception is sometimes secondary to a lymphoma of the small intestine or to Henoch-Schönlein purpura.

109. **(C)** A barium enema may be of both diagnostic and therapeutic value in such patients.

110. **(B)** Collapse in the first 3 hours after injury is most likely due to shock. At 3 days fat embolism is most likely, and at 3 weeks pulmonary embolus is likely. Immediate manifestation is uncommon.

111. **(E)** ITP is a disease of young women caused by a circulating antiplatelet antibody that tags the platelets for destruction by the reticuloendothelial system, particularly in the spleen. Hyaline subendothelial and intraluminal deposits of platelets and fibrin in capillaries and arterioles are characteristic of thrombotic thrombocytopenic purpura, which carries a higher mortality. Primary or secondary hypersplenism is not associated with ITP. Splenic vein thrombosis, most often secondary to pancreatitis, does increase platelet destruction.

112. **(A)** If a blind loop is created by repeated bypass surgery for intestinal obstruction, stagnation occurs. In this stagnant area, the bacterial flora changes, and the new bacteria compete for and produce a deficiency of vitamin $B_{12.}$

113. **(A)** The anemia in the blind loop syndrome is similar to pernicious anemia. It differs in that in patients with true pernicious anemia, the excretion of vitamin B_{12} rises to normal with the administration of intrinsic factor, but it remains unchanged in the blind loop syndrome.

114. **(B)** Tetracyclines and vitamin B_{12} will relieve the anemia of the blind loop syndrome, but surgery effects a permanent cure and is, therefore, preferred.

115. (D) The findings are characteristic of an atrial septal defect, a left-to-right shunt without cyanosis.

116. (E) A chest x-ray will confirm the fractures of the ribs and show the status of the heart, lungs, and mediastinum.

117. (B) Pericardiotomy is required for cardiac tamponade. This is not present in this patient.

118. (E) Atelectasis and pneumonia are likely complications of this injury, the likelihood rising with the age of the patient.

119. (A) It is important not to overload the circulation in patients with pulmonary injuries.

120. (E) Provided that the margin is adequate, a pulmonary lobectomy is the preferred treatment for pulmonary carcinoma.

121. (D) It is probable that this patient has pulmonary arteriovenous malformations. Pulmonary angiography is diagnostic.

122. (A) Segmental resection is best reserved for single pulmonary lesions of·this type, but two localized and symptomatic lesions can be excised.

123. (B) The more common histologic types of Hodgkin's disease, lymphocyte predominance and nodular sclerosis, have a better prognosis, whereas the less common mixed cellularity and lymphocyte depletion have a worse prognosis and are more likely to be found in the more advanced stages. The spleen is considered a lymph node in the Ann Arbor staging of Hodgkin's disease and is indicated as stage III when there is disease above and below the diaphragm with splenic involvement. Its involvement is usually a precursor of diffuse hematogenous spread and carries a poorer prognosis. Stage IV consists of involvement of nonlymph node areas, such as bone marrow or liver, and not contiguous extension from a single node group. The latter is staged as Ie and is treatable with radiotherapy. The posttreatment 5-year survival for both stage I and II is 85%, and it drops to 50 to 70% in stage III and 40 to 50% in stage IV.

124. (E) Since 1970, it has been appreciated that because the vagal innervation of the gastric antrum and pylorus is preserved, the operation of highly selective vagotomy need not be accompanied by a gastric drainage procedure.

125. (A) Hypesthesia of the medial side of the foot is produced by an L4–L5 disc. An L5–Sl lesion produces hypesthesia on the lateral side of the foot.

126. (C) The skeletal changes of hyperparathyroidism are less common now because of early treatment of this problem. The jaws are an important location for bone cysts and tumors in hyperparathyroidism. These giant cell tumors are partly cystic and brown or red-brown on section. They contain giant cells in a fibrous stroma.

127. (A) In the final analysis, the diagnosis of hyperparathyroidism rests on the biochemical changes, and of these, the serum calcium and phosphorus levels are the most significant.

128. (E) Congenital adrenal hyperplasia showing symptoms at birth is by far the most common cause of the adrenogenital syndrome. In the female, a pseudohermaphrodite is produced and, in the male, macrogenitosomia praecox. The adrenogenital syndrome appearing in adult life is usually due to an adrenal tumor.

129. (B) Endometriosis becomes quiescent during pregnancy and hormonally induced pseudopregnancy.

130. (D) Carcinomas of the breast, lung, thyroid, prostate, and kidney are especially liable to metastasize to bone.

131. (C) Surgery is scheduled at 10 weeks provided that the child weighs at least 10 pounds and has at least 10 g of hemoglobin.

132. (B) Non-Hodgkin's lymphoma, usually of monoclonal B cell origin, disseminates in an aggressive manner similar to a carcinoma and carries a worse prognosis than Hodgkin's disease. It is frequently already disseminated at diagnosis and rarely requires staging laparotomy before chemotherapy and radiotherapy are instituted. The disease behaves more aggressively in patients under 35 and over 65 years of age.

133. (E) The pain of the muscle spasms associated with a black widow spider bite can be controlled by 10 ml of a 10% solution of calcium gluconate.

134. (C) Erysipelas usually responds well to penicillin.

135. (C) Dupuytren first described this condition in 1832. Sir Astley Cooper suggested the etiology about 10 years before.

136. (E) Inheritance of Dupuytren's contracture is well accepted, but the cause is not known.

137. (C) Fibrosis and thickening of the palmar aponeurosis is the cause of Dupuytren's contracture.

138. (D) Radical excision of the palmar fascia is still the method of choice in severe cases of Dupuytren's contracture.

139. (E) The 5-year survival for stage I (T1,N0,M0) gastric carcinoma is excellent at 90%. Survival for succeeding stages is: stage II 50%, stage III 10%, stage IV rare. Unfortunately, most patients in the USA are stage III or IV at diagnosis.

140. (B) Gradual atherosclerotic narrowing of the major splanchnic vessels (celiac, superior mesenteric, inferior mesenteric) causes the syndrome of postprandial cramps, weight loss, malabsorption, and diarrhea referred to as "intestinal angina." Embolism, usually from a postinfarct mural thrombus, causes catastrophic occlusion of a major visceral vessel, usually the superior mesenteric because of the flow dynamics of its oblique takeoff. Embolism presents a sudden diffuse pain that may progress to intestinal gangrene and an acute abdomen. Ischemic colitis usually is localized to the splenic flexure or sigmoid, frequently resolves spontaneously, but may result in late fibrotic stricture. Low flow states due to pump failure, shock, or drugs, such as vasopressors, steroids, and digitalis, can cause massive bowel compromise, with mortality reaching 80%. Vasculitis may compound the risk when other causes of bowel ischemia supervene but is not a major primary factor and is unrelated to intestinal angina.

141. (D) Patients with insulin-producing tumors often give a history of episodes of loss of consciousness.

142. (A) Most patients with an insulinoma fail to show an abnormality on arteriography, but if the tumor is seen, it is accurately located and the operation is simplified.

143. (A) In Whipple's triad for hyperinsulinism, a

fasting blood sugar of less than 50 mg per 100 ml is one of the three findings.

144. (C) Donovan bodies are present in granuloma inguinale not lymphogranuloma venereum.

145. (C) Hypertension tends to occur in tumor-induced virilism.

146. (E) Limited early infection of the subphrenic spaces may resolve with antibiotics, but once an abscess has formed, drainage will be required as soon as the abscess has been localized.

147. (D) Approximately 75% of patients with esophageal carcinoma have lymph node metastasis at the time of diagnosis. The extensive plexus of freely communicating mediastinal lymphatics allows easy spread to any level rather than to localized segmental nodes. Longitudinal submucosal spread also is common, and margins must be checked for microscopic tumor spread. Transmural extension is the typical finding, and involvement of trachea, aorta, and recurrent laryngeal nerve occurs with upper esophogeal lesions.

148. (D) Classic hemophilia is due to failure to synthesize normal factor VIII. It is inherited as a sex-linked recessive trait.

149. (D) The central nervous system is not associated with extraintestinal manifestations of Crohn's disease. Erythema nodosum and pyoderma gangrenosum are the common skin disorders, uveitis and iritis affect the eye, arthritis and ankylosing spondylitis are associated joint disorders, and cholelithiasis and sclerosing cholangitis affect the biliary tree. There are also renal manifestations, vasculitides, and a variety of lesser associations. A variety of physiologic mechanisms may be involved in these conditions, ranging from nutritional derangements to immunologic problems.

150. (C) This is the typical history of a patient with trigeminal neuralgia.

151. (E) Amylase gains entry into the blood by regurgitation from the pancreas or by peritoneal absorption after leakage from dying bowel. It is not elevated in serum hepatitis.

152. (B) A sleeping pulse rate of over 80 is characteristic of thyrotoxicosis.

153. **(B)** The incidence of recurrent problems is 10 to 25%, not 50%.

154. **(D)** In this situation, the bowel sounds are increased.

155. **(A)** Adhesive bands are now the most common cause of intestinal obstruction in North America for all age groups combined.

156. **(C)** The principal factor in the mortality of acute appendicitis is whether or not the appendix has ruptured.

157. **(A)** The pain in the right lower quadrant in acute appendicitis is a somatic pain arising in the abdominal wall.

158. **(B)** Acute pancreatitis can usually be controlled without an operation. Severe pain is not an indication for surgery.

159. **(C)** Hemobilia is not characteristic of cancer of the head of the pancreas. Bleeding is frequent from cancer of the ampulla of Vater.

160. **(E)** Peritoneal lavage is indicated in all these situations. It is very inaccurate if the injury is retroperitoneal.

161. **(D)** The treatment of stomach cancer is surgical, and the preferred operation is subtotal gastrectomy.

162. **(E)** Gastric cancer spreads in the four ways listed.

163. **(B)** Mesenteric cysts occur as an abdominal mass not as an acute abdominal problem.

164. **(D)** Gas bloat syndrome is an inability to belch because of an overly tight fundoplication and is unrelated to ulcer surgery. Dumping, diarrhea (secondary to vagotomy), alkaline reflux gastritis, marginal ulcer, as well as anemia and steatorrhea, are all late complications of ulcer surgery.

165. **(D)** Condyloma accuminata, or anal warts, are usually transmitted by sexual contact.

166. **(C)** It is not possible to resect a carcinoma at this level with the mandatory margin of 4 cm and preserve fecal continence. Therefore, abdominoperineal excision is the preferred treatment.

167. **(A)** Cancers of the upper third of the rectum can be removed by anterior resection. The introduction of the stapler has made this easier.

168. **(B)** A pharyngoesophageal diverticulum (Zenker's) is an acquired abnormality associated with premature contraction of the cricopharyngeus muscle.

169. **(B)** Because of the high incidence of bleeding and volvulus in large paraesophageal hernias, surgical repair is usually indicated.

170. **(A)** The primary goal of the surgical treatment of gastroesophageal reflux is restoration of gastroesophageal competence.

171. **(C)** Richter's hernia is strangulation of an antimesenteric knuckle of bowel wall. It may lead to an abscess without obstruction.

172. **(C)** An incarcerated hernia is irreducible. If the blood supply is also compromised it becomes strangulated.

173. **(D)** In mesenteric infarction, the most striking and constant complaint is of extreme abdominal pain.

174. **(A)** The plane passing through gallbladder bed and inferior vena cava best represents the anatomic division between the right and the left lobes of the liver.

175. **(C)** The collateral vessels that become functional in the case of portal hypertension do not involve the renal veins.

176. **(A)** Hepatic adenomas, if asymptomatic, are best treated by discontinuing oral contraceptives.

177. **(B)** AFP is elevated significantly in the large majority of patients with hepatocellular carcinoma. Slight elevations are associated with other liver pathologic conditions, such as hepatitis, chronic liver disease, and some liver metastases. Levels may decrease after curative resection and may be monitered as a sign of recurrence. CEA is a marker for colorectal cancer that may be used to monitor recurrence and metastases, which occur most commonly in the liver. Haptoglobin, ceruloplasmin, and alpha-antitrypsin abnormalities are serum protein derangements associated with hepatocellular carcinoma.

178. **(C)** Fifty percent of the splenic mass must be preserved to maintain splenic immunologic benefits, and this can be accomplished in 30 to 50% of cases.

179. **(B)** Accuracy of preoperative diagnosis in acute appendicitis should be about 85%.

180. **(B)** The recognition of appendicitis as a clinical entity dates from 1886, when Reginald Fitz, Professor of Pathologic Anatomy, gave a paper "Perforating Inflammation of the Vermiform Appendix."

Sixth Examination
Questions

DIRECTIONS (Questions 1 through 107): Each of the numbered items or incomplete statements in this section is followed by answers or by completions of the statement. Select the <u>ONE</u> lettered answer or completion that is <u>BEST</u> in each case.

1. Which one of the following CANNOT be produced by a bronchogenic lesion?

   (A) ACTH
   (B) norepinephrine
   (C) antidiuretic hormone (ADH)
   (D) parathormone
   (E) gonadotropin   *(23:1001)*

2. The most severe disability follows dislocation of the

   (A) shoulder
   (B) knee
   (C) acromioclavicular joint
   (D) elbow
   (E) interphalangeal joint   *(3:1479)*

3. A 60-year-old man develops swelling and plethora of the head and neck. Obstruction of the superior vena cava is diagnosed. This obstruction is most likely secondary to

   (A) thymoma
   (B) chronic sclerosing mediastinitis
   (C) substernal goiter
   (D) lung carcinoma
   (E) chronic constrictive pericarditis   *(2:726)*

4. A 6-year-old female child has a fracture of the shaft of the femur with slight comminution. The treatment is

   (A) reduction and hip spica cast
   (B) open reduction and internal fixation with a plate
   (C) open reduction and intramedullary rod
   (D) Russell-type traction
   (E) Bryant suspension   *(2:1983)*

5. The LEAST likely fracture to occur in a 7-year-old child who falls on an outstretched arm is

   (A) fracture of both bones of the forearm
   (B) dislocation of the distal radial epiphysis
   (C) Colles' fracture
   (D) supracondylar fracture
   (E) Greenstick fracture of the ulna   *(2:1975)*

6. A 13-year-old girl who has never menstruated is examined because of pelvic discomfort and a sensation of pressure in the rectum. Rectal examination reveals a large cystic pelvic mass. You should immediately suspect the diagnosis of

   (A) functioning ovarian tumor
   (B) nonfunctioning ovarian tumor
   (C) imperforate hymen
   (D) extrarectal hemangioma
   (E) presacral tumor   *(2:1734)*

7. Which one of the following symptoms is NOT found in approximately 50% or more of patients with lung carcinoma?

   (A) cough
   (B) weight loss
   (C) dyspnea
   (D) chest pain
   (E) hemoptysis   *(23:1000)*

8. A patient with a past history of right upper quadrant pain and fatty food intolerance who has several episodes of crampy midabdominal pain over a 2-week period may have

   (A) acute cholecystitis
   (B) biliary colic
   (C) subacute pancreatitis
   (D) gallstones ileus
   (E) hydrops of the gallbladder   (3:1160)

9. On the sixth postoperative day after a right upper lobectomy, the patient has developed a moderate subcutaneous emphysema over the right chest wall and has an apical pneumothorax. Management of this condition should consist of

   (A) bronchoscopy
   (B) bed rest and close observation
   (C) aspiration of air and instillation of an antibiotic into the pleural cavity
   (D) intermittent positive pressure breathing
   (E) closed drainage of the pleural cavity
                                        (3:2066)

10. A 50-year-old white farmer presents with an indurated lesion of the lower jaw with multiple draining sinuses. The most likely diagnosis is

    (A) tuberculous lymphadenitis
    (B) carcinoma
    (C) sarcoma
    (D) actinomycosis
    (E) histoplasmosis   (2:191)

11. Hypoprothrombinemia in patients with obstructive jaundice is due to

    (A) inability of liver to convert thrombin to prothrombin
    (B) failure of calcium absorption
    (C) failure of absorption of vitamin K
    (D) decrease in intestinal bacteria
    (E) anemia   (2:101)

12. A patient has a mallet finger. Which of the following lesions causes this abnormality?

    (A) disruption of the extensor mechanism at its insertion into the distal phalanx
    (B) division of the long flexor tendon
    (C) division of the sublimis tendon
    (D) division of the long extensor tendon
    (E) paralysis of the lumbrical muscle   (2:2076)

13. The treatment of choice for an infected pancreatic pseudocyst is

   (A) internal drainage
   (B) external drainage
   (C) dependent on whether the cyst wall is mature (4 to 6 weeks)
   (D) percutaneous ultrasound-guided pigtail catheter drainage
   (E) high-dose antibiotics and fluid resuscitation until the toxicity subsides
                                        (3:1190-1192)

Questions 14 through 16

A 65-year-old man is bronchoscoped and esophagoscoped for possible tumor. One hour later, he develops substernal pain and crepitation in the suprasternal region of the neck. Chest x-ray shows no widening of the mediastinum. There is no fluid level and no pneumothorax.

14. The most likely diagnosis is

    (A) perforation of the cervical esophagus
    (B) perforation of the thoracic esophagus
    (C) perforation of the trachea or bronchus
    (D) perforation of the stomach
    (E) ruptured emphysematous bleb   (2:1099)

15. The next diagnostic procedure should be

    (A) lateral, anterior, and posterior x-rays of the neck
    (B) methylene blue by mouth
    (C) repeat esophagoscopy
    (D) upper gastrointestinal x-ray series
    (E) abdominal erect and supine x-rays   (2:1099)

16. The treatment of choice is

    (A) drainage of the cervical esophagus
    (B) posteromedial sternotomy
    (C) left thoracotomy and drainage
    (D) right thoracotomy and drainage
    (E) Levine tube aspiration and antibiotics
                                        (2:1100)

17. The most common source of lung metastasis is

    (A) colon
    (B) kidney
    (C) breast
    (D) testis
    (E) uterus   (23:1006)

18. Which of the following is NOT a major factor leading to delayed or nonunion of a fracture?

(A) damage to the blood supply
(B) insufficient traction to restore physiologic lengths
(C) inadequate immobilization
(D) interrupted immobilization
(E) shearing and rotational strains at the fracture site *(2:1955)*

19. After 3 years, a completely healed skin wound

(A) is as strong as unwounded skin
(B) becomes stronger than unwounded skin
(C) is weaker than unwounded skin
(D) is still weaker than unwounded skin but will become as strong as unwounded skin
(E) becomes weaker over the next 3 years *(2:289)*

20. A female, age 60, who is 1 year postmastectomy, develops one solitary bone metastasis, which is very painful. The best way to reduce her pain is with

(A) estrogens
(B) androgens
(C) radiation therapy
(D) adrenalectomy
(E) hypophysectomy *(2:1948)*

21. The incidence of squamous cell carcinoma is increased in areas of

(A) old chronic radiation scars
(B) chronic osteomyelitis sinuses
(C) leukoplakia
(D) chronic venous ulcers
(E) all of the above *(2:514)*

Questions 22 through 24

A 7-year-old male child, who was asymptomatic but known to have a heart murmur, was found on a routine examination to have a blood pressure in the arms of 160/90 and in the lower extremities 85/60. A systolic murmur is heard widely over the left chest. The chest x-ray shows moderate hypertrophy of the left ventricle.

22. The most likely diagnosis is

(A) coarctation of the aorta
(B) atrioseptal defect
(C) double aortic arch
(D) coarctation of the abdominal aorta
(E) tetralogy of Fallot *(2:752)*

23. The best treatment for this patient is

(A) bypass graft
(B) an arterioplasty: longitudinal incision and transverse closure
(C) excision with graft reconstruction
(D) excision and end-to-end anastomosis
(E) wait until the child is aged 10 years *(2:752)*

24. After satisfactory operative correction, the blood pressure will probably

(A) rapidly fall to normal level
(B) slowly fall to a normal level over several weeks
(C) rise and then rapidly fall to normal
(D) not change
(E) fluctuate over a wide range *(2:754)*

25. Murphy's sign is

(A) development of acute cholecystitis when the patient is least able to tolerate it
(B) right upper quadrant pain while the surgeon is palpating and the patient is inspiring
(C) resistance to passive dorsiflexion of the foot
(D) arrest of inspiration while the surgeon is palpating the right upper quadrant
(E) a nontender, palpable gallbladder *(3:1139)*

26. Which of the following is the LEAST likely to be found in a patient with mitral stenosis?

(A) atrial fibrillation
(B) arterial emboli
(C) left ventricular hypertrophy
(D) a presystolic murmur
(E) hemoptysis *(2:821)*

27. Which of the following is NOT associated with coarctation of the aorta in the adult?

(A) hypertension in the upper extremities and hypotension in the lower extremities
(B) absent femoral pulses
(C) murmur over the left chest
(D) hematuria
(E) notching of the ribs *(2:752)*

28. The percent decrease in cross-sectional area in acquired aortic valvular stenosis necessary to decrease resting cardiac output and create a significant increase in pressure gradient is

(A) 15%
(B) 35%
(C) 55%
(D) 75%
(E) 95%   *(3:2338)*

29. The etiology of chronic constrictive pericarditis includes all of the following EXCEPT

(A) trauma
(B) tuberculosis
(C) syphilis
(D) viral pericarditis
(E) idiopathic pericarditis   *(3:2126)*

30. A 2-week-old cyanotic infant has a large right ventricle and right atrium. The pulmonary markings are increased. Which of the following is the most likely diagnosis?

(A) tetralogy of Fallot
(B) transposition of the great vessels
(C) atrial septal defect
(D) ventricular septal defect
(E) pulmonary stenosis   *(2:782)*

31. Which of the following nerves is the most likely to show complete return of function following accurate reapproximation?

(A) sciatic nerve
(B) ulnar nerve
(C) digital nerve
(D) median nerve
(E) perineal nerve   *(24:145)*

32. Which of the following systemic collagen diseases most frequently involves the esophagus?

(A) periarteritis nodosa
(B) rheumatoid arthritis
(C) lupus erythematosus
(D) scleroderma
(E) erythema multiforme   *(2:1074)*

33. Mitral stenosis and mitral regurgitation share many pathophysiologic features. The most significant difference between the two aside from the mechanics of the valve defect is

(A) mitral stenosis is associated with greater dyspnea

(B) death by acute pulmonary edema is more likely with mitral regurgitation
(C) left atrial enlargement is greater with stenosis
(D) the left ventricle is normal with stenosis
(E) right ventricular failure is more common with regurgitation   *(3:2353)*

34. All of the following contribute to the formation of renal calculi EXCEPT

(A) hyperparathyroidism
(B) hyperthyroidism
(C) high urinary pH
(D) infection of the urinary tract
(E) dehydration   *(2:1697)*

35. A patient with chronic pancreatitits has had a sphincterotomy and T-tube drainage of the common bile duct. He also now completely abstains from alcohol. He still has severe symptoms, and an x-ray shows pancreatic calcification. The best treatment is

(A) pancreaticojejunostomy
(B) lumbar dorsal sympathectomy and splanchnicectomy
(C) vagotomy
(D) total pancreatectomy
(E) ligature of the pancreatic ducts   *(2:1354)*

36. The most frequent site of coronary artery narrowing by artherosclerosis is

(A) left main
(B) left anterior descending
(C) left circumflex
(D) right   *(3:2285)*

Questions 37 through 39

A 62-year-old man is admitted with a history of nocturia times four, urgency, and terminal dribbling. On rectal examination, the median sulcus of the prostate is present, the lateral lobes are well defined, and all lobes are enlarged to about three times the normal size.

37. Which of the following is the most likely diagnosis?

(A) carcinoma of the prostate
(B) median bar hypertrophy
(C) chronic prostatitis
(D) median lobe hypertrophy
(E) benign prostatic hypertrophy   *(2:1715)*

38. The most useful investigation in the patient is

(A) cystoscopy
(B) cystoscopy after voiding
(C) intravenous pyelography
(D) a metastatic survey of the bony skeleton
(E) urethral catheterization   *(2:1715)*

39. The best treatment for the patient is

(A) transurethral prostatectomy
(B) suprapubic prostatectomy
(C) retropubic prostatectomy
(D) perineal prostatectomy
(E) cryosurgery   *(2:1716)*

Questions 40 and 41

A 66-year-old white, male, retired executive is found on biopsy to have a squamous cell carcinoma localized to the right vocal cord. The cord has normal motion, and there is no evidence of extension beyond the vocal cord.

40. The best treatment is

(A) electrocautery excision
(B) radiotherapy
(C) laryngofissure and excision of the tumor
(D) laryngectomy
(E) laryngectomy with right neck dissection
          (2:578)

41. The probability of a 5-year survival with the treatment you should recommend is

(A) 90%
(B) 80%
(C) 70%
(D) 60%
(E) 50%   *(2:578)*

42. Most true polyps of the colon are

(A) juvenile
(B) hyperplastic
(C) tubular
(D) tubulovillous
(E) villous   *(3:1025–1027)*

43. The most common mediastinal neoplasm is

(A) lymphoma
(B) primary carcinoma
(C) germ cell neoplasm
(D) neurogenic tumor
(E) mesenchymal tumor   *(23:1027)*

44. Which of the following germ cell tumors found in the mediastinum is notably radiosensitive?

(A) embryonal cell carcinoma
(B) seminoma
(C) choriocarcinoma
(D) yolk sac tumor
(E) teratocarcinoma   *(23:1031)*

Questions 45 through 49

You are operating on a 5-year-old boy for an inguinal hernia when the anesthetist states that the patient has no blood pressure or pulse.

45. Which of the following should you do first?

(A) listen to the heart
(B) feel the femoral artery
(C) inject adrenalin
(D) look at the patient's pupils
(E) order an electrocardiogram   *(2:436, 817)*

46. The next step should be to

(A) commence closed-chest cardiac massage
(B) confirm that the patient is intubated and has adequate pulmonary ventilation
(C) inject epinephrine into the heart
(D) open the chest and perform cardiac massage
(E) defibrillate the heart   *(2:818)*

47. The patient is now known to have cardiac arrest and satisfactory pulmonary ventilation. The correct procedure is

(A) closed-chest cardiac massage
(B) to open the chest and perform cardiac massage
(C) to inject sodium bicarbonate
(D) to start a blood transfusion
(E) to inject calcium   *(2:819)*

48. The surgeon is using closed-chest cardiac massage. Which of the following assist the surgeon to estimate if he or she is performing satisfactorily?

(A) an easily palpable peripheral pulse
(B) a peripheral pulse rate of about 60
(C) the presence of a well-oxygenized patient, including the appearance of the hernia incision
(D) evidence that the patient is entering a lighter plane of anesthesia
(E) all of the above   *(2:818–820)*

49. The closed cardiac massage is proceeding well and the patient is responding, but the electrocardiogram shows the presence of ventricular fibrillation. The next step is to

(A) open the chest and defibrillate the heart
(B) apply the electrodes externally to the base and apex of the heart and defibrillate
(C) place wet saline sponges or conductive jelly between the electrodes and the skin over the base and apex of the heart and defibrillate
(D) make a small epigastric incision through the diaphragm and pericardium so that the heart may be inspected and the presence of ventricular fibrillation confirmed
(E) inject lidocaine   *(2:819)*

50. A 17-year-old girl has very severe primary dysmenorrhea not relieved by nonnarcotic analgesics. An appropriate treatment is

(A) psychotherapy
(B) cyclic oral contraceptives
(C) progesterone
(D) desiccated thyroid
(E) ibuprofen   *(2:1742)*

51. A patient, age 48, is admitted. He is known to have cirrhosis of the liver and portal hypertension. Six weeks before, he had been in the hospital suffering from hematemesis and tarry stools. An x-ray demonstrated esophageal varices but no peptic ulcer. The serum albumin is 2.7 g per 100 ml, the prothrombin time is prolonged, and the SGOT and SGPT are elevated. The patient has clinically obvious but not massive ascites. The treatment should be

(A) a splenorenal shunt
(B) an H-graft portacaval shunt
(C) transesophageal ligature of varices
(D) inpatient medical management
(E) a side-to-side portacaval shunt   *(2:1285)*

52. A 38-year-old man has a history of mild, chronic dyspnea and, on physical examination, has telangiectasia of the nasal and buccal mucosa and spider telangiectasia over his upper arms and chest. There is mild clubbing and cyanosis. A gastrointestinal series is negative, and the chest x-rays show a peripheral lesion of the left midlung field and a second lesion in the lower left lung field behind the heart. The most likely diagnosis is

(A) metastatic carcinoma
(B) bronchogenic carcinoma
(C) pulmonary arteriovenous fistula
(D) tuberculosis
(E) cirrhosis of the liver   *(2:668)*

53. The primary treatment of anal carcinoma of squamous cell origin is

(A) radical abdominoperineal resection
(B) radiation and chemotherapy
(C) fulguration
(D) topical 5-FU
(E) local excision   *(3:1009)*

54. Colitis associated with antibiotic therapy has been recognized as an increasing problem. This pseudomembranous-like condition is usually caused by overgrowth of

(A) *Escherichia coli*
(B) *Bacteroides*
(C) *Serratia*
(D) *Clostridium difficile*
(E) *Enterococcus*   *(3:999)*

Questions 55 and 56

A woman has had a right lower lobectomy 24 hours previously. She is dyspneic and coughs poorly. The chest tube does not bubble, but the water level in the chest tube moves markedly.

55. The likely diagnosis is

(A) tension pneumothorax
(B) left lobar pneumonia
(C) atelectasis of the right lung
(D) hemothorax
(E) hemopneumothorax   *(3:331)*

56. The best treatment of this patient is

(A) antibiotic therapy
(B) positive pressure respiration
(C) tracheobronchial aspiration
(D) chest aspiration
(E) oxygen   *(3:331)*

57. The risk of perforation increases significantly when the cecum exceeds a diameter of

(A) 10 cm
(B) 12 cm
(C) 14 cm
(D) 16 cm
(E) 18 cm   *(3:996)*

58. In which of the following circumstances is local anesthesia LEAST likely to be effective?

(A) when used for a breast biopsy
(B) in the skin of the back
(C) anesthetizing over an abscess
(D) in the skin of the buttock
(E) in the scalp   *(3:164)*

59. The leading cause of large bowel obstruction is

(A) volvulus
(B) intussusception
(C) diverticulitis
(D) carcinoma
(E) hernia   *(3:996)*

60. A chordoma

(A) occurs at the sphenoccipital and sacrococcygeal regions
(B) grows rapidly
(C) occurs more frequently in females than in males
(D) usually occurs in childhood
(E) does not invade bone   *(2:1944)*

61. The majority of female patients who complain of bleeding from the nipple are eventually found to have

(A) infiltrating duct carcinoma of the breast
(B) chronic cystic mastitis
(C) intraductal papilloma
(D) Paget's disease
(E) residual lactation mastitis   *(2:536)*

62. The major difference between intussusception in children and in adults is

(A) spontaneous reduction is more likely in a child
(B) sudden intermittent cramping pain is seen only in children
(C) barium enema reduction is safe for long-standing obstruction in adults but not in children
(D) most adult intussusceptions have a pathologic lesion as a lead point
(E) operative reduction is rarely required in children   *(3:995)*

63. A crush fracture of the zygoma may give rise to all of the following EXCEPT

(A) diplopia
(B) trismus
(C) malocclusion of the teeth

(D) opacity of the maxillary antrum on x-ray
(E) anesthesia of the upper lip   *(2:2077)*

64. Among the leukemias, splenectomy performed as initial therapy provides a clear survival advantage in

(A) chronic hairy cell leukemia (leukemic reticuloendotheliosis)
(B) acute myelogenous leukemia
(C) chronic myelogenous leukemia
(D) acute lymphocytic leukemia
(E) chronic lymphocytic leukemia *(3:1218–1219)*

65. Myeloid metaplasia is characterized by all of the following EXCEPT

(A) progressive bone marrow fibrosis
(B) a long history of rheumatoid arthritis
(C) extramedullary hematopoiesis
(D) immature erythrocytes and granulocytes in the peripheral blood
(E) massive splenomegaly   *(5:1223)*

66. The two most prevalent organisms normally found in the colon are

(A) *Enterococcus* and *Streptococcus*
(B) *Aerobacter* and *Staphylococcus*
(C) *Escherichia coli* and *Bacteroides*
(D) *Clostridium* and *Staphylococcus*
(E) *Aerobacter* and *Clostridium*   *(5:992)*

67. A quarterback, age 34, is sacked during a game and suffers an open fracture of the shafts of tibia and fibula. His optimal management 4 hours after injury would include, in addition to prophylactic antibiotic and antitetanus

(A) reduction, wound debridement, wound closure, and a padded and molded plaster cast from the thigh to the toes
(B) reduction, wound debridement, and padded and molded plaster cast from the thigh to the toes
(C) wound debridement, wound closure, and insertion of pins above and below the fracture to control bone length and maintain reduction
(D) wound debridement, wound closure, and the insertion of an intramedullary Küntscher nail
(E) reduction, wound debridement, wound closure, and the application of an unpadded plaster cast   *(2:1990)*

68. A 22-year-old male is brought to the emergency room after a head-on collision. He is responsive to shouted commands, is semicomatose and hypotensive, and has a bruise on his chest. Which treatment regimen has first priority?

(A) Trendelenburg position, immediate laboratory tests, and x-ray
(B) obtain supine chest x-ray to determine pathology
(C) insert endotracheal tube and place on ventilator
(D) establish patent airway and institute fluid for shock
(E) insert a chest tube on suction   *(9:147)*

69. Management of pyloric stenosis in an infant includes all of the following EXCEPT

(A) gastrojejunostomy
(B) extramucosal pyloromyotomy
(C) preoperative correction of fluid and electrolyte abnormalities
(D) gastric decompression via nasogastric tube
(E) barium swallow only when necessary for diagnosis   *(2:1648)*

70. Complication of a persistent omphalomesenteric duct include all of the following EXCEPT

(A) obstruction
(B) perforation
(C) hemorrhage
(D) cancer
(E) abdominal mass   *(2:1862)*

71. Surgical intervention is indicated in each of the following instances EXCEPT

(A) failed hydrostatic reduction of an ileocolic intussusception
(B) simple meconium ileus
(C) aganglionosis coli documented in newborn period
(D) perforated necrotizing enterocolitis
(E) malrotation with intestinal volvulus *(2:1653)*

72. A patient is seen in the emergency room who is unresponsive and has a 3-inch abrasion over the frontal area of the skull. Your primary concern for early management would be determined by

(A) blood alcohol levels
(B) spinal tap to rule out intracranial bleeding
(C) skull x-rays to rule out a depressed skull fracture

(D) lateral cervical spine film
(E) giving mannitol and dexamethasone *(9:253)*

73. The mother of a 4-year-old child says that for 2 days he has been cranky and refuses to walk. He has a low grade fever, 101°F, and has an ear ache. Left hip motion is decreased and tender. The course of action most likely to benefit this patient would be

(A) oral antibiotics to cover *Haemophilus influenzae* as the most likely organism
(B) ENT consultation
(C) aspiration of the left hip joint
(D) start intravenous antibiotics
(E) blood cultures and traction to the left leg   *(2:2011)*

74. A 40-year-old woman is seen in the emergency room after an automobile accident with a rigid belly and respiratory difficulty. Her left lower extremity shows the hip to be flexed, internally rotated, and painful on manipulation. You would suspect

(A) infected hip joint
(B) fractured femoral neck
(C) posterior dislocation of the hip
(D) anterior dislocation of the hip
(E) retroperitoneal bleeding with psoas irritation   *(2:1996)*

75. The most likely cause of hematemasis associated with severe colicky right upper quadrant pain in a 21-year-old male 1 month after closed trauma is

(A) duodenal hematoma
(B) arteriovenous malformation of the common duct
(C) hemobilia
(D) duodenal ulcers
(E) necrotizing hepatitis   *(2:1047)*

76. A pancreatic pseudocyst

(A) is usually malignant
(B) never resolves spontaneously
(C) is seldom related to alcohol ingestion or trauma
(D) displaces the stomach posteriorly
(E) has a wall consisting of surrounding structures instead of pancreas   *(2:1359)*

77. The most important muscle for maintaining anal continence during sleep is the

(A) internal sphincter
(B) external sphincter
(C) transverse perineii
(D) ischiorectal muscle
(E) puborectalis muscle   *(2:1231)*

78. The best medical management for bleeding hemorrhoids without prolapse is

(A) high fiber diet (bran)
(B) steroid creams
(C) silver nitrate
(D) Preparation H
(E) anesthetic ointments   *(2:1223)*

79. Hepatic encephalopathy is best treated by

(A) blood transfusions
(B) side-to-side protacaval shunt
(C) H graft mesocaval shunt
(D) distal splenorenal shunt
(E) nonspecific supportive measures   *(2:1287)*

80. In the routine follow-up of cirrhotics for the development of hepatocellular carcinoma, the most constant finding will be

(A) sudden variceal bleeding
(B) enlarging spleen
(C) fever of unknown origin
(D) enlarging liver
(E) rising alkaline phosphatase   *(2:1273)*

81. Which burns are blistered, moist, and painful?

(A) first degree
(B) second degree
(C) third degree
(D) fourth degree
(E) all of the above   *(2:271)*

82. The best test to determine need for escharotomy of an extremity is

(A) Doppler examination of the extremity
(B) tissue gram stain
(C) percutaneous oxygen monitoring
(D) electromyelography
(E) nerve conduction studies   *(2:274)*

83. Electrical burns

(A) are an uncommon type of childhood burn
(B) often appear less severe than they actually are
(C) never involve more than one location on the body

(D) infrequently involve the hands
(E) never involve deep muscle or bone   *(2:270)*

84. The most common cause of acute massive colonic bleeding (2 units) in the list below is

(A) carcinoma
(B) polyps
(C) diverticulae
(D) volvulus
(E) hemangioma   *(2:1186)*

85. In the patient with a colovesical fistula secondary to diverticulitis, the most definitive clinical symptom of the fistula is which of the following?

(A) melena
(B) dysuria
(C) hematuria
(D) pneumaturia
(E) hematochezia   *(2:1189)*

86. The most common cause of sigmoid colon to vaginal fistula is which of the following?

(A) colon carcinoma
(B) foreign body
(C) carcinoma of the uterus
(D) radiation therapy
(E) diverticulitis   *(2:1189)*

87. The most common site for diverticula of the colon is

(A) cecum
(B) transverse colon
(C) descending colon
(D) sigmoid colon
(E) rectum   *(2:1185)*

88. Optimal treatment for prevention of cancer in familial polyposis is

(A) close follow-up, with yearly colonoscopy
(B) close follow-up, with yearly air contrast barium enema
(C) colonoscopic removal of all polyps larger than 4 cm
(D) perineal resection with sigmoid colostomy
(E) total colectomy   *(2:1194)*

89. Anal lesions most commonly are associated with

    (A) ulcerative colitis
    (B) Crohn's disease
    (C) diverticular disease
    (D) sigmoid cancer
    (E) hepatoma   *(2:1150)*

90. The most common cause of primary hyperparathyroidism is

    (A) parathyroid adenoma
    (B) parathyroid hyperplasia
    (C) chief cell hyperplasia
    (D) parathyroid carcinoma
    (E) none of the above   *(2:1585)*

91. A 25-year-old woman has been prepared for subtotal thyroidectomy with propylthiouracil 150 mg every 6 hours for 4 weeks and Lugols' iodine solution 5 drops three times a day for 1 week. She is clinically euthyroid preoperatively. The thyroid is removed, and hemostasis is being attained; bleeding is not excessive. Temperature at 1½ hours after induction of anesthesia with narcotic, curare, and nitrous oxide is 37.2°C, pulse rate is 80, and blood pressure is 130/60. Fifteen minutes later, temperature is noted to be 39.4°C, pulse rate is 130, and blood pressure is 160/90. There have been no signs of swallowing or coughing. At this point, appropriate management of this patient would consist of

    (A) increasing the concentration of anesthesia
    (B) administration of intravenous sodium or potassium iodide
    (C) administration of reserpine
    (D) administration of intravenous propranolol
    (E) initiation of hypothermia with no additional drugs   *(2:1575)*

92. In patients with which of the following diseases of the thyroid is a high titer of autoantibodies to thyroglobulin most likely to be found?

    (A) adolescent goiter
    (B) Hashimoto's disease
    (C) toxic nodular goiter
    (D) papillary carcinoma
    (E) acute thyroiditis   *(2:1562)*

93. All of the following statements concerning follicular carcinoma of the thyroid are true EXCEPT

    (A) it may be difficult to diagnose on frozen section

    (B) metastases take up ^{131}I
    (C) it is usually well differentiated, with a good prognosis
    (D) it characteristically spreads by lymph nodes
    (E) it usually presents as a solitary nodule   *(2:1570)*

94. Medullary carcinoma of the thyroid is a hallmark of the endocrine abnormality called

    (A) MEA type I or MEN-1
    (B) Wermer's syndrome
    (C) Cushing's syndrome
    (D) Sipple's syndrome or MEN-2
    (E) Hazard's syndrome   *(2:1571)*

95. A symptomatic pulmonary embolus usually arises from

    (A) deep calf vein
    (B) arm
    (C) ileofemoral veins
    (D) superficial calf veins
    (E) superficial thigh veins   *(2:962)*

96. Which of the following parameters is most frequently seen with pulmonary embolus?

    (A) normal chest examination
    (B) hypoxia
    (C) decreased systemic vascular resistance
    (D) atrial fibrillation
    (E) elevated alkaline phosphatase   *(2:983)*

97. Universal donor blood for males and females (beyond the child bearing age) is

    (A) AB positive
    (B) O positive
    (C) O negative
    (D) pooled, washed red cells
    (E) none of the above   *(2:104)*

98. Chronic venous insufficiency is

    (A) frequently treated surgically
    (B) rarely treated surgically
    (C) usually the result of trauma
    (D) unrelated to obesity
    (E) rarely an etiology of leg ulcers   *(2:991)*

99. Superficial thrombophlebitis in an outpatient usually is treated with

    (A) surgery
    (B) elevation and rest
    (C) heparin

(D) steroids
(E) anti-inflammatory drugs   *(2:976)*

100. A 30-year-old weekend athlete sustains a twisting injury of his left knee while skiing in Colorado. At your clinic 1 week later, he is using crutches and has a mildly swollen knee. During your examination of his knee you note that he has a positive anterior drawer sign at 90° and 30° of knee flexion. He has most likely injured what ligament?

(A) medial collateral
(B) lateral collateral
(C) anterior cruciate
(D) posterior cruciate
(E) deep medial collateral only   *(2:1986)*

101. All of the following are true of knee arthroscopy EXCEPT

(A) the incidence of infection is low
(B) no anesthesia is required for the procedure
(C) torn meniscus tissue may be excised
(D) the technique is applicable as an outpatient procedure
(E) postoperative recovery usually is shorter than that of arthrotomy   *(2:1988)*

102. What precaution should be taken for a dental procedure involving a patient with an aortofemoral bypass graft in place?

(A) the dental procedure should not be done
(B) the graft should be removed first
(C) all teeth should be extracted
(D) the patient should be admitted to the hospital
(E) prophylactic antibiotics should be given   *(4:423)*

103. The primary factor in assessing abdominal injury is to

(A) make an accurate diagnosis of a specific type of injury
(B) perform a peritoneal lavage
(C) determine the presence of an acute abdomen and the need for surgical intervention
(D) get early acute abdominal series x-rays
(E) get a liver–spleen scan   *(9:223)*

104. The following statements concerning pelvic abscess are correct EXCEPT

(A) usually few symptoms or signs are present on examination of the abdomen
(B) the abscess usually can be palpated by rectal or vaginal examination
(C) it is important to distinguish between an inflammatory mass involving the fallopian tube and uterus and a true pelvic abscess
(D) in general, pelvic inflammatory masses involving the fallopian tubes bulge into the rectum
(E) drainage of a true pelvic abscess should be through the rectum and vagina   *(2:1415)*

105. Vasopressors are indicated in patients with hypovolemic shock under the following conditions.

(A) when the patient's blood pressure is not responding to fluids
(B) when the patient's urine output does not respond to fluids
(C) as an adjunct to fluid therapy when the patient has continuing internal bleeding
(D) to ensure better perfusion of the kidneys before surgery
(E) vasopressors are not indicated in hypovolemic shock   *(2:1502)*

106. Appropriate therapy for volvulus of the sigmoid colon is

(A) immediate sigmoid colectomy with colostomy
(B) decompression per rectum and colectomy if volvulus recurs
(C) transverse loop colostomy with planned colectomy following an adequate bowel preparation
(D) rectal decompression and pexy of the sigmoid colon
(E) long tube decompression from above and observation   *(2:1212)*

107. Diverticulitis of the sigmoid colon should be treated initially with

(A) sigmoid colectomy with primary reanastomosis
(B) diverting colostomy and antibiotics
(C) bowel rest, antibiotics, and observation
(D) sigmoid colectomy with colostomy
(E) exteriorization of the involved segment with planned second-stage sigmoid colectomy   *(2:1187)*

DIRECTIONS (Questions 108 through 180): Each question consists of an introduction followed by five statements. Mark T (true) or F (false) after each statement.

108. Torsion of the testicle

    (A) causes abdominal pain, nausea, and vomiting
    (B) should be operated on as an emergency
    (C) when treated, operation includes exploring the contralateral scrotum
    (D) often occurs spontaneously, even during sleep
    (E) causes testicular atrophy   *(2:1685)*

109. In the course of operating for presumed appendicitis, you discover inflammatory bowel disease localized to the terminal ileum. You should

    (A) remove the appendix
    (B) not resect the terminal ileum
    (C) resect the terminal ileum
    (D) do an ileocecal resection
    (E) do an ileocolic bypass   *(3:925)*

110. Which of the following are associated with Meigs' syndrome?

    (A) lymphedema of the leg
    (B) fibroma of the ovary
    (C) liver metastases
    (D) ascites and hydrothorax
    (E) ovarian carcinoma   *(2:1771)*

111. Of the following coagulation factors, which are present in banked blood?

    (A) factor IX (Christmas factor)
    (B) factor V (proaccelerin)
    (C) fibrinogen
    (D) factor VIII (antihemophilic factor A)
    (E) prothrombin   *(2:106)*

112. A patient has suffered a massive pulmonary embolus with reflex bronchial constriction. The following statements concern heparin therapy.

    (A) a large dose of heparin should be given initially (e.g., 10,000 units)
    (B) subcutaneous heparinization is preferable to intravenous heparinization
    (C) a large total dose of heparin should be given in the first 24 hours
    (D) heparinization is contraindicated
    (E) coumadin is given often before the completion of heparin therapy   *(1:741)*

113. The indications for surgery in Crohn's disease include

    (A) fistula
    (B) obstruction
    (C) failure of medical therapy
    (D) abscess
    (E) risk of carcinoma   *(3:926)*

114. The following statements refer to peritoneal lavage for abdominal trauma.

    (A) pregnancy is an absolute contraindication
    (B) a patient who will be unavailable for monitoring should have lavage
    (C) a negative lavage rules out retroperitoneal injury
    (D) 100,000 WBC/mm is a negative lavage
    (E) Foley catheter and nasogastric tube should be passed before lavage   *(9:228-229)*

115. Which of the following statements is/are true concerning a patient who is undergoing anticoagulation therapy?

    (A) the prothrombin time should be determined before beginning heparin therapy
    (B) the one-stage prothrombin time is the preferred method of controlling anticoagulation with coumarins
    (C) the partial thromboplastin time can be used as the method of controlling anticoagulation with heparin
    (D) an accurate prothrombin time cannot be carried out in a patient who has received heparin three hours earlier
    (E) with the coumarins keep the prothrombin time five times normal   *(2:100)*

116. Lymphangiogram, when used as a diagnostic aid for Hodgkin's disease

    (A) has an 80 to 90% accuracy rate for involvement of retroperitoneal lymph nodes
    (B) is equally accurate for all retroperitoneal lymph node sites
    (C) eliminates the need for staging laparotomy when positive
    (D) if positive, is associated with a 40% incidence of another intraabdominal site of Hodgkin's disease
    (E) is a good indicator of splenic involvement   *(3:1216)*

117. Which of the following statements about craniosynostosis is/are correct?

    (A) operative correction is not indicated if only the sagittal suture is involved
    (B) the sagittal suture is involved more frequently than other sutures
    (C) eye abnormalities indicate sagittal suture involvement
    (D) operation is sometimes indicated during the first 2 months of life
    (E) it leads to compression of the brain
    (2:1824)

118. When the hymen is imperforate at puberty

    (A) the menstrual blood will not be retained in the uterus
    (B) other vaginal anomalies are usually also found
    (C) uterine discharge into the vagina does not occur until the condition is corrected
    (D) the condition is treated by cruciate incisions of the mucous membrane
    (E) the uterus is distended   *(2:1734)*

119. Which of the following statements about Wilms' tumor is/are correct?

    (A) the prognosis is better in younger patients
    (B) treatment is a combination of surgery, radiotherapy, and chemotherapy
    (C) bilateral lesions occur in 5% of patients
    (D) usually presents as a flank mass
    (E) may contain calcium   *(2:1668)*

120. The following statements refer to burns.

    (A) airway injuries are evident immediately
    (B) alkali burns are more serious than acid burns
    (C) the most reliable measure of extremity circulation is capillary filling
    (D) a normal urine output indicates a systolic pressure of at least 90 mm Hg
    (E) the amount of fluid needed in the first 24 hours is roughly 2 to 4 ml/kg/percent area burned   *(9:284–286)*

121. The following statements refer to electrical burns.

    (A) the extent of burn is judged by surface area
    (B) muscles, nerves, and blood vessels commonly are injured

    (C) renal failure is more a common complication of electrical burns than of surface burns.
    (D) myoglobinuria is treated by increasing fluid volume
    (E) mannitol and sodium bicarbonate are given if the urine does not clear with increased fluids   *(9:287)*

122. The following statements relate to blood transfusion.

    (A) frozen red cells have a lower oxygen-carrying capacity when thawed than they had when frozen
    (B) 20% of transfusion-related hepatitis is non-A, non-B
    (C) most transfusion reactions are caused by human error in administration
    (D) multiple transfusions compound the acidosis of shock
    (E) most patients develop some hyperkalemia after transfusion   *(3:109)*

123. The following statements refer to the barbiturate anesthetic agents.

    (A) they cause myocardial stimulation
    (B) they cause peripheral vasoconstriction
    (C) they increase coronary blood flow
    (D) they are good agents to use in trauma
    (E) they cross the placental barrier   *(3:162)*

124. Staging laparotomy for Hodgkin's disease has become the most common indication for splenectomy. In this procedure

    (A) 20% of patients will have splenic involvement that was not detected clinically
    (B) isolated liver involvement is common
    (C) 40% of patients have their clinical stage changed
    (D) splenic involvement is related to size
    (E) information useful for determining therapy for all stages of Hodgkin's disease is obtained   *(3:1216–1217)*

125. The following statements are in regard to gas gangrene (diffuse clostridial myonecrosis).

    (A) there is marked tachycardia
    (B) the wound is not painful
    (C) give penicillin in large doses
    (D) give antitoxin in large doses
    (E) the patient is hypothermic   *(2:185)*

126. The following statements are about carcinoma of the oral cavity.

(A) carcinoma of the oral cavity is more differentiated and less aggressive than is carcinoma of the oropharynx
(B) the symptoms are minimal in the early stages
(C) carcinoma of the tongue metastasizes to the cervical lymph nodes only after many years
(D) the most common malignant tumor of the lower lip is a basal cell carcinoma
(E) the so-called verrucous carcinoma of the buccal mucosa occurs in tobacco chewers and is highly malignant   (2:570)

127. The conservative management of a patient with thrombosis of the superficial femoral artery should include

(A) stopping smoking
(B) treating anemia
(C) weight reduction in the obese
(D) control of diabetes
(E) no alcoholic beverages   (2:911)

128. A man, age 60, has a hard lymph node in the neck. He is examined by a surgeon who considers it to be malignant. Which of the following statements are correct?

(A) metastatic cervical nodes appearing below and behind the ear and along the border of the sternomastoid muscle are likely to come from the nasopharynx and lateral pharyngeal walls
(B) metastatic nodes near the angle of the mandible or in the area of the submandibular gland are rarely from metastases from the tonsillar area, the buccal mucosa, or the floor of the mouth
(C) squamous cell carcinoma found in a cervical node in a patient in whom no primary can be found has almost certainly arisen in a branchial cleft remnant
(D) metastatic nodes in the submental area often come from the tip of the tongue, the lower lip, and the anterior gingivobuccal gutter
(E) nodes in the middle third of the neck are often due to carcinomas arising in the hypopharynx, piriform sinus, larynx, or thyroid gland   (2:560)

129. Gardner's syndrome differs from familial polyposis in that Gardner's patients

(A) have adenomatous colon polyps
(B) have a 100% incidence of malignancy if untreated
(C) exhibit epidermoid cysts
(D) have benign osteomas
(E) may exhibit cortical thickening of tubular bones   (3:1028)

130. Classic hemophilia (factor VIII deficiency)

(A) occurs chiefly in males
(B) seldom causes hemarthrosis
(C) is associated with contractures of the elbows and knees
(D) is inherited as a sex-linked dominant
(E) results in a high incidence of peptic ulcer disease   (2:91–95)

131. Acute gastric mucosal erosions with hemorrhage occur with

(A) bony trauma
(B) burns
(C) sepsis
(D) stress
(E) steroid therapy   (2:1046)

132. Chronic insufficiency of the deep veins of the lower limb is recognized by

(A) stasis pigmentation
(B) subcutaneous edema of the distal leg and ankle
(C) relief of pain on standing
(D) ulceration of the lateral calf
(E) dermatitis   (2:987)

133. These methods of sterilizing surgical instruments are considered quite reliable.

(A) autoclaving (saturated steam at 75 mm Hg and 120°C)
(B) boiling in water for 30 minutes
(C) dry heat at 170°C for 1 hour
(D) soaking in 2% aqueous alkaline glutaraldehyde
(E) gas sterilization in 12% ethylene oxide and 88% freon for 105 minutes at 410 mm Hg and 55°C   (1:21)

134. The following statements concern the explanation of the cranial nerves in a patient who is seen in the emergency department soon after a head injury.

(A) a dilated nonnegative pupil on one side in a semiconscious patient indicates compression of the 3rd nerve

(B) the corneal reflex involves the 5th and 7th nerves

(C) the oculocephalic reflex (Doll's eye movement) should be performed at once

(D) the oculocephalic reflex depends on the integrity of the 3rd, 4th, 6th, and 8th cranial nerves

(E) the 3rd nerve passes through the incisura in the tentorium   *(9:239-243)*

135. Fecal impaction after surgery commonly occurs in association with

(A) old age
(B) diarrhea
(C) dehydration
(D) a gastrointestinal series
(E) prolonged, severe pain   *(2:1214)*

136. All of the following statements concern tetanus

(A) the first symptom is usually limitation of movement of the jaws

(B) the infected site must be debrided before initiating other measures of treatment

(C) tracheostomy often is required

(D) the injection of human immune globulin should precede surgery

(E) an attack of tetanus confers lasting immunity   *(2:186)*

137. The following statements concern the criteria for the establishment of brain death.

(A) the decision is a clinical one

(B) the decision is based primarily on signs of irreversible brainstem damage

(C) the decision should be made by physicians not associated with the transplant team

(D) the exact criteria vary from institution to institution

(E) the President's Commission for the Study of Ethical Problems in Medicine issued in 1981 a list of guidelines for the determination of death   *(2:415)*

138. About 4000 persons die in the United States each year from heat stroke. The following statements are in regard to that condition.

(A) heat stroke should be suspected in anyone in a hot environment who develops coma without an apparent cause. The diagnosis

is definite if the patient's temperature rises above 40°C.

(B) the rate of breathing may reach 60 per minute

(C) sweating is excessive

(D) rapid cooling is dangerous

(E) exercise-induced heat stroke often affects young people   *(1:243)*

139. The following statements concern an infection of the terminal pulp space of a finger or the thumb.

(A) the usual cause is a puncture wound
(B) the usual organism is a streptococcus
(C) the movements of the digit are full
(D) treatment includes incision and drainage
(E) if untreated, bone necrosis can occur
                    (2:2080)

140. Clinical manifestations of tentorial herniation may include

(A) ipsilateral (side of the lesion producing herniation) mydriasis

(B) contralateral hemiparesis
(C) decerebrate rigidity
(D) ipsilateral hemiparesis
(E) contralateral hemianopsia   *(9:239)*

141. The following are commonly associated with increased physiologic dead space and increased dead space-to-tidal volume ratio.

(A) atelectasis
(B) arterial hypotension
(C) pulmonary embolism
(D) high mean airway pressure
(E) fat embolism   *(1:26-27)*

142. The following statements refer to amebic hepatitis abscess.

(A) they are usually multiple

(B) metronidazole 750 mg orally three times a day for 10 days usually cures this abscess

(C) incision and drainage often are necessary

(D) the right lobe of the liver is the usual site

(E) the pus from the abscess contains the trophozoites of *Entamoeba histolytica*
                    (2:1265)

143. When a prosthetic arterial graft becomes infected, which of the following occurs?

(A) fever and peripheral septic emboli
(B) false aneurysm
(C) local wound infection
(D) hemorrhage
(E) septicemia   *(4:413)*

144. The following are indications for coronary artery bypass grafting.

(A) single-vessel disease with stable angina
(B) single-vessel disease with refractory angina
(C) proximal left anterior descending lesion with minimal angina
(D) left main lesion with 50% occlusion
(E) double-vessel disease, minimal angina, and abnormal exercise test   *(3:2292)*

145. The following statements deal with coronary artery bypass grafting.

(A) the only effective way to arrest the damage of an acute evolving myocardial infarction (MI) is coronary artery bypass grafting
(B) grafts can be performed safely only to vessels greater than 2 mm in diameter
(C) all vessels large enough to take a graft that have greater than 50% narrowing should be grafted
(D) internal mammary artery is superior to saphenous vein for grafting
(E) pericarditis is a rare complication of coronary artery bypass grafting
                                              (3:2294-2304)

146. The following statements are in regard to duodenal ulcer.

(A) plain water by mouth affords temporary relief of pain
(B) only 30% of patients with duodenal ulcer have normal gastric acid secretion
(C) the ulcer pain often awakens a sleeping patient
(D) the symptoms of duodenal ulcer usually occur when the stomach is full
(E) the symptoms of duodenal ulcer tend toward periodicity   *(3:822)*

147. Adynamic ileus of the alimentary tract usually lasts 2 to 4 days following laparotomy unless special measures are used to prevent it. Recovery may be prolonged in which of the following?

(A) fracture of the lumbar spine
(B) peritonitis
(C) hypokalemia
(D) lower lobe pneumonia
(E) starvation   *(2:1044)*

148. The following statements relate to Mallory-Weiss syndrome, bleeding lower esophageal tears.

(A) most cases are associated with vomiting
(B) most cases are associated with alcohol
(C) endoscopic cauterization usually is required to stop bleeding
(D) surgical oversewing of the tear from the stomach side is required in 50% of patients
(E) vagotomy should be performed after oversewing the tear   *(3:846)*

149. The following statements relate to duodenal trauma.

(A) paraduodenal hematomas should not be opened for fear of pancreatic fistula
(B) retroperitoneal rupture of the duodenum results in rapid sepsis
(C) the prognosis for duodenal rupture is related directly to the severity of associated injuries
(D) the most common associated organ injury is to the liver
(E) the majority of duodenal injuries are due to blunt trauma   *(3:847)*

150. The following are true of liver abscess.

(A) untreated liver abscess is associated with a 50% mortality
(B) pyogenic liver abscess is more likely to rupture than amebic abscess
(C) the prognosis for pyogenic abscess is better than for amebic abscess
(D) the most common complication of amebic liver abscess is extension into the chest
(E) death from liver abscess usually is due to secondary brain abscess   *(3:1072)*

151. The following are indications for admitting a patient to a burn unit.

(A) an adult with greater than 15% burn
(B) all burns of face, eyes, ears, hands, feet, and perineum
(C) burns associated with other major injuries
(D) high-voltage electrical burns
(E) inhalation injury   *(9:287)*

152. The following statements refer to hemorrhagic shock.

(A) a capillary filling time under 2 seconds indicates a patient is normovolemic
(B) of the femoral, carotid, and radial pulses, the femoral can be palpated at the lowest systolic pressure
(C) for emergency transfusion, low-titer type O blood is preferred
(D) urine output is significantly decreased in class II hemorrhage (15 to 30% of blood volume)
(E) femoral fractures are commonly associated with hematomas up to 1500 ml in volume
(9:181)

153. The following statements refer to coagulopathy that develops during resuscitation.

(A) early coagulopathy is usually due to fibrinogen depletion
(B) platelets, if indicated, should be administered after every 10 units of blood
(C) depletion of labile clotting factors usually requires 2 units of fresh frozen plasma to restore levels
(D) hypothermia and acidosis make microvascular bleeding worse
(E) the majority of patients receiving blood transfusions do not require supplemental calcium
(9:188)

154. Typical signs and symptoms of fat embolism include

(A) nausea
(B) hypotension
(C) confusion
(D) dyspnea
(E) petechiae
(3:1768)

155. The pulmonary manifestations of fat embolism

(A) appear slowly and insidiously
(B) are sudden and catastrophic
(C) require immediate intubation
(D) may be benefited by steroids
(E) are best assessed by P_{CO_2}
(3:1768)

156. The following bacterial factors favor the development of wound infection.

(A) virulent organism
(B) unshaved skin hair
(C) devitalized tissue

(D) foreign body
(E) large inoculum of bacteria
(3:262)

157. Phagocytosis is impaired by the following factors.

(A) bacterial encapsulation
(B) uremia
(C) prematurity
(D) leukemia
(E) hyperglycemia
(3:262)

158. The following statements refer to ketamine.

(A) it is a good muscle relaxant
(B) psychic disturbances are common in the recovery period
(C) it causes peripheral vasodilatation
(D) it increases cardiac output
(E) it increases myocardial oxygen consumption
(3:162)

159. The following statements refer to the muscle relaxants.

(A) curare causes fasciculation when administered
(B) curare is a depolarizing agent
(C) succinylcholine is a nondepolarizing agent
(D) succinylcholine is reversed by anticholinesterase drugs
(E) succinylcholine is broken down by cholinesterase
(3:163)

160. The following statements concern gallstone ileus.

(A) the average age of patients is about 70
(B) the patient has partial or complete intestinal obstruction
(C) the obstructing gallstone usually is at least 2.5 cm in diameter
(D) an x-ray film may show the gallstone in the intestine and gas in the biliary tree
(E) the treatment is an emergency operation and removal of the stone
(1:503)

161. The results of numerous clinical trials have demonstrated that much less aggressive surgical treatment of breast cancer than was previously thought necessary gives equivalent results to those obtained with total mastectomy.

    (A) axillary node disection is valuable therapy in preventing axillary recurrence
    (B) women with tumors less than 4 cm in diameter with or without axillary nodes can be treated by segmental mastectomy plus axillary dissection and radiotherapy
    (C) before operation, a full discussion with the patient of the rationale for treatment and the manner of coping with the cosmetic and psychologic effects of mastectomy is essential
    (D) treatment of the axillary nodes is indicated for noninfiltrating cancers
    (E) extended radical mastectomy is justified for patients with medial lesions   (1:265)

162. Achalasia of the esophagus is a neuromuscular disorder in which esophageal dilatation and hypertrophy occur without organic stenosis. The following statements concern the clinical findings in these patients.

    (A) weight loss is a prominent feature
    (B) dysphagia is the dominant symptom
    (C) the condition is painful
    (D) regurgitation is an important symptom
    (E) aspiration of regurgitated material during sleep may lead to repeated bouts of pneumonia   (1:372)

163. A patient coughs up large amounts of purulent, foul-smelling sputum. A lung abscess is considered to be a possible cause of this problem.

    (A) the most common cause of lung abscess is aspiration, with subsequent pneumonia
    (B) when the patient is supine, there is a tendency for aspirated material to enter either the posterior segment of the right upper lobe or the superior segment of the right lower lobe
    (C) alcoholism, dental caries, and diabetes predispose to the development of a lung abscess
    (D) initial treatment consists of culture of the sputum, the appropriate antibiotics, and regular, repeated bronchoscopy to maintain drainage
    (E) external surgical drainage or lobectomy is required in most patients   (1:301)

164. Cricopharyngeal (upper esophageal sphincter) motor dysfunction may be caused by

    (A) multiple sclerosis
    (B) superior laryngeal nerve injury
    (C) myasthenia gravis
    (D) gastroesophageal reflux
    (E) polymyositis   (3:706)

165. The following statements are about esophageal perforation.

    (A) the most common sites are cervical and above the cardia during instrumentation
    (B) the incidence of instrumental perforation is approximately 2%
    (C) dysphagia is the most remarkable symptom
    (D) perforation is more likely at the site of disease
    (E) the perforation rate during transabdominal vagotomy is 5%   (3:750)

166. The following statements refer to bile duct cancers.

    (A) they usually are detected late
    (B) they are likely to have metastasized by the time of diagnosis
    (C) most occur in the lower one third of the duct
    (D) a painless enlarged gallbladder is characteristic in distal lesions
    (E) most patients have jaundice   (3:1135)

167. The following statements are about choledochal cysts.

    (A) they are more common in adults than in children
    (B) they often are associated with intrahepatic ductal dilatation
    (C) the supraduodenal form is most common
    (D) cholangitis is a frequent manifestation
    (E) treatment of choice is drainage into a Roux-en-Y limb of jejunum   (3:1132)

168. The following are desirable effects of selective shunting for esophageal varices.

    (A) cessation of hepatopedal flow
    (B) maintenance of portal hypertension
    (C) reduction of variceal pressure
    (D) reduction of hepatic failure
    (E) reduction of encephalopathy   (3:1106)

169. The following are complications of type II para-esophageal hernia.

    (A) reflux esophagitis
    (B) gastric volvulus
    (C) gastric ulcer
    (D) gastric perforation
    (E) acute intrathoracic gastric dilatation *(3:757)*

170. The following statements refer to duodenal ulcer.

    (A) men are more often affected than women
    (B) the pain is exacerbated by eating
    (C) the patient is typically awakened by pain 2 to 3 hours after going to sleep
    (D) upper gastrointestinal series is the definitive diagnostic study
    (E) endoscopy is the most accurate diagnostic study *(3:822-825)*

171. The following statements are about pyloric outlet obstruction due to peptic ulcer disease.

    (A) the obstruction may resolve if it is due to an acute pyloric channel ulcer
    (B) these patients have a metabolic acidosis due to hypovolemia
    (C) a normal saline load test indicates that feeding may be resumed
    (D) vagotomy and drainage should be performed as soon as fluid, electrolyte, and acid-base derangements are corrected
    (E) anastomotic function is slower to occur in a stomach that has been obstructed than in one that has not *(3:830)*

172. A gastric ulcer that extends beyond the projected line of the stomach wall is likely

    (A) benign
    (B) malignant
    (C) to cause pain that is exacerbated by eating
    (D) to be located on the lesser curvature
    (E) to have a high rate of complications *(3:831)*

173. The surgical treatment of gastric ulcer should include

    (A) distal gastrectomy
    (B) excision of the ulcer
    (C) vagotomy
    (D) gastroenterostomy
    (E) splenectomy *(3:852)*

174. The following statements refer to echinococcal cysts of the liver.

    (A) most are solitary when they first occur
    (B) most are located in the right lobe
    (C) the Frei skin test has an 85% sensitivity
    (D) calcification of the cyst wall is rare
    (E) formalin is the scolicidal agent of choice *(3:1089)*

175. The better prognosis for variceal bleeding due to portal vein thrombosis results from

    (A) normal hepatocyte function
    (B) lower variceal pressure
    (C) normal sinusoidal pressure
    (D) extensive collaterals
    (E) hepatofugal flow *(3:1112)*

176. Sclerosing cholangitis is associated with

    (A) biliary cirrhosis
    (B) portal hypertension
    (C) ulcerative colitis
    (D) retroperitoneal fibrosis
    (E) a younger male population *(3:1136)*

177. The triad of symptoms associated with acute cholangitis includes

    (A) right upper quadrant mass
    (B) jaundice
    (C) fever and chills
    (D) hyperamylasemia
    (E) abdominal pain *(3:1156)*

178. Because bleeding from splenic trauma in children is more self-limited than in adults, selective non-operative management has been advocated if

    (A) initial shock is easily reversible
    (B) all associated organ injuries are identified
    (C) the patient is stable
    (D) the setting is an intensive care unit (ICU) experienced in such management
    (E) the patient stabilizes after several transfusions *(3:1208)*

179. The following are complications of pancreatic pseudocyst.

    (A) infection
    (B) obstruction of the gastrointestinal tract and common bile duct
    (C) renal failure
    (D) rupture
    (E) hemorrhage *(3:1190)*

180. Patients with three or more of Ransom's risk factors in acute pancreatitis have greater than 50% mortality. The initial risk factors include

(A) age under 55 years
(B) serum glucose less than 50 mg/100 ml
(C) leukocytosis greater than 16,000 WBC/mm³
(D) lactic dehydrogenase greater than 700 IU
(E) SGOT greater than 250 sigma-Frankel units

(3:1185)

Answers and Explanations

1. **(B)** Norepinephrine is one of the few hormones not known to be produced by bronchogenic lesions. ACTH has been isolated from small cell and carcinoid lesions, ADH is found in adenocarcinoma and small cell and carcinoid lesions, parathormone is found in squamous, small cell, and carcinoid lesions, and gonadotropin is found in small cell and carcinoid lesions. Other hormones, including serotonin, insulin, glucagon, and somatostatin, also are associated with these lesions.

2. **(B)** Dislocation of the knee is not common but is associated with injury to the popliteal vessels.

3. **(D)** Invasive malignant tumors, usually anaplastic lung cancers, are the most common cause of the superior vena cava syndrome.

4. **(D)** Russell's traction is used for older children. Bryant's traction is used for very young children. Open reduction is contraindicated because of potential damage to the epiphyseal plate.

5. **(C)** Colles' fracture usually occurs in patients over the age of 50.

6. **(C)** The history and the rectal examination should lead you to anticipate finding an imperforate hymen, and you can immediately confirm your diagnosis by inspection of the vagina.

7. **(E)** Hemoptysis represents bronchial erosion and is a presenting symptom in only 29% of patients. Cough (74%), weight loss (68%), dyspnea (58%), and chest pain (49%) are the most frequent symptoms. Significant weight loss is a common sign of metastasis.

8. **(D)** The picture of intermittent small bowel obstruction and a history of biliary symptoms is most suggestive of gallstone ileus. The majority (75%) of biliary-enteric fistulae that allow passage of a stone large enough to cause intestinal obstruction occur between gallbladder and duodenum. The tumbling effect of impaction and dislodgment is characteristic of this condition. The final point of impaction is terminal ileum in two thirds of patients. The frequency of this cause of intestinal obstruction in the elderly increases significantly. An associated diagnostic feature is air in the biliary tree.

9. **(E)** Closed drainage of the pleural cavity is used to overcome the effects of a bronchial stump leak.

10. **(D)** The cervicofacial type of actinomycosis is characterized by nodular granulomas that form sinus tracts.

11. **(C)** Bile salts are required for the absorption of vitamin K from the alimentary tract. Obstructive jaundice, therefore, reduces the absorption of vitamin K.

12. **(A)** Mallet or drop finger is caused by disruption of the extensor tendon to the distal phalanx.

13. **(B)** An infected pseudocyst is a surgical emergency requiring immediate effective drainage. Internal drainage in the presence of infection carries a high risk, so external drainage is the preferred treatment.

14. **(A)** Instrumental perforation of the esophagus occurs either adjacent to a pathologic process or at the sites of normal narrowing. The cervical esophagus is the most frequent site of esophageal perforation.

15. (A) Lateral, anterior, and posterior x-rays of the neck often demonstrate pathognomic features of perforation of the cervical esophagus. This study should, therefore, precede an upper gastrointestinal series using a contrast medium.

16. (A) Once diagnosed and localized, an instrumental perforation of the esophagus is best treated by urgent operation and drainage with repair if necessary. In this patient, the perforation appears to be in the cervical esophagus.

17. (A) Colon and rectum are the most frequent origin of lung metastases (23.4%), followed by kidney (16.5%), breast (14%), testis (12.1%), and uterus (11.6%). Other lesions, such as osteogenic sarcoma, constitute a smaller percentage of lung metastases but have a strong predilection for going to lung when they do metastisize. Beneficial results have been obtained with resection of single or even multiple lung metastases. Thyroid and breast cancer and melanoma have a tendency to seed multiple metastases.

18. (B) fractures unite well when there is some overlap of the bone ends.

19. (C) Using the rat as a model, the tensile strength of a healing skin wound increases rapidly for 17 days, more slowly for the next 10 days, and then almost imperceptibly for 2 years or more, but it never quite reaches the tensile strength of unwounded skin.

20. (C) Radiotherapy in doses of 6 to 10 Gy may produce rapid symptomatic relief for a solitary painful bone metastasis.

21. (E) A number of lesions, including the four listed, may develop squamous cell carcinomas.

22. (A) In patients with coarctation, the coarctation usually is distal to the left subclavian artery.

23. (D) In these patients, excision and end-to-end anastomosis usually is possible. It should be performed if possible before the child starts to attend school.

24. (B) The blood pressure may fall immediately. More often it falls gradually over a period of several weeks.

25. (D) Choice A may be an example of Murphy's law, but Murphy's sign is arrest of inspiration while the surgeon is palpating the right upper quadrant. When inspiration forces the inflamed gallbladder to descend and contact the examining fingers, pain causes an involuntary catch in the breath. Resistance to passive dorsiflexion of the foot is an indicator of calf thrombophlebitis, known as Homans' sign. A nontender, palpable gallbladder (Courvoisier's sign) signifies distal bile duct obstruction by carcinoma.

26. (C) The mitral valve is the left atrioventricular valve, and, therefore, the left ventricle is not enlarged in mitral stenosis.

27. (D) All except hematuria are present in adult patients with coarctation of the aorta.

28. (D) A 75% reduction in cross-sectional area of the aortic orifice is required to cause a significant reduction in resting cardiac output and a significant increase in the pressure gradient across the valve. The systolic gradient may rise to as much as 150 mm Hg. Cardiac output remains normal in the absence of failure but does not increase with exercise if the stenosis is severe. When stenosis is severe enough to cause congestive heart failure, angina, or syncope, surgery should be performed without delay. Without surgery, the life expectancy for such patients is only 2 to 3 years.

29. (C) In most patients, the cause of constrictive pericarditis is unknown, but syphilis plays no part.

30. (B) These findings strongly suggest a diagnosis of transposition of the great vessels.

31. (C) In 1927, Sterling Bunnell wrote, "Of all nerve sutures throughout the body, those that are the most uniformly, promptly, and completely successful are of the hand and fingers." Subsequent experience has confirmed the truth of this statement. After accurate approximation, very good regeneration occurs in the digital nerve.

32. (D) Scleroderma can produce symptomatic esophageal stricture and also can involve other parts of the gastrointestinal tract.

33. (D) The most important pathophysiologic difference between mitral stenosis and mitral regurgitation is that, with stenosis, the left ventricle is protected and remains normal, whereas regurgitation results in left ventricular failure.

Although both share the common feature of pulmonary venous hypertension and congestion, one results from valvular obstruction, and the other results from hemodynamic backpressure and ventricular failure.

34. **(B)** There is no increased incidence of renal stones in patients with hyperthyroidism.

35. **(A)** These patients have multiple strictures of the pancreatic ducts. Lateral pancreaticojejunostomy, or distal pancreatectomy followed by pancreaticojejunostomy, provides drainage of the pancreatic duct system and returns the pancreatic juice to the intestine.

36. **(B)** The most frequent site of coronary artery narrowing due to atherosclerosis is the left anterior descending branch, which is involved 43% of the time. The next most common site is the right (28%), followed by the left circumflex (24%). The least common site is the left main (5%).

37. **(E)** The history and findings are characteristic of benign prostatic hypertrophy. The size of the prostate is not of diagnostic importance, since the correlation between the size of the gland and degree of symptoms is poor.

38. **(B)** Cystoscopy after voiding permits the urologist to estimate the residual urine, examine the urine, and inspect the interior of the bladder.

39. **(A)** The transurethral procedure should be used when possible because the disability is less.

40. **(B)** If the cancer remains confined to the vocal cord, a high percentage of patients are cured by radiotherapy, and the larynx is preserved.

41. **(A)** When the lesion does not extend beyond the vocal cord, 90% of patients are cured.

42. **(C)** Approximately 75% of true colon polyps are tubular adenomas, followed by tubulovillous (15%) and villous (10%). Juvenile or retention polyps are rare benign lesions usually seen in the first decade of life. Hyperplastic polyps are nonneoplastic in nature, and their etiology is unclear.

43. **(D)** Neurogenic tumors are the most common mediastinal neoplasms (25 to 31%). They usually arise in the paravertebral gutter from sympathetic ganglia or intercostal nerves, and the majority are benign (80 to 90%). Those arising in infants are more likely to be malignant. These tumors include neurilemmomas and neurofibromas, either of which may degenerate into a neurosarcoma in 25 to 30% of cases—gangliomas, ganglioneuroblastomas, neuroblastomas, and pheochromocytomas. Neuroblastomas, which occur primarily in children, are the most poorly differentiated neurogenic malignancy but are known to undergo spontaneous regression.

44. **(B)** Seminoma is very radiosensitive and has a good prognosis with excision or radiation alone (up to 75% 5-year survival). The other germ cell tumors have a dismal prognosis but with some improvement using current chemotherapy regimens.

45. **(B)** The confirmation of the fact that the patient has no pulse can be made rapidly by feeling the femoral pulse in the incision.

46. **(B)** The most urgent step in cardiac arrest is to provide adequate oxygenation.

47. **(A)** In this emergency, once good ventilation is established, closed-chest cardiac massage usually restores a satisfactory blood circulation. During the whole episode of cardiac arrest, prompt, efficient action is required to prevent irreversible brain damage.

48. **(E)** Closed-chest cardiac massage usually is satisfactory, and in a patient of this type, recovery can be expected if the cardiac arrest had been recognized immediately.

49. **(C)** If the patient is well oxygenated and the heart muscle is well perfused, defibrillation should succeed if the electrodes have been applied properly.

50. **(E)** The treatment of choice is a prostaglandin inhibitor, such as ibuprofen. Prevention of ovulation frequently also will relieve primary dysmenorrhea.

51. **(D)** Ascites is best treated medically, if possible. This patient has bled mildy but is not now bleeding. At present, a portacaval shunt is recommended only for those patients with ascites who cannot be managed on a strict low-sodium diet and diuretic therapy, an unusual circumstance.

52. **(C)** The presence of telangiectasia indicates that this patient may have an arteriovenous malformation. The x-ray findings plus clubbing and cyanosis make it likely to be a pulmonary arteriovenous fistula.

53. **(B)** The recent trend in treatment of anal carcinoma is combination radiation and chemotherapy, which has met with considerable success for these mostly squamous lesions. If the lesion disappears, it can be closely followed. Persistence requires radical abdominoperineal resection. Squamous cancer of the perianal skin can be excised like any other squamous cell carcinoma of the skin.

54. **(D)** Antibiotic-related colitis is now often caused by overgrowth of *C. difficile* after administration of ampicillin, clindamycin, or a cephalosporin. The condition is diagnosed by proctoscopy and treated by stopping the antibiotic and giving fluid replacement.

55. **(C)** Atelectasis of the residual portion of a lung is an important early complication of pulmonary lobectomy.

56. **(C)** The first step in the treatment of postoperative pulmonary atelectasis is tracheobronchial aspiration followed by breathing and coughing exercises.

57. **(C)** The tension in the cecal wall dictated by LaPlace's law begins to reach a critical level when the cecal diameter reaches 14 cm as measured on a plain abdominal x-ray.

58. **(C)** Inflammation is associated with a low pH, at which local anesthesia is less effective. Local anesthetic is stored in an acidic medium for solubility and stability but becomes effective when neutralized by tissue fluids.

59. **(D)** Carcinoma is the leading cause of large bowel obstruction (58%), followed by volvulus (16%), diverticulitis (7%), hernia (4%), and intussusception (1%).

60. **(A)** Chordoma is a rare, low-grade malignant tumor found at either end of the spinal axis. Chordomas are locally invasive and tend to recur after removal. Nevertheless, an attempt at complete surgical excision of a sacral tumor should be made. Inaccessible and recurrent tumors are treated by irradiation.

61. **(C)** The hallmark of an intraductal papilloma is an abnormal excretion from the breast, which is usually blood-stained. Carcinoma must be excluded.

62. **(D)** Most adult intussusceptions have a pathologic lead point, usually a benign lesion in the small bowel and a malignancy in the colon. Intussusception most commonly occurs in children (84%) and is a common cause of intestinal obstruction, in contrast to adults, in whom it is a rare cause of obstruction. In children, there is rarely a pathologic lead point. Spontaneous reduction and asymptomatic intervals are more typical of the adult manifestation, whereas sudden crampy pain is characteristic at any age. When symptoms have been present less than 24 hours and there is no sign of complications, hydrostatic barium enema reduction may be attempted in children. No obstruction should be treated in this way when symptoms have been present for a longer period, and failure of reduction does require operative management.

63. **(C)** The alignment of the teeth is not altered by a fracture of the zygoma.

64. **(A)** Splenectomy for hairy cell leukemia not only alleviates cytopenias but frequently results in long-term survival. In contrast, splenectomy in chronic myelogenous and lymphocytic leukemia is only palliative. Splenectomy has no role in the acute form of these diseases.

65. **(B)** Rheumatoid arthritis, granulocytopenia, and splenomegaly is the triad that characterizes Felty's syndrome, in which granulocytopenia predisposes to recurrent infections until splenectomy is performed. Marrow fibrosis, extramedullary hematopoiesis, immature formed elements, and massive splenomegaly are attributes of myeloid metaplasia.

66. **(C)** *E. coli* and *Bacteroides* are found as normal flora in virtually all colons, whereas *Aerobacter* and *Enterococcus* are found in approximately 70% of the population. Clostridia, streptococci, staphylococci, and a variety of other organisms are found with decreasing frequency. The average count of the four major organisms is in the range of 10^6 to 10^{10} organisms/g feces.

67. **(B)** An open fracture of the tibia and fibula should be immediately debrided and the fracture immobilized. Occasionally, the wound may be

closed primarily, but the indications for this are extremely rare. Delayed primary closure 3 to 5 days later or leaving the open wound to granulate is a safer alternative.

68. **(D)** This patient requires a patent airway and intravenous fluids.

69. **(A)** Gastrojejunostomy is not used for the treatment of this condition.

70. **(D)** Persistence of the omphalomesenteric duct is not a cause of cancer.

71. **(B)** Uncomplicated meconium ileus usually can be resolved by Gastrografin enemas repeated at 12-hour intervals and hydration.

72. **(D)** A cervical spine injury should be assumed in any patient with an injury above the clavicle.

73. **(C)** The most likely diagnosis is septic arthritis of the hip joint.

74. **(C)** A patient with a dislocation of the hip may have other serious injuries, particularly within the abdomen or pelvis.

75. **(C)** Liver trauma may produce a central or subcapsular hematoma that discharges into the biliary tree and is a cause of moderate to massive bleeding.

76. **(E)** The wall of a pancreatic pseudocyst consists of the surrounding structures.

77. **(A)** The external sphincter and puborectalis are primarily responsible for voluntary control. The internal sphincter maintains continence at rest.

78. **(A)** The initial treatment for bleeding hemorrhoids is emphatic diet regulation.

79. **(E)** Hepatic coma is best treated by reducing nitrogenous material in the intestine, reducing the production of ammonia from this material, and increasing ammonia metabolism.

80. **(E)** A rising alkaline phosphatase in the absence of bone disease and significant hepatic dysfunction is considered presumptive evidence of a liver tumor.

81. **(B)** Second degree burns are blistered, moist, and painful.

82. **(A)** The most accurate monitoring device in this situation is the Doppler, used repeatedly on the digital arteries and veins.

83. **(B)** Electrical burns usually produce minimal skin loss often with considerable deep tissue destruction.

84. **(C)** Diverticulosis is responsible for about two thirds of all cases of lower gastrointestinal bleeding.

85. **(D)** Pneumaturia and fecaturia are diagnostic of colovesical fistulae.

86. **(E)** In about 5% of patients with diverticulitis, fistulae develop between the colon and adjacent organs: bladder and vagina.

87. **(D)** The sigmoid colon is the site of diverticulosis in about 50% of patients with this problem.

88. **(E)** The average age at death for patients with cancer secondary to familial polyphosis is 41.5 years, compared with 68 years for patients with large bowel cancer in the general population.

89. **(B)** Anal abscesses and fistulae are common in patients with Crohn's disease.

90. **(A)** Parathyroid adenoma is the most common cause of hyperparathyroidism.

91. **(B)** Large doses of intravenous sodium or potassium iodide supplemented with cortisol should be the first treatment of a thyroid storm.

92. **(B)** Hashimoto's disease (lymphadenoid goiter) is an autoimmune process in which the thyroid gland appears to be sensitive to its own thyroglobulin and cell constituents.

93. **(D)** Although there may be spread to the regional lymph nodes in 15% of patients, hematogenous spread to distant sites predominates.

94. **(D)** Medullary carcinomas occur in families as part of a syndrome called multiple endocrine neoplasia type 2. This is MEN-2, or Sipple's syndrome.

95. **(C)** The lower extremity veins are the source of 85% of pulmonary emboli. Symptomatic emboli usually arise in the larger veins, such as the ileofemoral.

96. **(B)** Classically, the patient with pulmonary emboli complains of dyspnea. This is due to hypoxia.

97. **(B)** Emergency blood transfusion can be performed with group O, Rh-negative blood.

98. **(B)** Careful education of the patient in the nonoperative management of this problem is of the utmost importance.

99. **(E)** In these patients, pulmonary embolization almost never occurs, and the late morbidity is insignificant. Therefore, bedrest, surgery, heparin, and steroids are not required.

100. **(C)** In such an injury, the anterior cruciate ligament may be ruptured in association with a tear of the medial collateral ligament.

101. **(B)** Regional or spinal anesthesia is required for arthroscopic surgery of the knee.

102. **(E)** In such a patient, antibiotics should be given prophylactically before a dental procedure.

103. **(C)** Although an accurate diagnosis is of help, the primary factor is to determine that an abdominal operation is required.

104. **(D)** In general, pelvic inflammatory masses involving the fallopian tubes do not bulge into the rectum.

105. **(E)** It is doubtful if the use of vasopressors in hypovolemic shock is ever warranted.

106. **(B)** At this time, nonoperative detorsion followed by elective resection has emerged as the preferred treatment of nonstrangulated volvulus of the sigmoid.

107. **(C)** Nonoperative therapy should be employed for the treatment of the first attacks of diverticulitis.

108. **(A) (T), (B) (T), (C) (T), (D) (T), (E) (T)** Prompt surgical treatment is necessary to preserve the testis. At operation, the contralateral scrotum should be explored. Abdominal symptoms and even fever are common.

109. **(A) (T), (B) (T), (C) (F), (D) (F), (E) (F)** Unless the cecum is grossly involved and friable, the appendix should be removed to avoid con-

fusion with later appendicitis. If a fistula develops, it will most likely be from the adjacent involved bowel. Involvement of cecum as well as ileum would mitigate for iliocecal resection. Inflammation of terminal ileum alone may represent the nonrecurring form of ileitis, and the ileum should not be resected. The older operation of bypass for Crohn's disease has been abandoned because of blind loop, perpetuation of extraintestinal manifestations, progression of disease, and development of carcinoma.

110. **(A) (F), (B) (T), (C) (T), (D) (T), (E) (T)** Meigs' syndrome is classically the association of ascites and hydrothorax with an ovarian fibroma. Removal of the fibroma cures the ascites and hydrothorax. Other ovarian tumors, particularly ovarian malignant tumors, may cause a similar syndrome.

111. **(A) (T), (B) (F), (C) (T), (D) (F), (E) (T)** Factors V and VIII are present in fresh blood but not in banked blood.

112. **(A) (T), (B) (F), (C) (T), (D) (F), (E) (T)** An initial dose of heparin (e.g., 10,000 units) is given intravenously. This is followed by a continuous intravenous infusion of heparin. The course of heparin is tapered after coumadin by mouth is started. When the one-stage prothrombin time has reached 2 to 2.5 times normal, heparin is discontinued.

113. **(A) (T), (B) (T), (C) (T), (D) (T), (E) (F)** Obstruction is the most frequent indication for surgery in Crohn's disease and usually occurs when a bowel segment has developed a rigid fibrous stricture after repeated bouts of inflammation. Fistula and abscess formation may require surgery, and in extreme cases, perianal disease may require abdominoperineal resection. Enterovesical fistula is one of the more urgent internal fistulae requiring surgery. Failure of medical therapy and control of extraintestinal manifestations are additional indications. The risk of malignancy in long-standing Crohn's colitis is significantly increased but is not believed to be as high a risk as in ulcerative colitis, and for this reason, prophylactic colectomy is not recommended.

114. **(A) (F), (B) (T), (C) (F), (D) (F), (E) (T)** Multiple prior abdominal operations is the only absolute contraindication to peritoneal lavage. Pregnancy is a relative contraindication. In the

face of obvious surgical indications (free air, penetrating injury, peritonitis), lavage is not indicated. Patients who will be unavailable for monitoring (e.g., who must undergo other surgical procedures) should have peritoneal lavage first. Lavage is not a sensitive test for retroperitoneal injuries (pancreas, duodenum, urologic, or major vessel injury). The criterion for negative lavage in terms of WBCs is less than 500, and 100,000 RBC/mm in unspun lavage fluid is the red cell criterion. Other indices are gross blood, spun hematocrit >2, bile, bacteria, or fecal matter. Stomach and bladder should be decompressed before lavage, taking care to rule out cribriform plate and urethral injuries before intubation.

115. (A) (T), (B) (T), (C) (T), (D) (T), (E) (F)
The prothrombin time will be prolonged in the presence of even minute amounts of heparin. Even though the prothrombin time will not be used in following a heparinized patient, the prothrombin time should be determined before initiating heparinization.

116. (A) (T), (B) (F), (C) (F), (D) (T), (E) (F)
Lymphangiography is the most sensitive noninvasive test of retroperitoneal lymph node involvement in Hodgkin's disease, with an 80 to 90% accuracy rate and a 10 to 15% false negative rate. The removal of suspect nodes can be confirmed by intraoperative x-ray. Celiac, splenic hilar, and portal nodes are not readily visualized by lymphangiography, and splenic involvement cannot be predicted by this means. Confirmation that nodes with filling defects are diseased must still be obtained at laparotomy. Forty percent of patients with positive lymphangiograms have an additional intraabdominal disease site.

117. (A) (F), (B) (T), (C) (F), (D) (T), (E) (T)
The sagittal suture is involved five times more frequently than is the coronal suture. When the coronal suture is involved, eye abnormalities frequently are present. Operation is indicated to prevent constriction of the brain and to prevent a cosmetic deformity. Cosmetic restoration is best achieved by operations performed during the first 2 months of life.

118. (A) (F), (B) (F), (C) (F), (D) (T), (E) (T)
Imperforate hymen may result in both hematocolpos (a distended vagina) and hematometra (a distended uterus). Although other vaginal anomalies also may be found, this is uncommon. The correct treatment is given in choice **D**. One

must guard against secondary infection after treatment if there is a significant hematocolpos and hematometra.

119. (A) (T), (B) (T), (C) (T), (D) (T), (E) (T)
Bilateral lesions occur in 5 to 10% of patients. The survival rate is 73% under the age of 2 but only 18% over the age of 2.

120. (A) (F), (B) (T), (C) (F), (D) (T), (E) (T)
Airway injuries may not be clinically apparent for 24 hours. Facial burns, carbonaceous sputum, and bronchoscopy may give warning of impending respiratory distress. Alkali burns penetrate more deeply and are more serious than acid burns. They require flushing with water for longer periods, especially when the eye is involved. Doppler evaluation of the distal palmar arch and posterior tibial artery is the most reliable indicator of extremity circulation. Systolic pressure must be at least 90 to produce a normal urine output (50 ml/hour for an adult; 0.7 to 1 ml/kg/hour for a child). The most commonly used burn formula administers 2 to 4 ml/kg/percent burn in the first 24 hours, half in the first 8 hours and the rest over the next 16 hours.

121. (A) (F), (B) (T), (C) (T), (D) (T), (E) (T)
Unlike surface burns, electric current travels through the entire volume of tissue between the entrance point and the exit point (ground), damaging the muscles, nerves, and vessels it travels along. A serious complication is the release of myoglobin from damaged muscle. The myoglobin can block kidney tubules, causing renal failure. If myoglobinuria appears, fluids should be increased to maintain a urine output of 100 ml/hour. If the urine fails to clear, mannitol should be added (25 g immediately, followed by 12.5 g/L). Counteracting acidosis with sodium bicarbonate also may be beneficial.

122. (A) (F), (B) (F), (C) (T) (D) (F), (E) (F)
Frozen red cells retain the same capabilities they were frozen with. Eighty percent of transfusion related hepatitis is non-A, non-B. Stored blood is acidotic, and patients in shock have lactic acidosis, but when perfusion is restored, the acids are burned off rapidly. In fact, as the citrate from the sodium citrate preservative is consumed, sodium bicarbonate is formed. Persistent acidosis is more likely due to hypoperfusion rather than transfused blood. Potassium is released from stored red cells and may be as high as 30 mEg/L in banked blood, but the transfused cells take

up as much as they lost, and most patients become hypokalemic due to transfusion-induced alkalosis.

123. **(A) (F), (B) (F), (C) (F), (D) (F), (E) (T)**
The barbiturates cause myocardial depression and peripheral vasodilatation, which results in reduced coronary blood flow. For these reasons, they must be used cautiously in shock. They do cross the placental barrier and may cause depression in the newborn.

124. **(A) (T), (B) (F), (C) (T), (D) (T), (E) (F)**
Staging laparotomy will increase the stage in 25% of patients and decrease the stage in 15%, for a total reclassification of 40%. Twenty percent of patients will have splenic involvement that was clinically undetected, and the size of the spleen is directly related to the probability of involvement. Spleens weighing over 400 g are invariably diseased and have characteristic gray-white nodules. The liver rarely harbors disease when the spleen is normal. Proven stages IIIB and IV are treated with combination chemotherapy, and this therapy will not be altered by staging. Therefore, the procedure is not indicated for these stages.

125. **(A) (T), (B) (F), (C) (T), (D) (T), (E) (F)**
Tachycardia of a very rapid rate, fever, and pain are signs and symptoms of clostridial myositis. Penicillin is given in large doses. Gas gangrene antitoxin is not effective.

126. **(A) (T), (B) (T), (C) (F), (D) (F), (E) (F)**
Early in their course, carcinomas of the floor of the mouth often cause few or no symptoms and for this reason may be neglected. Carcinomas of the oropharynx are usually less differentiated and are more difficult to control than are carcinomas of the oral cavity. Lower lip carcinomas are usually squamous cell carcinomas.

127. **(A) (T), (B) (T), (C) (T), (D) (T), (E) (F)**
The majority of patients with thrombosis of the superficial femoral artery never require an operation. A number of measures, in addition to the true statements given in the answer, are useful in overcoming vascular insufficiency. Alcohol, if not contraindicated for other reasons, can be helpful if used in moderation.

128. **(A) (T), (B) (F), (C) (F), (D) (T), (E) (T)**
Although there is some evidence that branchiogenic cysts may become malignant, the reported

probable cases number only a handful. Metastatic nodes near the angle of the mandible are commonly from the tonsillar area, buccal mucosa, or floor of the mouth.

129. **(A) (F), (B) (F), (C) (T), (D) (T), (E) (T)**
Familial polyposis and Gardner's syndrome are variants of the syndrome of adenomatous colonic polyposis that are determined by an autosomal dominant gene. If untreated, both conditions result in malignancy and death at an average age of 41. Gardner's syndrome is characterized by the additional findings of sebaceous cysts (usually large ones of the face and extremities), benign osteomas, and cortical thickening of tubular bones.

130. **(A) (T), (B) (F), (C) (T), (D) (F), (E) (F)**
Classic hemophilia is inherited as a sex-linked recessive. Hemarthroses are a fairly common complication in poorly controlled patients.

131. **(A) (T), (B) (T), (C) (T), (D) (T), (E) (T)**
Stress of all varieties increases the incidence of gastric mucosal erosions unless preventive measures are used. Aspirin can cause mucosal erosions and does interfere with normal platelet function. Sometimes stress ulcers occur with no apparent cause.

132. **(A) (T), (B) (T), (C) (F), (D) (F), (E) (T)**
The maximum effect of chronic insufficiency of the veins of the legs occurs above the malleoli. Ulcers occur chiefly on the medial calf. Pain usually is accentuated when the patient stands.

133. **(A) (T), (B) (F), (C) (T), (D) (F), (E) (T)**
Boiling in water for 30 minutes and soaking in 2% aqueous alkaline glutaraldehyde may disinfect instruments, but instruments treated in this fashion are not considered sterile.

134. **(A) (T), (B) (T), (C) (F), (D) (T), (E) (T)**
The 3rd oculomotor nerve can be compressed as it passes through the tentorium. The oculocephalic reflex (Doll's eye) is best left to a neurosurgeon because this maneuver can produce spinal cord injury even when the cervical spine x-ray is normal.

135. **(A) (T), (B) (T), (C) (T), (D) (T), (E) (T)**
Barium is particularly likely to cause fecal impaction in the elderly patient and is associated with dehydration. Measures should be taken to prevent fecal impaction from barium given in the early postoperative period. Impaction should

be prevented in patients receiving narcotics. Stool softeners are helpful and should be given to patients receiving large or frequent doses of narcotics. Small diarrheal stools may occur because of impaction.

136. **(A) (T), (B) (F), (C) (T), (D) (T), (E) (F)**
Debridement of the wound, if the site is known, is important but not as urgent as other modes of treatment. Tetanus does not confer lasting immunity.

137. **(A) (T), (B) (T), (C) (T), (D) (T), (E) (T)**
The procurement of cadaver organs for transplantation has raised serious moral, ethical, legal, and psychologic problems. Death may be cardiopulmonary or neurologic. The neurologic category has been considered here.

138. **(A) (T), (B) (T), (C) (F), (D) (F), (E) (T)**
In heat stroke, the patient does not sweat, and the skin is dry. Rapid cooling to about 39°C is important.

139. **(A) (T), (B) (T), (C) (T), (D) (T), (E) (T)**
The usual infecting organism is a streptococcus. Incision and drainage should be performed before tissue and bone necrosis occur.

140. **(A) (T), (B) (T), (C) (T), (D) (T), (E) (T)**
All of these abnormalities occur if the medial aspect of the temporal lobe is forced through the incisura in the tentorium. This compresses the third nerve and the cerebral peduncles.

141. **(A) (T), (B) (T), (C) (T), (D) (T), (E) (T)**
The physiologic dead space is that portion of each tidal volume that does not exchange gas.

142. **(A) (F), (B) (T), (C) (F), (D) (T), (E) (F)**
Metronidazole given for 10 days cures most amebic liver abscesses. Most do not require drainage. They occur most often in the right lobe of the liver, as do bacterial pyogenic hepatic abscesses.

143. **(A) (T), (B) (T), (C) (T), (D) (T), (E) (T)**
Infected prosthetic materials placed as arterial grafts produce the signs and symptoms of any other infection and they also cause hemorrhage when the resulting false aneurysm ruptures.

144. **(A) (F), (B) (T), (C) (T), (D) (T), (E) (T)**
For single-vessel disease, bypass is palliative and is indicated only for refractory angina that interferes with the patient's lifestyle. The two ex-

ceptions to this are the proximal left anterior descending lesion and a left main lesion occluding more than 50% of the lumen; these once had a dismal prognosis and have been benefited dramatically by surgery. Double- and triple-vessel disease with significant angina or with left ventricular dysfunction or abnormal exercise test are candidates for surgery. The major contraindications to coronary artery bypass are unresponsive class IV congestive heart failure and pulmonary edema from a fixed myocardial deficit. Only 1 to 2% of patients fall into this category.

145. **(A) (F), (B) (F), (C) (T), (D) (T), (E) (F)**
The benefit of intervention in an evolving MI is not yet defined, but thrombolysis, balloon angioplasty, and coronary bypass all have been tried. The lower limit of vessel diameter practical for grafting is 1.2 mm, and all vessels of such size with greater than 50% occlusion should be grafted. An average of four grafts now are placed, with jump anastomoses to intervening vessels. The internal mammary arteries have proven superior to saphenous vein grafts in patency, longer relief of angina, fewer reoperations, and improved survival. Pericarditis is a common complication of bypass grafting and is treated with steroids and anti-inflammatory agents.

146. **(A) (T), (B) (F), (C) (T), (D) (F), (E) (T)**
The symptoms of duodenal ulcer tend to develop when the stomach is empty. At least half of the patients have gastric acid secretions that are considered to be within the normal limits.

147. **(A) (T), (B) (T), (C) (T), (D) (T), (E) (T)**
When an operation has been performed for generalized peritonitis or for prolonged, high-grade intestinal obstruction, the bowel does not regain its motility rapidly. Some causes of prolonged ileus can be corrected but others respond only to prolonged gastric suction.

148. **(A) (T), (B) (T), (C) (F), (D) (F), (E) (F)**
Ninety percent of cases are associated with vomiting, usually forceful in nature, and alcohol is implicated in 60% of cases. The great majority of patients stop bleeding spontaneously. Endoscopic cauterization has been used successfully for the few patients who do not stop bleeding, and surgical oversewing rarely is required. Vagotomy is not indicated.

149. **(A) (F), (B) (F), (C) (T), (D) (T), (E) (F)**
The large majority of duodenal injuries are due

to penetrating trauma. Duodenal rupture due to blunt trauma is particularly insidious because the leak of gastric juice, bile, and pancreatic enzymes is contained in the retroperitoneum. Symptoms may not appear for 24 to 36 hours, and the first signs may be sepsis and shock. All paraduodenal hematomas should be explored to verify duodenal integrity. For the deeply placed duodenum to be injured, it is inevitable that surrounding organs also are injured. These associated injuries influence the prognosis, and the liver is the organ most commonly involved (38%), followed by pancreas (28%) and inferior vena cava (17%).

150. (A) (F), (B) (F), (C) (F), (D) (T), (E) (F)
One hundred percent of patients with untreated liver abscess will die, usually from sepsis and multiple organ failure. Age, multicentricity, multiple organisms, and associated malignancy make the prognosis worse. Amebic abscesses are prone to grow to a larger size and are more likely to rupture. The most common route of amebic abscess rupture is from the dome of the right lobe into the right chest cavity. Large left lobe lesions are more prone to rupture into the pericardium and peritoneal cavity. Despite these complications, the prognosis for amebic abscess is better than for pyogenic abscess.

151. (A) (F), (B) (T), (C) (T), (D) (T), (E) (T)
An adult with any burns over 25% of body surface area, over 20% second degree, or over 10% third degree should be admitted to a burn unit. Children under 10 and adults over 40 should be admitted with smaller percent burns. Special area burns, burns associated with major injuries, electrical burns, and inhalation injury are all indications for burn unit care. Preexisting disease also should lower the admission standard.

152. (A) (T), (B) (F), (C) (F), (D) (F), (E) (T)
The lowest systolic pressure at which a pulse is palpable in the carotid is 60, whereas the femoral pulse requires a systolic pressure of 70, and for a radial pulse to be palpable, a pressure of 80 is necessary. Unmatched type-specific blood (ABO and Rh saline cross-matched blood usually available in 10 minutes) is preferred over type O for emergency transfusion. Type O, Rh-negative is the second choice. Urine output does not drop significantly until class III hemorrhage (30 to 40% blood volume loss). Up to 1500 ml of blood is commonly sequestered in the hematoma around

a femoral fracture. This alone constitutes a class II hemorrhage.

153. (A) (F), (B) (T), (C) (F), (D) (T), (E) (T)
Early coagulopathy is usually due to dilution of platelets. If platelets are found to be low, a 500 ml platelet pack (concentrated from 6 to 10 donors) is given and repeated after every 10 units of blood. Depletion of labile clotting factors (factor VIII, fibrinogen) is a more serious problem, which may require 6 or more units of fresh frozen plasma. Hypothermia and acidosis aggravate microvascular bleeding. Although calcium is chelated by EDTA in banked blood, patients can mobilize enough calcium for coagulation for long periods unless the transfusion rate is greater than 100 ml/minute. If calcium supplement is required, 0.2 g of calcium chloride (2 ml of 10% solution) is given through a separate line.

154. (A) (F), (B) (F), (C) (T), (D) (T), (E) (T)
The classic triad of signs and symptoms related to fat embolism include confusion, dyspnea, and petechiae, especially following long bone fracture.

155. (A) (T), (B) (F), (C) (F), (D) (T), (E) (F)
The manifestations of fat embolism usually appear insidiously, with tachypnea and tachycardia without apparent distress. Confusion, initially without hypoxia, is typical. Only one third of patients exhibit fluffy pulmonary densities initially. With time, dyspnea and cyanosis may ensue, confusion may progress to agitation, stupor, and coma, and all patients develop x-ray findings resembling pulmonary edema. The Pao_2 is the most sensitive indicator of severity, and a value below 60 is considered critical enough to warrant intubation and volume ventilator support with PEEP. High-dose steroids (30 mg/kg methylprednisolone every 24 hours) may be beneficial in controlling the inflammatory component and stabilizing lung surfactant.

156. (A) (T), (B) (F), (C) (T), (D) (T), (E) (T)
A large inoculum of bacteria ($>10^5$) strongly favors the development of wound infection. Fewer organisms are required to cause infection if the organism is virulent (e.g., *Streptococcus pyogenes*) or if there is devitalized tissue or foreign body, as in traumatic wounds. Hair per se does not predispose to infection, and breaks in the skin caused by preoperative shaving may be more detrimental than the hair itself. The predominant sources of bacterial contamination in elective surgical wounds are the surgeon and the

patient, and the risk is proportional to the duration of surgery. Violating bacteria-containing cavities during surgery compounds the risk.

157. **(A) (T), (B) (T), (C) (T), (D) (T), (E) (T)**
Encapsulated bacteria, such as *Klebsiella* and the pneumococcus, are more difficult to phagocytize. Uremia, hyperglycemia, ketosis, prematurity, and old age are associated with impairment of phagocytosis. Some malignancies, particularly the leukemias, also result in deficiencies. Phagocytes are inhibited by foreign body, seroma, hematoma, high-dose steroids, chemotherapy, and radiotherapy. In severe burns, trauma, and malnutrition, there also may be impairment of intracellular killing.

158. **(A) (F), (B) (T), (C) (F), (D) (T), (E) (T)**
Ketamine is a potent intravenous dissociative agent that has two significant side effects: it increases muscle tone, and it causes psychic disturbances during recovery. The adjunctive use of muscle relaxants and benzodiazepine drugs has made it widely useful. It is the only intravenous anesthetic agent that causes cardiovascular stimulation. By a combination of vagal inhibition and adrenergic stimulation, it raises blood pressure, increases cardiac output, and increases myocardial oxygen consumption. These factors make its usefulness limited in patients with cardiac compromise.

159. **(A) (F), (B) (F), (C) (F), (D) (F), (E) (T)**
Succinylcholine is a depolarizing muscle relaxant that causes initial fasciculations on administration. There is no reversing agent, and it is rapidly broken down by tissue cholinesterase. Curare competes with acetylcholine for receptor sites and does not cause depolarization when it binds to those sites. Anticholinesterase drugs, such as neostigmine and pyridostigmine, allow a buildup of acetylcholine at the synapse and cause competitive reversal by the law of mass action equilibrium.

160. **(A) (T), (B) (T), (C) (T), (D) (T), (E) (T)**
All statements are correct.

161. **(A) (T), (B) (T), (C) (T), (D) (F), (E) (F)**
It is not necessary to treat the axillary nodes in patients with noninfiltrating cancers because nodal metastases are present in only 1% of such patients. Extended radical mastectomy is rarely if ever appropriate.

162. **(A) (F), (B) (T), (C) (F), (D) (T), (E) (T)**
Weight loss is not usually severe even though the functional obstruction may appear to be severe. Pain is infrequent even in the presence of shallow ulceration.

163. **(A) (T), (B) (T), (C) (T), (D) (T), (E) (F)**
Less than 5% of patients require a surgical operation unless a carcinoma is present. Medical therapy succeeds in most patients.

164. **(A) (T), (B) (T), (C) (T), (D) (T), (E) (T)**
All of the conditions listed can be associated with cricopharyngeal dysfunction. Several of the CNS conditions are multiple sclerosis, Parkinson's disease, bulbar polio, and stroke. Injuries to the recurrent and superior laryngeal nerves, myasthenia gravis, and myogenic conditions, such as polymyositis, also have been implicated. Reflex spasm is associated with gastroesophageal reflux. With the multitude of organic etiologies to explain cricopharyngeal dysfunction, the once common diagnosis of psychogenic disorder (globus hystericus) should be a last resort diagnosis of exclusion.

165. **(A) (T), (B) (F), (C) (F), (D) (T), (E) (F)**
During instrumentation of the esophagus, spasm of the cricopharyngeus and angulation at the cardia may pose mechanical difficulties that make these likely sites of perforation. The incidence of such perforation is 0.2%. The most dramatic and consistent symptom of perforation is pain related to the level of perforation. This is commonly attributed to other conditions. Because of destruction of the strong submucosal layer, perforation is more likely at the site of pathology. The incidence of perforation during transabdominal vagotomy is 0.5%.

166. **(A) (T), (B) (F), (C) (F), (D) (T), (E) (T)**
Late diagnosis of extrahepatic bile duct cancers is usual, but they have a low probability of metastasizing. The majority of these lesions are found in the upper one third of the duct (50 to 75%), followed by middle one third (10 to 25%) and lower one third (10 to 20%). Painless enlargement of the gallbladder (Courvoisier gallbladder) is characteristic of lesions on the duodenal side of the cystic duct junction. Ninety percent of patients have jaundice.

167. **(A) (F), (B) (T), (C) (F), (D) (T), (E) (F)**
Eighty percent of choledochal cysts are seen in childhood and classically occur with abdominal

pain, mass, and jaundice. Solitary fusiform dilatation is most common, and the supraduodenal variety is most rare. Recent attention has focused on associated intrahepatic cystic bile duct dilatation, a condition given the name Caroli's disease. Cholangitis is a frequent complication. The former practice of biliary enteric drainage has been abandoned because of recurrent pancreatitis (33%) and development of carcinoma (25%). Current preferred treatment is excision and Roux-en-Y hepaticojejunostomy.

168. **(A) (F), (B) (T), (C) (T), (D) (T), (E) (T)**
Selective shunting for esophogeal varices achieves decreased variceal pressure while permitting maintenance of portal hypertension. The head of pressure in the portal system is necessary to continue perfusion through the deranged hepatic architecture. This, in turn, reduces the incidence of hepatic failure and encephalopathy that caused increased mortality with the end-to-side shunt. The most popular selective shunt is the distal splenorenal.

169. **(A) (F), (B) (T), (C) (T), (D) (T), (E) (T)**
The esophagogastric junction usually remains in its normal intraabdominal position with type II paraesophageal hernia, and reflux is not part of the clinical picture. Stasis in an incarcerated stomach can lead to ulceration, which may bleed or perforate. When the entire stomach is within the sac (a so-called upside-down stomach), volvulus may lead to strangulation, with catastrophic results. Obstruction with acute intrathoracic gastric dilatation may occur and cause respiratory insufficiency. For a very large type II paraesophageal hernia, the best approach may be through the chest because of chronic adhesions of the sac. The sac is resected, a fundoplication is performed to prevent reflux, and the crura are sutured together.

170. **(A) (T), (B) (F), (C) (T), (D) (F), (E) (T)**
Men are affected with duodenal ulcer four times as frequently as women. The pain is typically relieved by eating or taking antacid (although spicy foods, fatty foods, and alcohol may exacerbate the pain). Being awakened by pain, relief by antacid, and absence of pain in the morning is a typical pattern. Upper gastrointestinal series is 75 to 80% accurate for diagnosing duodenal ulcer and is the preferred screening procedure because it is less expensive and less invasive than endoscopy. If the upper gastrointestinal series does not explain the symptoms, endoscopy

is the definitive test, with a 95% accuracy rate. In addition, endoscopy identifies bleeding sites that x-rays cannot.

171. **(A) (T), (B) (F), (C) (F), (D) (F), (E) (T)**
The edema associated with an acute pyloric channel ulcer may subside with conservative therapy and open the outlet, whereas a scarred pylorus from recurrent ulcer disease is incapable of opening. The vomiting that follows obstruction results in a hypochloremic, hypokalemic alkalosis. Hypovolemia is a part of the picture but does not alter the alkalosis. A negative saline load test does not mean the patient will tolerate solid food. A several-day period of gastric decompression is necessary to allow the dilated stomach to shrink and regain some tone before surgery is performed. The lack of gastric tone also predisposes to delayed function of the gastroenterostomy after definitive surgery.

172. **(A) (T), (B) (F), (C) (T), (D) (T), (E) (T)**
The radiologic sign of ulcer penetration beyond the projected line of the adjacent stomach wall is approximately 95% accurate in identifying a benign gastric ulcer. The less frequent malignant ulcers generally appear at the apex of a mass effect impinging on the gastric lumen. Most gastric ulcers (95%) occur on the lesser curvature, usually near the incisura. In contrast to duodenal ulcer, gastric ulcers are often more painful with eating. Gastric ulcers in general have a high rate of complications.

173. **(A) (T), (B) (T), (C) (F), (D) (F), (E) (F)**
The mainstay of gastric ulcer surgical treatment is excision of the ulcer and distal gastrectomy. It usually is possible to include the ulcer with the specimen, since 95% are found on the lesser curve, usually near the incisura. The occasional high lesser curve lesion may need to be excised separately or included in a lesser curve wedge from the margin of the gastrectomy. Vagotomy generally is considered unnecessary. Gastroenterostomy and splenectomy usually are not indicated.

174. **(A) (T), (B) (T), (C) (F), (D) (F), (E) (F)**
On initial presentation, most echinococcal cysts are solitary, and 80% are found in the right lobe. The Casoni skin test has an 85% sensitivity for echinococcus. The Frei skin test is diagnostic for lymphogranuloma venereum. Calcification of the cyst wall can be seen on plain abdominal film in over half of the cases. Formalin is no

longer used to kill scolices because of its toxicity. Hypertonic saline and 80% alcohol are two of the agents currently used and are 80 to 90% effective.

175. **(A) (T), (B) (F), (C) (T), (D) (T), (E) (F)**
The normal hepatic architecture and sinusoidal pressure with portal vein thrombosis make variceal bleeding less devastating than when it results from cirrhosis. The extensive collaterals between splanchnic veins and the low pressure liver bed help maintain liver function. Lower variceal pressure is not a distinguishing feature of this condition. Treatment of choice is distal splenorenal shunt.

176. **(A) (T), (B) (T), (C) (T), (D) (T), (E) (T)**
Sclerosing cholangitis is a progressive inflammatory process leading to segmental strictures of intrahepatic and extrahepatic bile ducts. Slow progression to biliary cirrhosis and portal hypertension is the natural history. Seventy percent of cases are associated with ulcerative colitis, which supports an autoimmune etiology. Two thirds of cases are seen in patients under age 45, and the male/female ratio is 3:2. There is an association with retroperitoneal and mediastinal fibrosis. Medical therapy with steroids, immunosuppressants, and antibiotics has little effect on the course of the disease, and surgical palliation is limited.

177. **(A) (F), (B) (T), (C) (T), (D) (F), (E) (T)**
The triad of symptoms described by Charcot includes fever and chills, jaundice, and abdominal pain. These symptoms are manifestations of infection within the bile ducts and pressure elevation sufficient to produce bacteremia (20 cm H_2O experimentally). Pressure elevation results from the fact that this condition invariably is associated with partial or complete bile duct obstruction. Abdominal pain may be absent (20%) or less severe than in acute cholecystitis and may help differentiate the two conditions.

178. **(A) (F), (B) (F), (C) (T), (D) (T), (E) (F)**
Selective management of pediatric splenic trauma is based on firm criteria, including a stable patient, isolated splenic injury, and an experienced ICU staff. Shock, significant transfusion requirement, and multiple organ injury (seen in 30% of splenic injuries caused by blunt trauma and 100% with penetrating trauma) all dictate urgent laparotomy.

179. **(A) (T), (B) (T), (C) (F), (D) (T), (E) (T)**
Of the listed complications, only renal failure is not directly related to pseudocyst. Rupture may release cyst contents into the peritoneal or pleural cavities or into adjacent organs. Hemorrhage, the most catastrophic of the complications, may result from the cyst causing portal hypertension, from irritation of contiguous mucosa, and from intracystic rupture of a pseudoaneurysm.

180. **(A) (F), (B) (F), (C) (T), (D) (T), (E) (T)**
Older patients, those over 55, rather than younger patients tend to do worse. Insulin release is inhibited, and the serum glucose rises, becoming a risk factor at greater than 200 mg/100 ml.